AF614698

Methods in Molecular Biology™

Series Editor
John M. Walker
School of Life Sciences
University of Hertfordshire
Hatfield, Hertfordshire, AL10 9AB, UK

For further volumes:
http://www.springer.com/series/7651

Cellular Cardiomyoplasty

Methods and Protocols

Edited by

Race L. Kao

Department of Surgery, East Tennessee State University, Johnson City, TN, USA

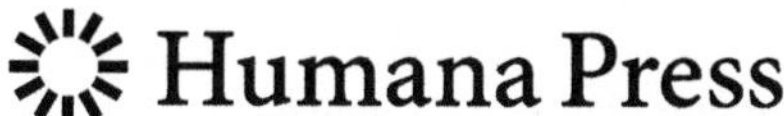

Editor
Race L. Kao
Department of Surgery
East Tennessee State University
Johnson City, TN, USA

ISSN 1064-3745 ISSN 1940-6029 (electronic)
ISBN 978-1-62703-510-1 ISBN 978-1-62703-511-8 (eBook)
DOI 10.1007/978-1-62703-511-8
Springer New York Heidelberg Dordrecht London

Library of Congress Control Number: 2013941035

Printed on acid-free paper

Humana Press is a brand of Springer
Springer is part of Springer Science+Business Media (www.springer.com)

Preface

Ventricular muscle cells of adult mammals are terminally differentiated cells that have lost their ability to replicate for the repair or reconstitution of damaged myocardium. Adult mammalian ventricular myocardium lacks adequate regeneration capability, and an injured heart is normally repaired by scar formation, hypertrophy of surviving myocytes, and hyperplasia of non-muscle cells. Cellular cardiomyoplasty is to use stem cells or progenitor cells for angiogenesis and myogenesis of injured heart to replace, repair, maintain, and enhance ventricular function of an ailing heart. Since we first reported cellular cardiomyoplasty in 1989, successful outcomes have been confirmed by experimental and clinical studies with exponential growth in the last two decades.

Embryonic stem cells and adult stem cells are the two major types of stem cells that have been used for experimental and clinical studies. Embryonic stem cells are totipotent cells that have the capability to differentiate into any type of cell in the body. However, their application in regenerative medicine is limited due to ethical concerns, formation of teratoma, and possible rejection after utilization. Adult stem cells are undifferentiated cells residing in differentiated tissues capable of self-renewal and proliferation to produce differentiated cells. Adult stem cells can yield the specialized cell types of the tissue from which it originated and are capable of developing into cell types that are characteristic of other tissues (plasticity). Self-renewal and plasticity of adult stem cells have been well established. Recently, the induction of pluripotent stem cell lines from adult cells has been successfully achieved in different laboratories. If autologous cells are used to develop the induced pluripotent stem cells, the ethical concerns and immune rejection will not limit their application. For this volume of cellular cardiomyoplasty, only adult stem cells or adult progenitor cells are included.

The methods covered in this volume are contributed by pioneers and internationally well-known experts in cellular cardiomyoplasty. Not only the step-by-step detailed description of the methods and procedures but also invaluable insight information to safeguard against potential pitfalls are provided. This volume will benefit the cardiologist, cardiothoracic surgeons, biologist (cell, molecular, or structural), biochemist, and physiologist who are interested in understanding and treating damaged myocardium and failing heart. I would like to express my sincere gratitude to all the contributing authors who have made this book possible. I also want to thank Professor Emeritus John M. Walker, the series editor, for his guidance, advice, and encouragement in editing this volume.

Johnson City, TN, USA *Race L. Kao*

Contents

Contributors

MOHAMMAD R. AFZAL • *Division of Cardiovascular Diseases, Cardiovascular Research Institute, University of Kansas Medical Center, Kansas City, KS, USA*
PAYAM AKHYARI • *Department for Cardiovascular Surgery, Heinrich Heine University, Duesseldorf, Germany*
MIRIAM ARAÑA • *Laboratory of Cell Therapy, Division of Cancer, Foundation for Applied Medical Research, Clínica Universidad de Navarra, University of Navarra, Pamplona, Spain*
PABLO ARANDA • *Laboratory of Cell Therapy, Division of Cancer, Foundation for Applied Medical Research, Clínica Universidad de Navarra, University of Navarra, Pamplona, Spain*
RONY ATOUI • *Division of Cardiac Surgery, Health Sciences North Sudbury, Greater Sudbury, ON, Canada*
HUG AUBIN • *Department for Cardiovascular Surgery, Heinrich Heine University, Duesseldorf, Germany*
PAUL W. BURRIDGE • *Department of Medicine, Institute of Stem Cell Biology and Regenerative Medicine, Stanford Cardiovascular Institute, Stanford University School of Medicine, Stanford, CA, USA; Department of Radiology, Institute of Stem Cell Biology and Regenerative Medicine, Stanford Cardiovascular Institute, Stanford University School of Medicine, Stanford, CA, USA*
JUAN CARLOS CHACHQUES • *Department of Cardiovascular Surgery and Laboratory of Biosurgical Research, Pompidou Hospital, University of Paris Descartes, Paris, France*
LIJUAN CHEN • *Division of Cardiovascular Disease, Department of Internal Medicine, College of Medicine, University of Cincinnati, Cincinnati, OH, USA*
RAY C.J. CHIU • *Department of Surgery, McGill University Health Center, McGill University, Montreal, QC, Canada*
JARED M. CHURKO • *Department of Medicine, Institute of Stem Cell Biology and Regenerative Medicine, Stanford Cardiovascular Institute, Stanford University School of Medicine, Stanford, CA, USA; Department of Radiology, Institute of Stem Cell Biology and Regenerative Medicine, Stanford Cardiovascular Institute, Stanford University School of Medicine, Stanford, CA, USA*
BUDDHADEB DAWN • *Division of Cardiovascular Diseases, University of Kansas Medical Center, Cardiovascular Research Institute, Kansas City, KS, USA*
RENATE DE JONG • *Molecular Cardiology Laboratory & Intervention Cardiology, Thoraxcenter Rotterdam, Rotterdam, The Netherlands*
HENRICUS J. DUCKERS • *Department of Interventional Cardiology, Division of Cardiology & Pulmonology, University Medical Center Utrecht, Utrecht, The Netherlands*
MINH NGOC DUONG • *Department of Surgery, McGill University Health Center, McGill University, Montreal, QC, Canada*

JÖRN HÜLSMANN • *Department for Cardiovascular Surgery, Heinrich Heine University, Duesseldorf, Germany*
VINODH JEEVANANTHAM • *Division of Cardiovascular Diseases, Cardiovascular Research Institute, University of Kansas Medical Center, Kansas City, KS, USA*
GRACE W. KAO • *Department of Surgery, James H. Quillen College of Medicine, East Tennessee State University, Johnson City, TN, USA*
RACE L. KAO • *Department of Surgery, James H. Quillen College of Medicine, East Tennessee State University, Johnson City, TN, USA*
ISSEI KOMURO • *Department of Cardiovascular Medicine, Osaka University Graduate School of Medicine, Suita, Osaka, Japan; Department of Cardiovascular Medicine, The University of Tokyo Graduate School of Medicine, Tokyo, Japan*
ALEXANDER KRANZ • *Department for Cardiovascular Surgery, Heinrich Heine University, Duesseldorf, Germany*
ELIZABETH K. LAMB • *Department of Surgery, James H. Quillen College of Medicine, East Tennessee State University, Johnson City, TN, USA*
ALICE LE HUU • *Division of Cardiac Surgery, Department of Surgery, McGill University Health Center, McGill University, Montreal, QC, Canada; Division of Surgical Research, Department of Surgery, McGill University Health Center, McGill University, Montreal, QC, Canada*
RONGLIH LIAO • *Cardiovascular and Genetics Divisions, Department of Medicine, Brigham and Women's Hospital, Harvard Medical School, Boston, MA, USA*
ARTUR LICHTENBERG • *Department for Cardiovascular Surgery, Heinrich Heine University, Duesseldorf, Germany*
YU-TING MA • *Department of Surgery, McGill University Health Center, McGill University, Montreal, QC, Canada*
KATSUHISA MATSUURA • *Department of Cardiology, Institute of Advanced Biomedical Engineering and Science, Tokyo Women's Medical University, Tokyo, Japan*
MANUEL MAZO • *Hematology and Area of Cell Therapy, Clínica Universidad de Navarra, University of Navarra, Pamplona, Spain*
TOSHIO NAGAI • *Department of Cardiovascular Medicine, Chiba University Graduate School of Medicine, Chuo-ku, Chiba, Japan*
ANGELOS OIKONOMOPOULOS • *Cardiovascular Division, Department of Medicine, Brigham and Women's Hospital, Harvard Medical School, Boston, MA, USA*
YAOHUA PAN • *Department of Internal Medicine, Division of Cardiovascular Disease, College of Medicine, University of Cincinnati, Cincinnati, OH, USA*
ILIA ALEXANDER PANFILOV • *Molecular Cardiology Laboratory & Intervention Cardiology, Thoraxcenter Rotterdam, Rotterdam, The Netherlands*
ARGHYA PAUL • *Department of Biomedical Engineering, Biomedical Technology and Cell Therapy Research Laboratory, Artificial Cells and Organs Research Centre, McGill University, Montreal, QC, Canada*
BEATRIZ PELACHO • *Laboratory of Cell Therapy, Division of Cancer, Foundation for Applied Medical Research, Clínica Universidad de Navarra, University of Navarra, Pamplona, Spain*
SATYA PRAKASH • *Department of Biomedical Engineering, Biomedical Technology and Cell Therapy Research Laboratory, Artificial Cells and Organs Research Centre, McGill University, Montreal, QC, Canada*

FELIPE PROSPER • *Laboratory of Cell Therapy, Division of Cancer, Foundation for Applied Medical Research, Hematology and Area of Cell Therapy, Clínica Universidad de Navarra, University of Navarra, Pamplona, Spain*
KONSTANTINA-IOANNA SERETI • *Cardiovascular Division, Department of Medicine, Brigham and Women's Hospital, Harvard Medical School, Boston, MA, USA; University of Crete-Medical School, Heraklion, Greece*
DOMINIQUE SHUM-TIM • *Department of Surgery, Division of Cardiac Surgery, McGill University Health Center, McGill University, Montreal, QC, Canada; Department of Surgery, Division of Surgical Research, McGill University Health Center, McGill University, Montreal, QC, Canada*
SHIN-ICHIRO TAKASHIMA • *Molecular Cardiology Laboratory & Intervention Cardiology, Thoraxcenter Rotterdam, Rotterdam, The Netherlands*
YAOLIANG TANG • *Department of Internal Medicine, Division of Cardiovascular Disease, College of Medicine, University of Cincinnati, Cincinnati, OH, USA*
KAZUMASA UNNO • *Department of Medicine, Cardiovascular and Genetics Divisions, Brigham and Women's Hospital, Harvard Medical School, Boston, MA, USA*
YINGJIE WANG • *Department of Internal Medicine, Division of Cardiovascular Disease, College of Medicine, University of Cincinnati, Cincinnati, OH, USA*
NEAL WEINTRAUB • *Department of Internal Medicine, Division of Cardiovascular Disease, College of Medicine, University of Cincinnati, Cincinnati, OH, USA*
JOSEPH C. WU • *Department of Medicine, Institute of Stem Cell Biology and Regenerative Medicine, Stanford Cardiovascular Institute, Stanford University School of Medicine, Stanford, CA, USA; Department of Radiology, Institute of Stem Cell Biology and Regenerative Medicine, Stanford Cardiovascular Institute, Stanford University School of Medicine, Stanford, CA, USA*
LAN ZHANG • *Department of Internal Medicine, Division of Cardiovascular Disease, College of Medicine, University of Cincinnati, Cincinnati, OH, USA*
EWA K. ZUBA-SURMA • *Department of Cell Biology, Faculty of Biochemistry, Biophysics and Biotechnology, Jagiellonian University, Krakow, Poland*

Chapter 1

Cellular Cardiomyoplasty: Its Past, Present, and Future

Elizabeth K. Lamb, Grace W. Kao, and Race L. Kao

Abstract

Cellular cardiomyoplasty is a cell therapy using stem cells or progenitor cells for myocardial regeneration to improve cardiac function and mitigate heart failure. Since we first published cellular cardiomyoplasty in 1989, this procedure became the innovative method to treat damaged myocardium other than heart transplantation. A significant improvement in cardiac function, metabolism, and perfusion is generally observed in experimental and clinical studies, but the improvement is mild and incomplete. Although safety, feasibility, and efficacy have been well documented for the procedure, the beneficial mechanisms remain unclear and optimization of the procedure requires further study. This chapter briefly reviews the stem cells used for cellular cardiomyoplasty and their clinical outcomes with possible improvements in future studies.

Key words Cellular cardiomyoplasty, Skeletal muscle stem cell, Bone marrow stem cells, Adipose tissue stem cells, Cardiac stem cells, Induced pluripotent stem cells, Clinical trials

1 Introduction

Cardiovascular disease (heart disease and stroke) is the number one contributor to global mortality accounting for 17.3 million deaths per year (www.who.int/entity/cardiovascular_diseases/en/). There are 5.8 million heart failure patients in the United States alone with substantial morbidity, morality, and healthcare expenditure [1]. Congestive heart failure is not a disease per se but a pathophysiologic condition which the cardiac output cannot meet the demand for normal functioning of the body. Other than replacing the ailing heart (cardiac transplantation), there is no clinical therapy to cure the failing heart. Cellular cardiomyoplasty is a cell therapy using stem cells or progenitor cells to induce myogenesis and angiogenesis as well as to minimize scar formation and remodeling of an injured heart. The therapy is intended to regenerate the lost myocardium and to prevent or mitigate the progressive and irreversible loss of cardiac function and eventually heart failure.

Ventricular muscle cells of adult mammals are terminally differentiated cells that have lost their ability to replicate by cell division.

Race L. Kao (ed.), *Cellular Cardiomyoplasty: Methods and Protocols*, Methods in Molecular Biology, vol. 1036,
DOI 10.1007/978-1-62703-511-8_1,

This view has been challenged for more than 150 years; however, clear evidence of dividing ventricular cardiomyocytes produced from adult mammals remains lacking. The mammalian cell cycle is a highly conserved and regulated process that can be divided into gap, DNA synthesis, and mitotic phases (mitosis and cytokinesis). Although ventricular cardiac myocytes constitute about 80 % of the myocardial mass, they only contribute 20–30 % of the total cell number. In addition, the identification of true myocyte nuclei is very challenging [2], and the mitotic figures are extremely rare in normal myocardium which makes the finding of dividing heart muscle cells very difficult. DNA synthesis [3] using ^{3}H-thymidine incorporation in transgenic mice (cardiac myocytes nuclear LacZ to unambiguously locate cardiac myocyte nuclei) suggests a maximum labeling index of 0.00055 % (1/180,000). After the Limited Nuclear Test Ban Treaty in 1963, the ^{14}C in the atmosphere dropped exponentially by diffusion, the ^{14}C in cardiomyocyte nuclei can be used to date the age of cardiac myocytes, and by this method, it is estimated that adult heart muscle cells turn over at a rate of 0.45 % (age 75) to 1 % (age 25) per year [4]. Even DNA synthesis can be found in adult human heart, this cannot be considered as cardiomyocyte proliferation due to DNA repair, polyploid nucleus, and multinucleated cardiac myocytes all have DNA synthesis without cytokinesis [5–7]. New heart muscle cells can be derived from extracardiac sources as evidenced by the male cardiac transplant recipient with female donor heart showing Y chromosome containing cardiomyocytes [8, 9]. However, cell fusion can also produce Y chromosome-positive cardiomyocytes.

The lack of sufficient heart muscle cells to generate required pressure and output from the ventricles has been considered as the primary cause of heart failure. Myocardial infarction is normally repaired by scar formation associated with hyperplasia of non-muscle cells and hypertrophy of cardiac myocytes. Although stem cells in the ventricular myocardium have been identified in 1996 [10] and several types of stem or progenitor cells (c-kit^{+}, sca-1^{+}, isl-1^{+}, side population, and cardiac sphere) have been reported in recent years [11–17], however, functionally significant myocardial regeneration has not been documented in diseased or injured heart. A good question to ask would be: why does an organ with highly limited regeneration would have several types of stem cells? Although cardiac stem cells can give rise to cardiomyocytes, smooth muscle cells, endothelial cells, and other cell types, the cell surface markers are not specific to cardiac stem or progenitor cells, and the derived cardiomyocytes can be contaminants from the original tissue [7, 18]. Adult mammalian myocardium lacks adequate endogenous regenerative capability, and cellular cardiomyoplasty offers a viable approach to reconstitute damaged myocardium and prevent heart failure.

Adult stem cells are undifferentiated cells residing in differentiated tissues capable of self-renewal and proliferation to produce differentiated cells. Adult stem cell can yield the specialized cell types of the tissue from which it originated and is capable of developing into cell types that are characteristic of other tissue (plasticity). Although embryonic stem cells can be used for cellular cardiomyoplasty especially embryonic stem cell-derived cardiomyocytes [19]; however, due to the ethical, social, political, and religious concerns in addition to the formation of teratoma after their transplantation, we will not consider embryonic stem cells in this book. To avoid possible rejection, only autologous stem cells from adult individuals are covered in this chapter.

2 Different Stem Cells for Cellular Cardiomyoplasty

2.1 Skeletal Muscle Stem Cells

Skeletal muscle has several types of stem cells such as side population cells, pericytes, mesoangioblasts, myoendothelial cells, and satellite cells. However, satellite cell is the only type of stem cell that clearly proved for growth, maintenance, and repair of skeletal muscle. Our group is the first one using dog satellite cells for cellular cardiomyoplasty in 1989 [20]. Since then a number of research laboratories started the similar project to confirm the safety and efficacy of satellite cells for cellular cardiomyoplasty [21] and lead to the first clinical case in 2000 [22].

Satellite cells are mononucleated myogenic precursor cells located under the basal lamina but outside the sarcolemma of skeletal muscle [21, 23, 24]. They are 25 by 5 μm spindle-shaped cells containing a heterochromatic nucleus and scanty cytoplasm with few organelles. Satellite cell was first identified and named by Mauro in 1961 [25]; since then, many studies and reviews have been published [26, 27]. Satellite cells offer several advantages for cellular cardiomyoplasty: can be easily obtained without affecting one's function, can be vastly proliferated in culture, have high resistance to ischemic and hypoxic conditions, have no identified risk for tumor generation, and have more commitment to myogenic differentiation. Formation of new muscle tissue, improvement of local perfusion, augmentation of local and global contractility, enhancement of metabolic activities, maintenance of ventricular wall thickness, decrease of scar tissue, and increase of ejection fraction and cardiac output are the observed benefits using satellite cells for cellular cardiomyoplasty [5–7, 26, 28, 29].

2.2 Bone Marrow Stem Cells

Bone marrow contains multiple cell populations of differentiated and undifferentiated cells (stem cells) such as hematopoietic and mesenchymal stem cells and endothelial progenitor cells. The presence of mesenchymal stem cells in bone marrow was first suggested in 1867, and the ability of these cells differentiated into other mesenchymal cells was described in 1976 [30]. Mesenchymal stem cells are rare and most researches rely on the stromal cells derived from bone marrow by their adherent to culture flask [31]. The cell preparation contains multiple cell types and can also be derived from other tissues of the body. The term "MSC" has been used for mesenchymal stem cells, marrow stromal cells, marrow stem cells, mononuclear stem cells, etc. that adds additional confusion to the published results. The mesenchymal stem cells should be negative for the hematopoietic markers (CD34, CD54, CD14) or endothelial marker (CD133) and selection of cells positive to these markers are not mesenchymal stem cells [32]. Human multipotent mesenchymal stromal cells must (1) be plastic-adherent when maintained in standard culture conditions; (2) express CD105, CD73, and CD90 and lack expression of CD45, CD34, CD14 or CD11b, CD79α or CD19, and HLA-DR surface molecules; and (3) differentiate to osteoblasts, adipocytes, and chondroblasts in vitro [33].

Bone marrow stem cells especially mesenchymal stem cells are the most studied stem cell for cellular cardiomyoplasty. The cells can be easily obtained, proliferate to vast quantity, proved to differentiate into cardiomyocyte with or without 5-azacytidine, and has the potential to be universal donor cells (Chapters 3 and 10 of this book). Early experimental studies [34–36] using bone marrow cells clearly demonstrated the formation of muscle tissue, reduced scar tissue, as well as improved perfusion and cardiac function after myocardial infarction. Clinical trials followed shortly after these encouraging reports, but most are small-scale nonrandomized controlled trials and outcomes of both beneficial or no effect have been reported [37, 38]. Even double-blind randomized controlled trials show conflicting results [37, 38]. These conflicts arise mainly due to the differences in cell preparation procedures, route and time of stem cell delivery, patient selection, and end point applied to evaluate the outcomes.

The beneficial mechanisms of bone marrow mesenchymal stem cells are suggested to be their paracrine effects by releasing angiogenic factors, growth factors, cytokines, or chemokines to induce neovascular formation, anti-inflammatory and antiapoptotic effects, or activation of cardiac myocyte progenitor cells. Therefore, other stem or progenitor cells should have similar beneficial effects, and bone marrow $CD34^+$ cells but more commonly blood mononuclear cells or blood $CD34^+$ cells especially after granulocyte colony-stimulating factor (G-CSF) treatment to increase blood $CD34^+$ cells have been used for patient after myocardial infarction. Following the same reasoning, circulating endothelial progenitor cells have also been used for patients suffering myocardial infarction. Meta-analysis [39, 40] of randomized controlled trials revealed that left ventricular ejection fraction (LFEF) was moderate but significantly improved in both intracoronary autologous bone marrow stem cell group (8.4 %) and intracoronary autologous blood stem/progenitor cell group (3.72 %).

2.3 Adipose Tissue Stem Cells

Adipose tissue consists of various sizes of adipocytes and stroma, which is composed of endothelial cells, smooth muscle cells, fibroblasts, leukocytes, macrophages, and preadipocytes. Adipose tissue stem cells were first identified in 2001 [41, 42] and prepared as adipose stromal vascular fraction or adipose mesenchymal stem cells. Adipose tissue is an abundant and expandable tissue that can be easily harvested in large quantities with minimal morbidity in several regions of the human body. Adipose stem cells in addition to their easy obtainable in large quantities, they offer several advantages [43–46] as compared to other stem cells: (1) adipose tissue has significantly higher stem cells per gram tissue, (2) the adipose tissue stem cells are pluripotent stem cells, (3) they secrete significantly more angiogenic and growth factors, (4) they have excellent anti-inflammatory effects, (5) they can differentiate into muscle cells, and (6) they can be an excellent source for induced pluripotent stem cells.

Adipose tissue stromal cells can spontaneously differentiate into cardiomyocytes [47] and be induced by 5-azacytidine [48] or phorbol myristate acetate [49] to differentiate into cardiomyocytes. The earlier experimental studies using adipose tissue-derived stem cell for acute and chronic animal models of myocardial infarction are reviewed and summarized [50]. Adipose tissue stem cell transplantation improved neovascularization and perfusion, regenerated myocardium, reduced inflammation and apoptosis, and ameliorated ventricular remodeling. The possible beneficial mechanisms of adipose stem cells are (1) the secretion of angiogenic and growth factors; (2) differentiation of transplanted cells into myocytes, smooth muscle cells, and endothelial cells; and (3) secretion of antioxidant, free radical scavengers, and chaperone/heat-shock proteins. Both cultured and freshly isolated adipose tissue stem cells can be used for cellular cardiomyoplasty without causing arrhythmia or tumor genesis [51]. After standardization of isolation procedures and better characterization of adipose stem cells, they can be excellent cell for myocardial regeneration.

2.4 Cardiac Stem Cells

The presence of stem cells in the ventricular myocardium have been suggested since 1996 [10], and several types of stem or progenitor cells (c-kit$^+$, sca-1$^+$, isl-1$^+$, side population, and cardiac sphere) have been reported in recent years [11–17] by cell surface markers. The c-kit$^+$-positive cells are small interstitial cells of the myocardium that express the tyrosine kinase receptor protein. Cardiac c-kit$^+$ cells are self-renewing, clone-forming (cell proliferation after plating single cell per well), and multipotent cells. Cardiac c-kit$^+$ cells can be selected by magnetic-activated cell sorting or flow cytometer and used for myocardial regeneration after myocardial infarction with significant improvement in ventricular function [11, 12].

A population of cells isolated from mouse heart that express stem cell antigen 1 (sca-1) have been isolated by flow cytometer and magnetic enrichment [52]. The sca-1$^+$ cells do not spontaneously differentiate to cardiac myocytes in vitro but will form cardiac myocytes after 5-azacytidine treatment. When sca-1$^+$ cell transplanted into infarcted myocardium differentiation occurred in about half of the cells while the other half by cell fusion to host heart muscle cells [52] for myocardial regeneration. More than 93 % of cardiac side population cells are sca-1$^+$ cells [52]. Side population cells are cells that have the ability to actively efflux the DNA-binding dye "Hoechst 33342" [11]. This is done by an ATP-binding cassette (ABC) transporter-dependent manner and appeared to the "side" on fluorescence-activated cell sorting (FACS) analysis [53]. Cardiac side population cells differentiate into cardiomyocytes in vitro and in vivo and can be used for cellular cardiomyoplasty [14, 16].

The isl-1$^+$ cells have shown to contribute to the development of outflow tract, atria, right ventricle, and part of the left ventricle during embryonic development [13]. The presence of isl-1$^+$ cells in postnatal mouse, rat, and human heart has also been identified and considered as multipotent cardiac stem cells [13]. The isl-1$^+$ cells can contribute to cardiac muscle, smooth muscle, endothelial, and pacemaker cells during myocardial regeneration.

Cardiosphere can be developed from human and animal myocardium samples that contain a mixed population of stem cell expression of c-kit, sca-1, CD34, and CD31 [53] indicating cardiac myocyte and endothelial progenitor cells. When cardiosphere is dissociated into single cells, the isolated cells are clonogenic in vitro. Cardiosphere can be used as a source of cardiac stem cells [16], and the stem cells from cardiosphere formed new myocardium and improved ventricular ejection fraction after myocardial infarction [17].

Why would a highly regeneration-limited organ have several types of stem cells? Are cardiac stem cells true progenitor cells for repairing and maintaining homeostasis of heart muscle cells or are they stem cells for other cell types in the myocardium? Although cardiac stem cells can give rise to cardiomyocytes, smooth muscle cells, endothelial cells, and other cell types, the cell surface marker is not specific to cardiac stem or progenitor cells, and the derived cardiomyocytes can be contaminants from the original tissue [7, 18]. Despite all the unanswered questions, cardiac stem cells have been applied in clinical trials with highly encouraging early results.

2.5 Induced Pluripotent Stem Cells

Induced pluripotent stem cells (iPS) can be generated from mouse and human fibroblasts by retroviral-mediated introduction of four transcription factors (Oct3/4, Sox2, Klf4, c-Myc) to produce cells like embryonic stem cells [54, 55]. The iPS can also be reprogrammed from various differentiated cell types of different animals using several methods [56–58]. Pluripotent describes a cell that can generate cell types from each of the three embryonic germ layers (endoderm, mesoderm, and ectoderm). For a more strict sense, pluripotent describes a cell that can give rise to an entire organism. Other than avoiding the ethical concern of destroying an embryo for embryonic stem cells, the major advantage of iPS is to generate a customized, personalized pluripotent cell specific to each patient without immune rejection for regenerative medicine. The iPS can also be used for the investigation of disease mechanisms or in vitro drug screening, toxicity test, and therapeutic potential, as well as gene repair coupled with cell replacement therapy [56–60].

To reprogram somatic cells into iPS, either retroviruses or lentiviruses are commonly used to introduce the reprogramming factors. Viral integration into the host genome increases the risk of tumorigenicity; thus viral-free procedures can be used to reduce the risk of tumor formation [61]; however, this method substantially lowers the already very low efficiency of iPS generation. Alternatively, the non-integrative Sendai virus can be used to avoid viral integration into host genome (Chapter 7). Another important risk in the clinical application of human iPS is the teratoma formation by residual undifferentiated cells. Immunodepletion with antibodies against stage-specific embryonic antigen-5 and two pluripotency surface markers completely prevented teratoma formation [62].

The reprogramming efficiency remains very low and several adjunctive treatments have developed to improve the efficiency [56–58]. To avoid the risk of tumorigenicity from viral integration into the host genome, integration-free virus (adenovirus, Sendai virus), plasmid DNA, modified RNA, microRNA, and proteins have been used to produce iPS [56–58]. Numerous protocols also developed for differentiation of iPS to cardiac cells. Transplantation of iPS [63] or iPS-derived cardiac progenitor cells [64] regenerated smooth muscle cells, endothelial cells, and muscle cells that improved ventricular wall thickness, contractile function, electrical stability, and reduced scar tissue after myocardial infarction. Continuous refinement and standardization of reprogramming methods for production of iPS and their induced differentiation procedures will be necessary before full clinical application especially for cellular cardiomyoplasty.

3 Clinical Outcomes Using Different Stem Cells

A list of clinical trials can be found from http://www.ClinicalTrials.gov, and summaries of clinical trials have been reported in several recent reviews [37, 38, 65–69]. The stem cells have been delivered to the heart through coronary system or by direct injection into myocardium through the epicardial or endocardial route. The retention and engraftment rates of the cells are very low due to biological and mechanical losses [37, 70, 71]. Theoretically even a few stem cells survived at the transplant site, they should be able to proliferate to vast quantity in a reasonably short time, but the robust proliferation of transplanted stem cells has not been observed. A significant improvement in cardiac function, metabolism, and perfusion is generally observed in most clinical studies; but the improvement is mild and incomplete. Although safety, feasibility, and efficacy have been well documented for the procedure, the beneficial mechanisms remain unclear and optimization of the procedure requires further study.

3.1 Satellite Cells (Myoblasts)

Skeletal muscle stem cells (satellite cells, myoblasts) were the first type of cells applied for clinical cellular cardiomyoplasty in 2000 [22]. Since then a number of small-scale uncontrolled clinical studies have been reported by different groups. Early clinical applications produced highly encouraging results and are summarized in recent review papers [5, 26, 28, 29]. Although feasibility, safety, improved survival, and ventricular functions have been observed in long-term follow-up studies, definitive long-term efficacy requires large-scale placebo-controlled double-blind randomized trials as the MAGIC study [72]. The MARVEL trial is a double-blind, randomized, controlled, multicenter study for 330 patients but has been terminated after 23 enrollments due to financial reasons [73]. The SEISMIC trial is a randomized, open-label trial for only 40 patients with congestive heart failure [74] that proves the procedure is safe and may provide symptomatic relief. The MAGIC trial completed 97 patients but myoblasts treatment did not improve regional or global left ventricular function. However, the suspected complication of arrhythmia was not observed, and the high-dose cell group demonstrated significant better cardiac outcomes [29, 72]. The "study of the efficacy of percutaneous implantation of autologous myoblasts in patients with old infarction (PERCUTANEO) trial (NCT00908622)" will recruit 50 patients that have not reported their results.

3.2 Mesenchymal Stem Cells

Mesenchymal stem cells are present in most tissues as a rare population of cells that have the ability to differentiate into other mesenchymal cells. The bone marrow only contain about 0.01 % of mesenchymal stem cells, and bone marrow mononuclear cells isolated by density centrifugation after bone marrow aspiration are mixed population of cells with very few mesenchymal stem cells. Therefore, most investigators use bone marrow stromal cells, bone marrow mononuclear cells, or blood mononuclear cells for clinical studies. From recent reviews [5, 38, 65, 67, 68] and www.ClinicalTrials.gov site, we can identify only 14 clinical trials with 100 patients or more for their clinical trials.

There are seven completed clinical trials. The "autologous stem cell transplantation in acute myocardial infarction (ASTAMI) trial (NCT00199823)" with ($n = 50$) or without ($n = 50$) intracoronary injection of autologous mononuclear bone marrow cells in acute myocardial infarction is one. At 3 years after cell therapy, the treatment is safe with small improvements in exercise time without significant improvement in left ventricular function [75]. The "reinfusion of enriched progenitor cells and infarct remodeling in acute myocardial infarction (REPA*R*-AMI) trial (NCT00279175)" is a double-blind, placebo-controlled, multicenter trial with intracoronary infusion of bone marrow-derived progenitor cells ($n = 101$) or culture medium ($n = 103$) at 3 ~ 7 days after successful infarct reperfusion. At the 2-year follow-up, the procedure has been found to be safe with no undesired effects, while the major adverse cardiovascular events and progression toward heart failure are markedly decreased with significant improvement in left ventricular function [76]. The "efficacy of the endocardial stem cells implantation in ischemic heart failure patients (ESCAPE) trial (NCT00841958)" is an intramyocardial injection of bone marrow mononuclear cells ($n = 55$) or optimal medical therapy ($n = 54$) to patients with chronic myocardial infarction and end-stage chronic heart failure. A significant reduction in mortality, a market increase in left ventricular function, and significant improvement in NYHA functional classes without any complications due to cell therapy are observed [77]. The "autologous bone marrow derived CD133$^+$ and mononuclear cells in-patient with acute myocardial infarction during coronary artery bypass grafting: a randomized phase III clinical trial (NCT01167751)" is planned for 105 patients but only has a small number of patients completed [78]. The HEBE trial [79] is the intracoronary administration of autologous bone marrow mononuclear cells or peripheral blood mononuclear cells versus controls after primary percutaneous coronary intervention for 200 patients. Only 26 patients have been included in their report without improving left ventricular function but demonstrated to be beneficial to left ventricular remodeling. The BALANCE trial is with ($n = 62$) or without ($n = 62$) intracoronary administration of autologous bone marrow cells. The left ventricular ejection fraction, stroke volume index, ventricular function, and exercise capacity are all significantly improved in the cell therapy group with lower mortality rate during 3-, 12-, and 60-month follow-up [80]. The STAR-heart trial included 391 chronic heart failure patients with ($n = 191$) or without ($n = 200$) intracoronary bone marrow cell treatment. At 3 months and 5 years after cell therapy, a significant increase in left ventricular ejection fraction, cardiac index, exercise capacity, oxygen uptake, and left ventricular contractility was observed. Importantly, there was a significant decrease in long-term mortality in the cell-treated patients compared with the control group [81].

The ongoing trials are "intramyocardial transplantation of bone marrow stem cells in addition to coronary artery bypass graft surgery (PERFECT) trial (NCT00950274)" for 142 patients, "bone marrow derived AC 133+ and mononuclear cells implantation in myocardial infarction (NCT01187654)" for 100 patients, "use of adult autologous stem cells in treating people who have had a heart attack (The TIME Study) trial (NCT00684021)" for 120 patients, "bone marrow derived adult stem cells for chronic heart failure (REGEN-IHD) trial (NCT00747708)" for 148 patients, "effects of intracoronary progenitor cell therapy on coronary flow reserve after acute MI (REPAIR-ACS) trial (NCT00711542)" for 100 patients, and "Swiss multicenter intracoronary stem cell study in acute myocardial infarction (SWISS-AMI) trial (NCT00355186)" for 150 patients. Even with so many clinical trials of moderate size, a clear conclusion on the efficacy of mesenchymal stem cells remains debatable. This is mainly due the diverse cell preparation, number of cells given, the time of cell administration, patient selection, and follow-up evaluations. We will need a large, randomized controlled, multicenter long-term study like the "coronary artery bypass surgery off or on pump revascularization study (CORONARY) trial (NCT00463294)" that involved 4,700 patients [82] to have a better evaluation of using mesenchymal stem cells for cellular cardiomyoplasty.

To overcome this limitation, several meta-analyses have been used to determine the benefit of mesenchymal stem cells for cellular cardiomyoplasty. By including 33 randomized controlled trials that involved 1,765 patients, stem/progenitor cell improves left ventricular ejection fraction early after treatment and at 12–61 months follow-up [83] with some studies also showing improved left ventricular volume. The beneficial outcomes are associated with dose and time of cell treatment. Changes in mortality and morbidity are not statistically significant. Randomized controlled trials of bone marrow cells in combination with coronary artery bypass grafting or percutaneous coronary intervention include ten clinical trials with 422 patients [84]. Randomized controlled trials with blood-derived stem/progenitor cells include seven clinical trials with 343 patients [40]. Randomized controlled trials of intracoronary autologous bone marrow-derived stem cells include eight clinical trials with 307 patients [39]. Randomized controlled clinical trials of intramyocardial bone marrow stem cells during coronary bypass grafting include six clinical trials with 179 patients [85]. All indicate a moderate but statistically significant improvement in left ventricular ejection fraction. A standardized multicenter randomized controlled trial with sufficient patients is recommended from all meta-analyses.

3.3 Adipose Tissue Stem Cells

There are a total of six clinical trials using adipose tissue stem cells identified (www.ClinicalTrials.gov) with only three of them recruiting patients. The "mesenchymal stromal cell therapy in patients with chronic ischemic (MyStromalCell) trial (NTC01449032)" is a double-blind placebo-controlled trial in patients with coronary artery disease to test efficacy and safety of treatment with adipose-derived stem cells to improve perfusion in the heart muscle and exercise capacity and reduce the patient's symptoms [86]. The "safety and efficacy of adipose derived stem cells for non-ischemic congestive heart failure (NTC01502501)" and "safety and efficacy of adipose derived stem cells for congestive heart failure (NTC01502514)" trials are open-label, nonrandomized, multicenter studies to assess the safety and cardiovascular effects of intramyocardial and intravenous implantation of autologous adipose-derived stem cells in nonischemic or ischemic congestive heart failure patients.

The "randomized clinical trial of adipose-derived stem cell in the treatment of patients with ST-elevation myocardial infarction (APOLLO) trial (NTC00442806)" [87], the "a randomized clinical trial of adipose-derived stem cells in treatment of nonrevascularizable ischemic myocardium (PRECISE) trial (NTC00426868)," and the "safety and efficacy of ADRCs delivered via the intracoronary route in the treatment of patients with ST-elevation acute myocardial infarction (ADVANCE) trial (NCT01216995)" have not started recruiting patients at the moment. No clinical data are available with adipose tissue stem cells as this stem cell was only identified in 2001 [41, 42].

3.4 Cardiac Stem Cells

Cardiosphere-derived cells are superior in paracrine potency and myocardial repair efficacy as compared to bone marrow- and adipose tissue-derived cells in experimental animals [88]. The investigators started "cardiosphere-derived autologous stem cells to reverse ventricular dysfunction (CADUCEUS) trial (NCT00893360)." This is a prospective, randomized, dose escalation study to evaluate the safety and efficacy of intracoronary delivery of cardiosphere-derived stem cells in patients with ischemic left ventricular dysfunction and recent myocardial infarction for 31 eligible patients. No complications with 24 h of cell infusion, no patient death, no cardiac tumor, and no major adverse cardiac event have been observed within 6 months for all patients [89]. At 6 months compared with controls, cell treatment significantly decreased scar mass, increased viable myocardial mass, as well as increased regional contractility and regional systolic wall thickening. The safety of cell infusion, the significant reduce in scar mass (28 %), and small increase in ejection fraction (39–41 %) warrant phase 2 study [89].

The "cardiac stem cell infusion in patients with ischemic cardiomyopathy (SCIPIO) trial (NCT00474461)" is a phase 1, randomized, open-label trial of autologous c-kit$^+$ cardiac stem cells in patients with heart failure due to ischemia undergoing coronary artery bypass grafting [90]. A total of 33 patients (20 cell treated and 13 control) are enrolled in the clinical trial. The increase of left ventricular ejection fraction, decrease of infarct size, decrease of left ventricular nonviable mass, and increase of left ventricular viable mass are strikingly improved for the cell-treated group at 4- and 12- month follow-up [91]. The "autologous human cardiac-derived stem cell to treat ischemic cardiomyopathy (ALCADIA) trial (NCT01697033)" is recruiting patients but has not reported their results.

3.5 Induced Pluripotent Stem Cells

At the moment there are no clinical trials using induced pluripotent stem cells (iPS) for cellular cardiomyoplasty (www.ClinicalTrials.gov). The approved "Evaluating Cardiovascular Phenotypes Using Induced Pluripotent Stem Cells" (NCT01517425) is using iPS to determine the changes in phenotypes of patients developing coronary artery disease. Although iPS have the potential for cell therapy and regenerative medicine, at the moment they are mainly used for the investigation of disease models [56–58].

4 Future Directions in Cellular Cardiomyoplasty

Any molecular, genetic, or cellular therapies that can restore or regenerate the damaged myocardium and improve ventricular function to prevent end-stage heart failure will alleviate mortality and morbidity to the patients. Unfortunately, other than heart transplant there is no clinical procedure to restore cardiac function for the patients suffering end-stage heart failure, and cellular cardiomyoplasty may offer an alternative after its perfection. Although a number of different cell types have been investigated experimentally and clinically, the search for the ideal cell type or combination of cell types for cellular cardiomyoplasty is still ongoing. The method of cell delivery and enhance retention, timing and dosing of cells, survival and engraftment of cells, the adjunctive treatment, or combined therapies will not be optimized till a better understanding of the beneficial mechanisms on cellular cardiomyoplasty.

The possible beneficial mechanisms for cell therapy are many, and a general consensus is lacking among different groups of investigators. In general the beneficial mechanisms of cellular cardiomyoplasty can be divided into myogenesis (activate contraction, improve compliance, scaffold effect, wall thickening, cell fusion, rescue damaged cells, modify matrix), angiogenesis (neovascularization, improve perfusion, enhance metabolism, minimize remolding, reverse remolding, salvage hibernating cells, rescue at-risk cells), and paracrine or endocrine effects (growth factors, angiogenic factors, cytokines, activate stem cells, mobilize stem cells, homing stem cells). The outcomes of beneficial mechanisms can be seen as follows: prevent infarct expansion, minimize remodeling, avoid cell death, regenerate myocardium, decrease scar tissue, better blood perfusion, enhance metabolism, augment regional function, and improve global function [5, 92].

The primary beneficial mechanism after mesenchymal stem cell transplantation is due to its paracrine effect by releasing angiogenic factors, antiapoptotic factors, and growth factors to improve perfusion, enhance metabolism, salvage damaged cells, and mobilize or activate endogenous stem cells. The paracrine effect that regulates the cellular and molecular mechanisms of endogenous heart stem cells for myocardial regeneration and repair can offer another alternative to cellular cardiomyoplasty. Indeed, intracoronary injection of insulin-like growth factor and hepatocyte growth factor [93] in a dose-dependent manner improved cardiomyocyte survival, reduced fibrosis, and significantly increased cardiac stem/progenitor cells.

Improving cellular retention, survival, mobilization, homing, and differentiation are different areas that can improve the outcomes of cellular cardiomyoplasty. The retention and engraftment rates of the cells are very low due to biological and mechanical losses [37, 70, 71]. Microencapsulation (Chapter 11), nanobiotechnology (Chapter 12), tissue engineering (Chapter 13), and magnetic targeting [94] all significantly increased cell retention and engraftment of implanted cells. Preconditioning of cells, pharmacologic agent, and genetic modification of stem cells are additional procedures to improve survival, mobilization, homing, and differentiation of stem cells for cellular cardiomyoplasty [37, 95].

Before resolving the problems of cell retention and survival, the study of the dose and time of cell administration may be meaningless due to the extremely low retention and engraftment rate. Most studies indicate that high doses of cells ($>10^8$) are more beneficial than the lower doses. Although early cell therapy (≤ 7 days) after myocardial infarction seems more effective than delayed treatment [39, 40, 83, 85], the delayed treatment also provides significant improvement in left ventricular function. More importantly, timing of treatment from animal studies cannot directly translate to clinical study. The changes in pathologic state is faster in smaller animals than large animals and humans after myocardial infarction, and relative pathologic state rather than actual date should be considered. To overcome the lack of transdifferentiation for skeletal muscle and bone marrow stem cells, treating the cultured cells with retinoic acid, dimethyl sulfoxide, 5-azacytidine, or other compound [96] can induce them different into cardiomyocytes. Cardiomyogenic pretreatment significantly increased the formation of cardiac myocytes after their transplantation into the injured heart [97], and different stem cells may require different treatment [98].

Cellular cardiomyoplasty has been moved rapidly from animal experiment to clinical trials with highly encouraging results. Unfortunately, the beneficial mechanisms lack general consensus that limit the optimization of the procedure. Although cell therapy has proved to be significantly beneficial to acute myocardial infarction, to chronic ischemic cardiomyopathy, and to heart failure patients, the beneficial outcomes are moderate. After a better understanding regarding the mechanisms of cellular cardiomyoplasty, the ideal cell type or combination of cell types, the optimal dose and time of treatment, and the beneficial adjunct therapies can be devised.

References

1. Roger VL, Go AS, Lloyd-Jones DM et al (2011) Heart disease and stroke statistics—2011 update: a report from the American Heart Association. Circulation 123:e18–e209
2. Ang KL, Shenje LT, Reuter S et al (2010) Limitations of conventional approaches to identify myocyte nuclei in histologic sections of the heart. Am J Physiol Cell Physiol 298:C1603–C1609
3. Soonpaa MH, Field LJ (1997) Assessment of cardiomyocyte DNA synthesis in normal and injured adult mouse hearts. Am J Physiol 272:H220–H226
4. Bergmann O, Bhardwaj RD, Bernard S et al (2009) Evidence for cardiomyocyte renewal in humans. Science 324:98–102
5. Kao RL, Browder W, Li C (2009) Cellular cardiomyoplasty: what have we learned? Asian Cardiovasc Thorac Ann 17:89–101
6. Steinhauser ML, Lee RT (2011) Regeneration of the heart. EMBO Mol Med 3:701–712
7. Laflamme MA, Murry CE (2011) Heart regeneration. Nature 473:326–335
8. Laflamme MA, Myerson D, Saffitz JE, Murry CE (2002) Evidence for cardiomyocyte repopulation by extracardiac progenitors in transplanted human hearts. Circ Res 90:634–640
9. Müller P, Pfeiffer P, Koglin J et al (2002) Cardiomyocytes of noncardiac origin in myocardial biopsies of human transplanted hearts. Circulation 106:31–35
10. Warejcka DJ, Harvey R, Taylor BJ et al (1996) A population of cells isolated from rat heart capable of differentiating into several mesodermal phenotypes. J Surg Res 62:233–242
11. Hierlihy AM, Seale P, Lobe CG et al (2002) The post-natal heart contains a myocardial stem cell population. FEBS Lett 530:239–243
12. Beltrami AP, Barlucchi L, Torella D et al (2003) Adult cardiac stem cells are multipotent and support myocardial regeneration. Cell 114:763–776
13. Laugwitz KL, Moretti A, Lam J et al (2005) Postnatal isl1+ cardioblasts enter fully differentiated cardiomyocyte lineages. Nature 433:647–653
14. Oyama T, Nagai T, Wada H et al (2007) Cardiac side population cells have a potential to migrate and differentiate into cardiomyocytes in vitro and in vivo. J Cell Biol 176:329–341
15. Bearzi C, Rota M, Hosoda T et al (2007) Human cardiac stem cells. Proc Natl Acad Sci USA 104:14068–14073
16. Tang YL, Shen L, Qian K, Phillips MI (2007) A novel two-step procedure to expand cardiac Sca-1+ cells clonally. Biochem Biophys Res Commun 359:877–883
17. Smith RR, Barile L, Cho HC et al (2007) Regenerative potential of cardiosphere derived cells expanded from percutaneous endomyocardial biopsy specimens. Circulation 115:896–908
18. Andersen DC, Andersen P, Schneider M et al (2009) Murine "cardiospheres" are not a source of stem cells with cardiomyogenic potential. Stem Cells 27:1571–1581
19. Shiba Y, Fernandes S, Zhu WZ et al (2012) Human ES-cell-derived cardiomyocytes electrically couple and suppress arrhythmias in injured hearts. Nature 489:322–325
20. Kao RL, Rizzo C, Magovern GJ (1989) Satellite cells for myocardial regeneration. Physiologist 32:220
21. Kao RL, Chiu RCJ (1997) Satellite cell implantation. In: Kao RL, Chiu RCJ (eds) Cellular cardiomyoplasty: myocardial repair with cell implantation. Chapman & Hall, New York, pp 129–162
22. Menasché P, Hagège AA, Scorsin M et al (2001) Myoblast transplantation for heart failure. Lancet 357:279–280
23. Mauro A (1978) Muscle regeneration. Raven, New York

24. Pallafacchina G, Blaauw B, Schiaffino S (2012) Role of satellite cells in muscle growth and maintenance of muscle mass. Nutr Metab Cardiovasc Dis [Epub ahead of print]
25. Mauro A (1961) Satellite cells of skeletal muscle fibers. J Biophys Biochem Cytol 9:493–495
26. Usas A, Mačiulaitis J, Mačiulaitis R et al (2011) Skeletal muscle-derived stem cells: implications for cell-mediated therapies. Medicina (Kaunas) 47:469–479
27. Aziz A, Sebastian S, Dilworth FJ (2012) The origin and fate of muscle satellite cells. Stem Cell Rev 8:609–622
28. Menasché P (2011) Stem cell therapy for chronic heart failure: lessons from a 15-year experience. C R Biol 334:489–496
29. Menasche P (2011) Cardiac cell therapy: lessons from clinical trials. J Mol Cell Cardiol 50:258–265
30. Friedenstein AJ (1976) Precursor cells of mechanocytes. Int Rev Cytol 47:327–359
31. Prockop DJ (1997) Marrow stromal cells as stem cells for nonhematopoietic tissues. Science 276:71–74
32. Chamberlain G, Fox J, Ashton B, Middleton J (2007) Concise review: mesenchymal stem cells: their phenotype, differentiation capacity, immunological features, and potential for homing. Stem Cells 25:2739–2749
33. Dominici M, Le Blanc K, Mueller I et al (2006) Minimal criteria for defining multipotent mesenchymal stromal cells. The International Society for Cellular Therapy position statement. Cytotherapy 8:315–317
34. Tomita S, Li RK, Weisel RD et al (1999) Autologous transplantation of bone marrow cells improves damaged heart function. Circulation 100(19 Suppl):II247–II256
35. Wang JS, Shum-Tim D, Galipeau J et al (2000) Marrow stromal cells for cellular cardiomyoplasty: feasibility and potential clinical advantages. J Thorac Cardiovasc Surg 120:999–1005
36. Orlic D, Kajstura J, Chimenti S et al (2001) Bone marrow cells regenerate infarcted myocardium. Nature 410:701–705
37. Wu KH, Mo XM, Han ZC, Zhou B (2011) Stem cell engraftment and survival in the ischemic heart. Ann Thorac Surg 92:1917–1925
38. Hoover-Plow J, Gong Y (2012) Challenges for heart disease stem cell therapy. Vasc Health Risk Manag 8:99–113
39. Wen Y, Meng L, Xie J, Ouyang J (2011) Direct autologous bone marrow-derived stem cell transplantation for ischemic heart disease: a meta-analysis. Expert Opin Biol Ther 11:559–567
40. Wen Y, Meng L, Ding Y, Ouyang J (2011) Autologous transplantation of blood-derived stem/progenitor cells for ischaemic heart disease. Int J Clin Pract 65:858–865
41. Zuk PA, Zhu M, Mizuno H et al (2001) Multilineage cells from human adipose tissue: implications for cell-based therapies. Tissue Eng 7:211–228
42. Halvorsen YD, Franklin D, Bond AL et al (2001) Extracellular matrix mineralization and osteoblast gene expression by human adipose tissue-derived stromal cells. Tissue Eng 7:729–741
43. Zhu Y, Liu T, Song K et al (2008) Adipose-derived stem cell: a better stem cell than BMSC. Cell Biochem Funct 26:664–675
44. van Dijk A, Naaijkens BA, Jurgens WJ et al (2011) Reduction of infarct size by intravenous injection of uncultured adipose derived stromal cells in a rat model is dependent on the time point of application. Stem Cell Res 7:219–229
45. Sun CK, Yen CH, Lin YC et al (2011) Autologous transplantation of adipose-derived mesenchymal stem cells markedly reduced acute ischemia-reperfusion lung injury in a rodent model. J Transl Med 9(118):1–13
46. Cawthorn WP, Scheller EL, MacDougald OA (2012) Adipose tissue stem cells: the great WAT hope. Trends Endocrinol Metab 23:270–277
47. Planat-Bénard V, Menard C, André M et al (2004) Spontaneous cardiomyocyte differentiation from adipose tissue stroma cells. Circ Res 94:223–229
48. Rangappa S, Fen C, Lee EH et al (2003) Transformation of adult mesenchymal stem cells isolated from the fatty tissue into cardiomyocytes. Ann Thorac Surg 75:775–779
49. Chang W, Lim S, Song BW et al (2012) Phorbol myristate acetate differentiates human adipose-derived mesenchymal stem cells into functional cardiogenic cells. Biochem Biophys Res Commun 424:740–746
50. Madonna R, Geng YJ, De Caterina R (2009) Adipose tissue-derived stem cells: characterization and potential for cardiovascular repair. Arterioscler Thromb Vasc Biol 29:1723–1729
51. Bai X, Alt E (2010) Myocardial regeneration potential of adipose tissue-derived stem cells. Biochem Biophys Res Commun 401:321–326
52. Oh H, Bradfute SB, Gallardo TD et al (2003) Cardiac progenitor cells from adult myocardium: homing, differentiation, and fusion after infarction. Proc Natl Acad Sci USA 100:12313–12318
53. Messina E, De Angelis L, Frati G et al (2004) Isolation and expansion of adult cardiac stem cells from human and murine heart. Circ Res 95:911–921

54. Takahashi K, Yamanaka S (2006) Induction of pluripotent stem cells from mouse embryonic and adult fibroblast cultures by defined factors. Cell 126:663–676
55. Takahashi K, Tanabe K, Ohnuki M et al (2007) Induction of pluripotent stem cells from adult human fibroblasts by defined factors. Cell 131:861–872
56. Robinton DA, Daley GQ (2012) The promise of induced pluripotent stem cells in research and therapy. Nature 481:295–305
57. Oh SI, Lee CK, Cho KJ et al (2012) Technological progress in generation of induced pluripotent stem cells for clinical applications. ScientificWorldJournal 2012: 417809. Epub 2012 Mar 12
58. Yamanaka S (2012) Induced pluripotent stem cells: past, present, and future. Cell Stem Cell 10:678–684
59. Greenow K, Clarke AR (2012) Controlling the stem cell compartment and regeneration in vivo: the role of pluripotency pathways. Physiol Rev 92:75–99
60. Oh Y, Wei H, Ma D et al (2012) Clinical applications of patient-specific induced pluripotent stem cells in cardiovascular medicine. Heart 98:443–449
61. Okita K, Nakagawa M, Hyenjong H et al (2008) Generation of mouse induced pluripotent stem cells without viral vectors. Science 322:949–953
62. Tang C, Lee AS, Volkmer JP et al (2011) An antibody against SSEA-5 glycan on human pluripotent stem cells enables removal of teratoma-forming cells. Nat Biotechnol 29:829–834
63. Nelson TJ, Martinez-Fernandez A, Yamada S et al (2009) Repair of acute myocardial infarction by human stemness factors induced pluripotent stem cells. Circulation 120:408–416
64. Mauritz C, Martens A, Rojas SV et al (2011) Induced pluripotent stem cell (iPSC)-derived Flk-1 progenitor cells engraft, differentiate, and improve heart function in a mouse model of acute myocardial infarction. Eur Heart J 32:2634–2641
65. Choudry FA, Mathur A (2011) Stem cell therapy in cardiology. Regen Med 6(6 Suppl):17–23
66. Malliaras K, Marbán E (2011) Cardiac cell therapy: where we've been, where we are, and where we should be headed. Br Med Bull 98:161–185
67. Abdelli LS, Merino H, Rocher CM, Singla DK (2012) Cell therapy in the heart. Can J Physiol Pharmacol 90:307–315
68. Duran JM, Taghavi S, George JC (2012) The need for standardized protocols for future clinical trials of cell therapy. Transl Res 160(6):399–410
69. Durdu S, Deniz GC, Dogan A et al (2012) Stem cell mediated cardiovascular repair. Can J Physiol Pharmacol 90:337–351
70. Al Kindi A, Ge Y, Shum-Tim D, Chiu RC (2008) Cellular cardiomyoplasty: routes of cell delivery and retention. Front Biosci 13:2421–2434
71. Anderl JN, Robey TE, Stayton PS, Murry CE (2009) Retention and biodistribution of microspheres injected into ischemic myocardium. J Biomed Mater Res A 88:704–710
72. Menasché P, Alfieri O, Janssens S et al (2008) The myoblast autologous grafting in ischemic cardiomyopathy (MAGIC) trial: first randomized placebo-controlled study of myoblast transplantation. Circulation 117:1189–1200
73. Povsic TJ, O'Connor CM, Henry T et al (2011) A double-blind, randomized, controlled, multicenter study to assess the safety and cardiovascular effects of skeletal myoblast implantation by catheter delivery in patients with chronic heart failure after myocardial infarction. Am Heart J 162:654–662
74. Duckers HJ, Houtgraaf J, Hehrlein C et al (2011) Final results of a phase IIa, randomised, open-label trial to evaluate the percutaneous intramyocardial transplantation of autologous skeletal myoblasts in congestive heart failure patients: the SEISMIC trial. EuroIntervention 6:805–812
75. Beitnes JO, Hopp E, Lunde K et al (2009) Long-term results after intracoronary injection of autologous mononuclear bone marrow cells in acute myocardial infarction: the ASTAMI randomised, controlled study. Heart 95:1983–1989
76. Assmus B, Rolf A, Erbs S et al (2010) Clinical outcome 2 years after intracoronary administration of bone marrow-derived progenitor cells in acute myocardial infarction. Circ Heart Fail 3:89–96
77. Pokushalov E, Romanov A, Chernyavsky A et al (2010) Efficiency of intramyocardial injections of autologous bone marrow mononuclear cells in patients with ischemic heart failure: a randomized study. J Cardiovasc Transl Res 3:160–168
78. Ahmadi H, Farahani MM, Kouhkan A et al (2012) Five-year follow-up of the local autologous transplantation of CD133+ enriched bone marrow cells in patients with myocardial infarction. Arch Iran Med 15:32–35
79. van der Laan A, Hirsch A, Nijveldt R et al (2008) Bone marrow cell therapy after acute myocardial infarction: the HEBE trial in perspective, first results. Neth Heart J 16:436–439
80. Yousef M, Schannwell CM, Köstering M et al (2009) The BALANCE Study: clinical benefit and long-term outcome after intracoronary

autologous bone marrow cell transplantation in patients with acute myocardial infarction. J Am Coll Cardiol 53:2262–2269
81. Strauer BE, Yousef M, Schannwell CM (2010) The acute and long-term effects of intracoronary Stem cell Transplantation in 191 patients with chronic heARt failure: the STAR-heart study. Eur J Heart Fail 12:721–729
82. Lamy A, Devereaux PJ, Prabhakaran D et al (2012) Off-pump or on-pump coronary-artery bypass grafting at 30 days. N Engl J Med 366:1489–1497
83. Clifford DM, Fisher SA, Brunskill SJ et al (2012) Stem cell treatment for acute myocardial infarction. Cochrane Database Syst Rev 2, CD006536
84. Zhao Q, Ye X (2011) Additive value of adult bone-marrow-derived cell transplantation to conventional revascularization in chronic ischemic heart disease: a systemic review and meta-analysis. Expert Opin Biol Ther 11:1569–1579
85. Donndorf P, Kundt G, Kaminski A et al (2011) Intramyocardial bone marrow stem cell transplantation during coronary artery bypass surgery: a meta-analysis. J Thorac Cardiovasc Surg 142:911–920
86. Qayyum AA, Haack-Sørensen M, Mathiasen AB et al (2012) Adipose-derived mesenchymal stromal cells for chronic myocardial ischemia (MyStromalCell Trial): study design. Regen Med 7:421–428
87. Houtgraaf JH, den Dekker WK, van Dalen BM et al (2012) First experience in humans using adipose tissue-derived regenerative cells in the treatment of patients with ST-segment elevation myocardial infarction. J Am Coll Cardiol 59:539–540
88. Li TS, Cheng K, Malliaras K et al (2012) Direct comparison of different stem cell types and subpopulations reveals superior paracrine potency and myocardial repair efficacy with cardiosphere-derived cells. J Am Coll Cardiol 59:942–953
89. Makkar RR, Smith RR, Cheng K et al (2012) Intracoronary cardiosphere-derived cells for heart regeneration after myocardial infarction (CADUCEUS): a prospective, randomised phase 1 trial. Lancet 379:895–904
90. Bolli R, Chugh AR, D'Amario D et al (2012) Cardiac stem cells in patients with ischaemic cardiomyopathy (SCIPIO): initial results of a randomised phase 1 trial. Lancet 378:1847–1857
91. Tatooles A, Stoddard MF, Lima JA et al (2012) Administration of cardiac stem cells in patients with ischemic cardiomyopathy: the SCIPIO trial: surgical aspects and interim analysis of myocardial function and viability by magnetic resonance. Circulation 126(11 Suppl 1):S54–S64
92. Kao RL, Ganote E, Pennington DG, Borwder IW (2007) Myocardial regeneration, tissue engineering and therapy. In: Prakash S (ed) Artificial cells, cell engineering and therapy, 1st edn. Woodhead Publishing Ltd., Cambridge, England, pp 349–365
93. Ellison GM, Torella D, Dellegrottaglie S et al (2011) Endogenous cardiac stem cell activation by insulin-like growth factor-1/hepatocyte growth factor intracoronary injection fosters survival and regeneration of the infarcted pig heart. J Am Coll Cardiol 58:977–986
94. Cheng K, Li TS, Malliaras K et al (2010) Magnetic targeting enhances engraftment and functional benefit of iron-labeled cardiosphere-derived cells in myocardial infarction. Circ Res 106:1570–1581
95. Lu HH, Li YF, Sheng ZQ, Wang Y (2012) Preconditioning of stem cells for the treatment of myocardial infarction. Chin Med J (Engl) 125:378–384
96. Haider HK, Ashraf M (2005) Bone marrow stem cell transplantation for cardiac repair. Am J Physiol Heart Circ Physiol 288: H2557–H2567
97. Bittira B, Kuang JQ, Al-Khaldi A, Shum-Tim D, Chiu RC (2002) In vitro preprogramming of marrow stromal cells for myocardial regeneration. Ann Thorac Surg 74:1154–1159
98. Grajales L, García J, Geenen DL (2012) Induction of cardiac myogenic lineage development differs between mesenchymal and satellite cells and is accelerated by bone morphogenetic protein-4. J Mol Cell Cardiol 53:382–391

Chapter 2

Skeletal Muscle Stem Cells

Grace W. Kao, Elizabeth K. Lamb, and Race L. Kao

Abstract

Skeletal muscle satellite cells (myoblasts) are the primary stem cells of skeletal muscle which contribute to growth, maintenance, and repair of the muscles. Satellite cells are the first stem cells used for cellular cardiomyoplasty more than 20 years ago. The isolation, culture, labeling, and identification of satellite cells are described in detail here. The implantation and outcomes of cellular cardiomyoplasty using satellite cells have been summarized in the previous chapter (Chapter 1).

Key words Satellite cell, Stem cell, Skeletal muscle, Cell isolation, Cell culture, Cell transfection, GFP, Y chromosome FISH

1 Introduction

During embryonic life, myoblasts multiply and fuse to form multinuclear myotubes that mature into myofibers (muscle fibers) which are the functional units of skeletal muscle. Normal muscle growth takes place through increases in the length and diameter of existing muscle fibers with 2- to 4-fold increase in the number of muscle nuclei. Injured skeletal muscles regenerate both by the repair of surviving muscle fibers and the formation of new fibers [1–5]. True muscle nuclei are postmitotic and normally cannot produce additional muscle nuclei, while injured skeletal muscle is primary regenerated from satellite cells.

Satellite cells (Fig. 1) are mononucleated myogenic precursor cells located under the basal lamina but outside the sarcolemma of skeletal muscle [1, 6, 7]. They are 25 by 5 μm spindle-shaped cells containing a heterochromatic nucleus and scanty cytoplasm with few organelles. The cytoplasm is dominated by large quantities of free ribosomes with some rough endoplasmic reticulum [8–10]. Satellite cell was first identified and named by Mauro in 1961 [11], since then many studies and reviews have been published [12, 13]. Radioautographic studies reveal that dividing satellite cells are able to fuse with existing muscle fibers for providing new muscle nuclei

Race L. Kao (ed.), *Cellular Cardiomyoplasty: Methods and Protocols*, Methods in Molecular Biology, vol. 1036, DOI 10.1007/978-1-62703-511-8_2, © Springer Science+Business Media New York 2013

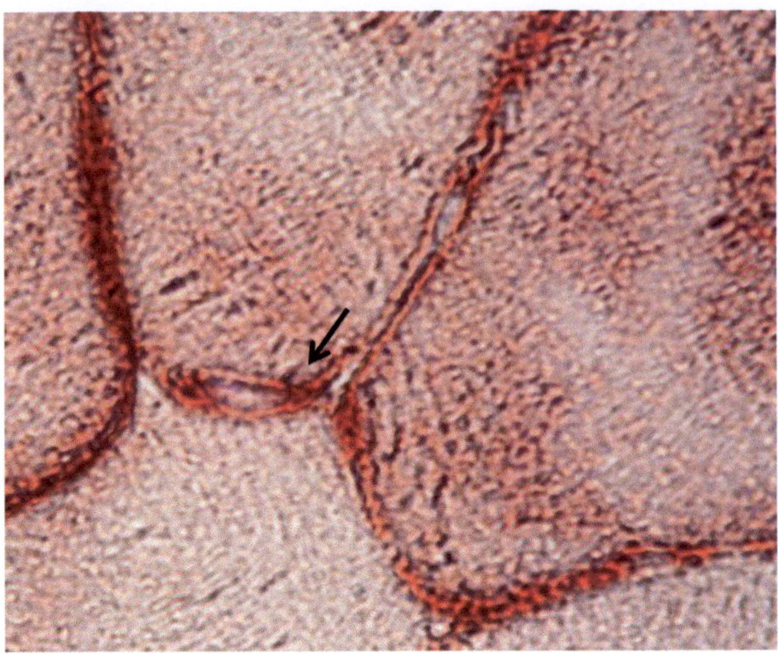

Fig. 1 Satellite cell (*arrow*) located under the basal lamina but outside of the sarcolemma associated with a muscle fiber. This picture represents a cross section sample from skeletal muscle

and to fuse with themselves for forming new muscle fibers [1, 4]. In adult skeletal muscles, satellite cell nuclei represent 3–6 % of all muscle nuclei, which are located under the basal lamina with higher frequency in slow fibers as compared to fast fibers [6].

Although other skeletal muscle stem cells such as side population cells, pericytes, mesoangioblasts, and myoendothelial cells have also been identified, their contribution to growth, maintenance, or repair of muscle requires further study. For this chapter, we will name the skeletal muscle stem cells as satellite cells, and the isolation, culture, labeling, and identification of satellite cells will be described in detail here. The implantation and outcomes of cellular cardiomyoplasty using satellite cells have been reviewed [14, 15] and summarized in Chapter 1.

2 Materials

2.1 Skeletal Muscle Sampling

1. Animals: dog, pig, rat, mouse, or others can be used (*see* **Note 1**).
2. Medication and anesthetic agents: atropine; pentobarbital sodium injection, 50 mg/mL (pentobarbital); telazol; xylazine; and isoflurane.
3. Clipper and shaver.
4. 70 % Ethanol: ethanol dilute with water to 70 % (v/v).

5. Betadine solution: 5 % povidone-iodine.
6. Hanks balanced salt solution without Ca^{++} or Mg^{++}.
7. Antibiotic antimycotic solution 100×: 10,000 U penicillin, 10 mg streptomycin, and 25 μg amphotericin B per mL (catalog number A 5955) (Sigma Chemical Co., St. Louis, MO, USA).
8. 50 ml sterile centrifuge tubes or sterile Petri dishes.
9. Sterile gauze and drapes.
10. Scalpel, scissors, forceps, hemostats, retractor, needle holders, and sutures.

2.2 Satellite Cell Culture

1. Sterile scalpel, scissors, forceps, hemostats, and gauze.
2. Laminar flow hood.
3. 70 % Ethanol.
4. Hanks balanced salt solution without Ca^{++} or Mg^{++}.
5. Collagenase and hyaluronidase (*see* **Note 2**).
6. Sodium bicarbonate solution: 7.5 % sodium bicarbonate, sterile filtered.
7. Rinsing solution: Hanks balanced salt solution without Ca^{++} or Mg^{++} equilibrated with 95 % O_2:5 % CO_2 containing 1 % antibiotic antimycotic solution.
8. Enzyme solution: Medium 199 equilibrated with 95 % O_2:5 % CO_2 containing 0.2 % collagenase, 0.1 % hyaluronidase, and 4 % sodium bicarbonate solution (adjusted per each lot of collagenase, *see* **Note 2**) follow by sterile filtration. Store the solution on ice if it is not used right away.
9. Culture medium: Medium 199 adding 1 % antibiotic antimycotic solution and 10 % fetal bovine serum (*see* **Note 3**).
10. Centrifuge tubes and culture flasks.
11. 37 °C shaking water bath.
12. Vacuum filter system (*see* **Note 4**).
13. Pipet system.
14. Protease or 2.5 %, 10× solution trypsin solution.
15. Detaching medium: Medium 199 with 1 % protease and sterile filtered or medium 199 with 10 % trypsin solution.
16. 95 % O_2:5 % CO_2 with inline filter and sterile end.
17. Differentiation medium: Medium 199 with 2 % horse serum and 1 % antibiotic antimycotic solution.
18. 5 % CO_2 incubator.

2.3 Labeling of Satellite Cells

In order to identify the satellite cells after implanted into injured heart, it is necessary to label the cells before implantation. We have compared different labeling procedures for satellite cells in our previous publication [16]. Although satellite cells can be labeled with fluorescent microspheres (0.49 μ, Polysciences Inc., Warrington, PA, USA), 4′-6-diamidino-2-phenylindole (DAPI), or pulse labeled with ^{3}H-thymidine, the major limitation of these procedures is that the labeling intensity will decrease as the cell divides. The mammalian reporter vectors lacZ (pCMVβ) from Clontech Laboratories, Inc. (Palo Alto, CA, USA), and green fluorescent protein (GFP) from Invitrogen (Carlsbad, CA, USA) can be transfected into satellite cells using Lipofectamine (Gibco BRL) (Gaithersburg, MD, USA). Transfection with Lipofectamine suffers the low-efficiency and losing labeling intensity after cell implantation.

AdenoLacZ and AdenoGFP from Quantum Biotechnologies (Montreal, Quebec, Canada) can be added directly into the culture medium and labeling the cultured satellite cells. The adenovectors offer high-efficiency labeling of satellite cells that can be detected even after 8 weeks in culture. However, to reveal β-galactosidase activity, labeled satellite cells need to be fixed, and false-positive X-gal reaction should be carefully avoided [17]. X-gal reaction at pH 7.4 and 37 °C for 6 h is recommended. AdenoGFP provides outstanding labeling efficiency with high specific and definition without interfering with the myogenic capability of labeled satellite cells. Recently retroviral and lentiviral vectors have been developed for labeling of cells and gene transfection. Their application will be described. In addition using male inbred animal donor cells and transplant into inbred female animals, the Y chromosome of donor cells can be an ideal preexisting marker for the donor cells.

2.3.1 Viral Transfection of Satellite Cells

1. Cultured satellite cells at 70–80 % confluent.
2. Certified biosafety cabinet.
3. Culture medium: Medium 199 adding 1 % antibiotic antimycotic solution and 10 % fetal bovine serum (heat inactivated).
4. Hexadimethrine bromide (Polybrene) stock solution: 6 mg/mL Polybrene dissolved in Medium 199 and sterile filtered (*see* **Note 5**).
5. Stratagene pFB-hrGFP retroviral supernatant (catalog number 972000-43) (Agilent Technologies, Inc., Santa Clara, CA, USA) or Invitrogen CMV-GFP lentiviral supernatant (catalog number A1357701) (Invitrogen, Grand Island, NY, USA).
6. Centrifuge tubes and culture flasks.
7. Pipet system.
8. 5 % CO_2 incubator.
9. 70 % Ethanol and bleach.
10. Transfection medium: culture medium (as **item 3**) adding

Polybrene stock solution to a final concentration of 6 μg/mL and proper amount of viral supernatant (*see* **Note 5**).

2.3.2 Y Chromosome FISH

Fluorescence in situ hybridization (FISH) can be used to identify specific chromosomes. Using inbred animals in cellular cardiomyoplasty, it is possible to use the male donor cells transplanted into female animals and identify the donor cells by the presence of Y chromosome. The differentiation fate of the transplanted cells can be determined by the specific cell markers by histologic or immunohistochemical procedures [18].

1. Saline sodium citrate solution (SSC): for 20× SSC use 500 mL of deionized distilled water containing 87.6 g NaCl and 44.1 g Na citrate at pH 7.0 adjusted by concentrated HCl (adjust pH before make up to final volume). Autoclaved or sterile filtered before aliquot and stored at 4 °C.
2. Absolute ethanol (100 %) and (v/v) 70 and 90 % ethanol.
3. Pipet system.
4. Coplin jars.
5. Phosphate buffer saline (PBS): containing 137 mM NaCl, 2.7 mM KCl, 10 mM Na_2HPO_4, and 2 mM KH_2PO_4 at pH 7.4.
6. Citrate buffer: 0.1 M citrate acid stock solution and 0.1 M trisodium citrate stock solution. Mix 9 mL of 0.1 M citrate acid stock solution and 41 mL of 0.1 M trisodium citrate stock solution and adjust to pH 6.0 and make up to 500 mL.
7. RNase solution: 100 μg/mL RNase in 2× SSC.
8. Pepsin solution: to 1 mL of 10 mM HCl adding 0.5 μL of pepsin stock solution (1 mg/mL) mix well.
9. Humidified chamber.
10. Water bath.
11. Incubator.
12. Biotin-labeled Y chromosome probe for mouse (catalog number 1697-MB-01) or for human (catalog number CPBR-70-00Y) (Cambio Ltd., Dry Drayton, Cambridge, UK).
13. Detergent wash solution: 500 mL 4× SSC add 250 μL Tween 20.
14. Detection reagent (catalog number 1124-Y1-50) (Cambio Ltd.) with Cy3 streptavidin.
15. Working reagent: 2.5 μL detection reagent mixed with 1247.5 μL of detergent wash solution.
16. DAPI if nuclear stain is preferred.
17. Confocal microscope.

3 Methods

3.1 Skeletal Muscle Sampling

1. After overnight fasting, the small animals (rat, mouse) were euthanized with an overdose of pentobarbital (100 mg/kg, intraperitoneally). The large animals were treated with atropine (0.05 mg/kg intramuscularly to reduce salivation for intubation) before induction with pentobarbital (dog, 20 mg/kg intravenously) or telazol (4.4 mg/kg) plus xylazine (1 mg/kg) intramuscularly for pig. After intubation, the anesthesia was maintained by 2–2.5 % isoflurane inhalation.
2. The surgical site was clipped and shaved before being cleaned with 70 % ethanol and followed by Betadine solution.
3. The hindquarter muscles were removed from the small animals, while the muscle sample from tibialis anterior (dog) or longissimus (pig) was obtained (*see* **Note 6**).
4. The muscle sample was placed in a 50 ml sterile centrifuge tube or a sterile Petri dish containing Hanks balanced salt solution without Ca^{++} or Mg^{++} but with 1 % antibiotic antimycotic solution.
5. For dog and pig, the wound was closed in layers, and subcuticular closure should be used for skin.

3.2 Culture of Satellite Cells

1. Quickly take the muscle to a laminar flow hood, and while holding the sample with forceps or hemostat, rinse it with 70 % ethanol followed by rinsing solution.
2. Place the muscle sample on a sterile cutting board and remove any connective tissue or adipose tissue before cutting the muscle into small pieces using the scalpel. Alternatively, the muscle can be teased into very thin bundles (<1 mm in diameter) using an 18-gauge hypodermic needle following the direction of muscle fibers. Transfer about 5 g of muscle tissue into a 50 mL centrifuge tube adding 40 mL rinsing solution and mix thoroughly.
3. Centrifuge at 145 ×*g* for 1 min to pellet the muscle pieces. After removal of the supernatant, the muscle pieces are further minced with a pair of scissors to about 1 mm^3 (*see* **Note 7**).
4. Repeat the washing of muscle slurry with rising solution for two additional times by resuspension and centrifugation (*see* **Note 8**).
5. Add 35 mL of enzyme solution to the muscle slurry and incubate at 37 °C in the shaking water bath with vigorous shaking for 10 min.
6. Centrifuge at 145 ×*g* for 1 min and filter the supernatant through layers of sterile gauze. Centrifuge the filtered supernatant at 580 ×*g* for 5 min to pellet the satellite cells.

After removal and discard of the supernatant, the pelleted satellite cells are vortexed (to avoid clumping) and resuspended in culture medium. Repeat the washing of satellite cells with culture medium for two additional times by resuspension and centrifugation.

7. The remaining muscle tissue is subjected to one or two (depending on the completeness of enzyme digestion) additional enzyme treatment to release the remaining satellite cells. The satellite cells are recovered and washed as above.
8. The isolated and washed satellite cells are cultured with the culture medium using culture flasks in the 5 % CO_2 incubator with humidified atmosphere at 37 °C.
9. Preplate technique [12, 19] can be used to reduce the fibroblasts in satellite cell preparation. However, if connective tissue has been carefully removed after muscle sampling, a high percentage of satellite cells in culture can be obtained.
10. After 3 days, replace the culture medium and discard the nonadherent cells. The cultured satellite cells are observed daily (Fig. 2a) and replaced with fresh medium twice a week.
11. When satellite cells reach 70–80 % confluent, the cells are recovered, and each flask is plated into two flasks to maintain continued multiplication without differentiation.
12. To detach the cultured satellite cells, remove the culture medium, rinse with Medium 199, and cover the cells with detaching medium (~2 mL). Observe under microscope frequently within 2–3 min. As soon as the cells are detached, add 5 mL of culture medium and pellet the detached cells by centrifugation. Repeat the washing of satellite cells with culture medium for two additional times by resuspension and centrifugation before subculturing in culture flasks.
13. To determine the myogenic capability of satellite cells, the culture medium will be replaced with differentiation medium, and the formation of myotubes can be observed (Fig. 2b).

3.3 Labeling of Satellite Cells

Recently retroviral and lentiviral vectors have been developed for labeling of cells and gene transfection. Replication-defective retroviral and lentiviral gene transfer systems are commercially available. After entering the cells, the viral reverse transcriptase synthesizes viral DNA from the viral RNA. The viral DNA will integrate into host genome and result in sustained expression of vector. Lentivirus is a member of the retroviral family and can efficiently infect both dividing and nondividing cells.

3.3.1 Viral Transfection of Satellite Cells

1. The day before transfection, satellite cells will be detached and plated as above (Subheading 3.2 **step 12**).

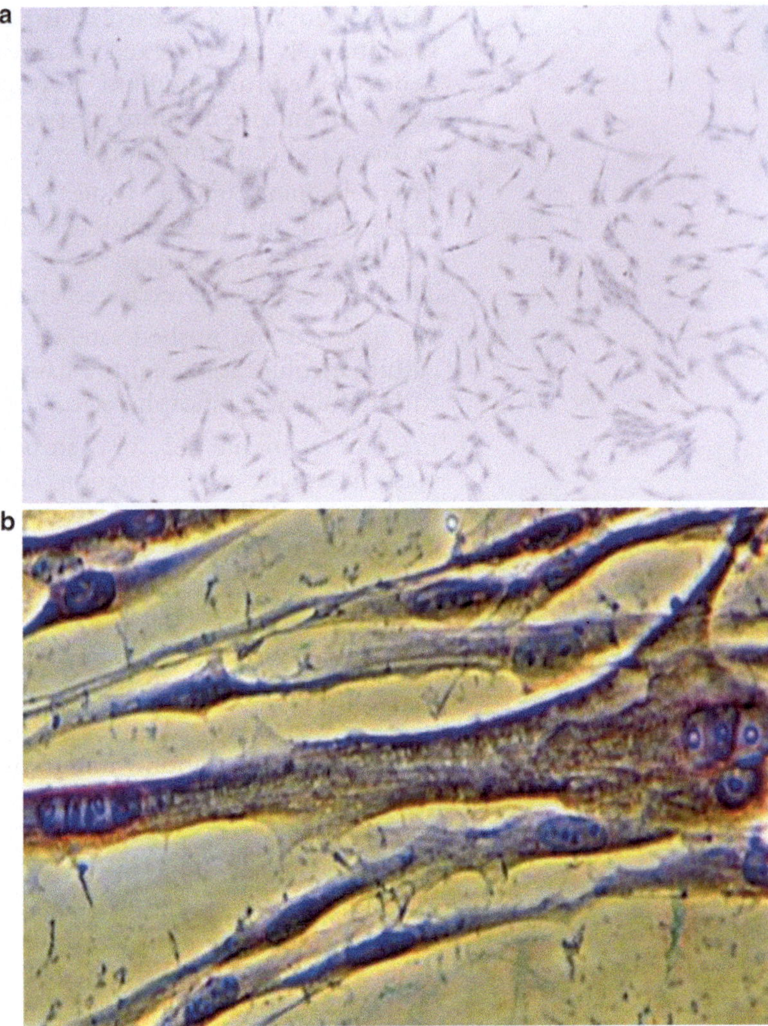

Fig. 2 Cultured satellite cells from skeletal muscle (**a**) and myotube formed from cultured satellite cells after being maintained in differentiation medium. Multiple nuclei can be observed in the myotube (**b**)

2. All procedures should perform in a certified biosafety cabinet. Wear gloves, laboratory coat, and safety glasses or goggles and following federal and institutional guidelines for working with infectious agents. The outside of tubes should be wiped with 70 % ethanol before opening. Treat used pipettes, pipette tips, tissue culture supplies, and used or remaining transfection medium with bleach and dispose as biohazardous waste (*see* **Note 9**).
3. After rinsing the cells with fresh culture medium and discard, the culture medium will be replaced by transfection medium at an amount just enough to cover the cells. Gently mix the transfection medium with the cells and put back into the 5 % CO_2 incubator.

4. After 12 h, the transfection medium will be replaced with regular culture medium (*see* **Note 5**).
5. The expression of GFP can be evaluated for the satellite cells under a fluorescence microscope at 24 or 48 h later (48 h will have higher GFP signal) (Fig. 3a).
6. The excitation/emission peaks for Stratagene pFB-hrGFP is 500/506 nm and for Invitrogen CMV-GFP (EmGFP) is 487/509 nm. Filter sets can be obtained from Omega Optical, Inc. (www.omegafilters.com), Chroma Technology Co. (www.chroma.com), or other sources.
7. Differentiation medium can be used to observe the myotube formation of the transfected satellite cells (Fig. 3b, c).

3.3.2 Y Chromosome FISH

1. For cells grown on slides, cells will be fixed in ethanol/acetic acid (3:1) and allowed to dry (*see* **Note 10**).
2. The slides are passed through a graded ethanol series of 70, 90, and 100 % for 2 min to remove acid residue and air-dry.
3. Bake the slides at 65 °C for 15 min to allow better attachment of cells on slides, cool to room temperature, and placed in acetone for 10 min before air-dry.
4. For frozen sections, equilibrate the slides to room temperature.
5. Wash in 2× SSC twice at 3 min each.
6. Incubate in 0.2 M HCl at room temperature for 10 min.
7. Wash again in 2× SSC twice at 3 min each.
8. Incubate in 1 M sodium thiocyanate (NaSCN) for 20 min at 75 °C.
9. Rinse in water and dehydrate in graded ethanol (70, 90, and 100 %) for 2 min each and air-dry.
10. For paraffin-embedded slides, the slides will be deparaffinized in xylene (twice), 100, 90, and 70 % ethanol for 5 min each.
11. Rinse in water and then wash with PBS for 5 min.
12. Boil the slide in citrate buffer for 10 min and let it stand in the buffer without heating for 20 min.
13. Wash in 2× SSC twice at 3 min each.
14. Incubate in 0.2 M HCl at room temperature for 10 min.
15. Wash again in 2× SSC twice at 3 min each.
16. Incubate in 1 M NaSCN for 20 min at 75 °C.
17. Rinse in water and dehydrate in graded ethanol (70, 90, and 100 %) for 2 min each and air-dry.
18. Wash slides in PBS for 5 min.
19. Dehydrate through graded ethanol.
20. Air-dry slides.

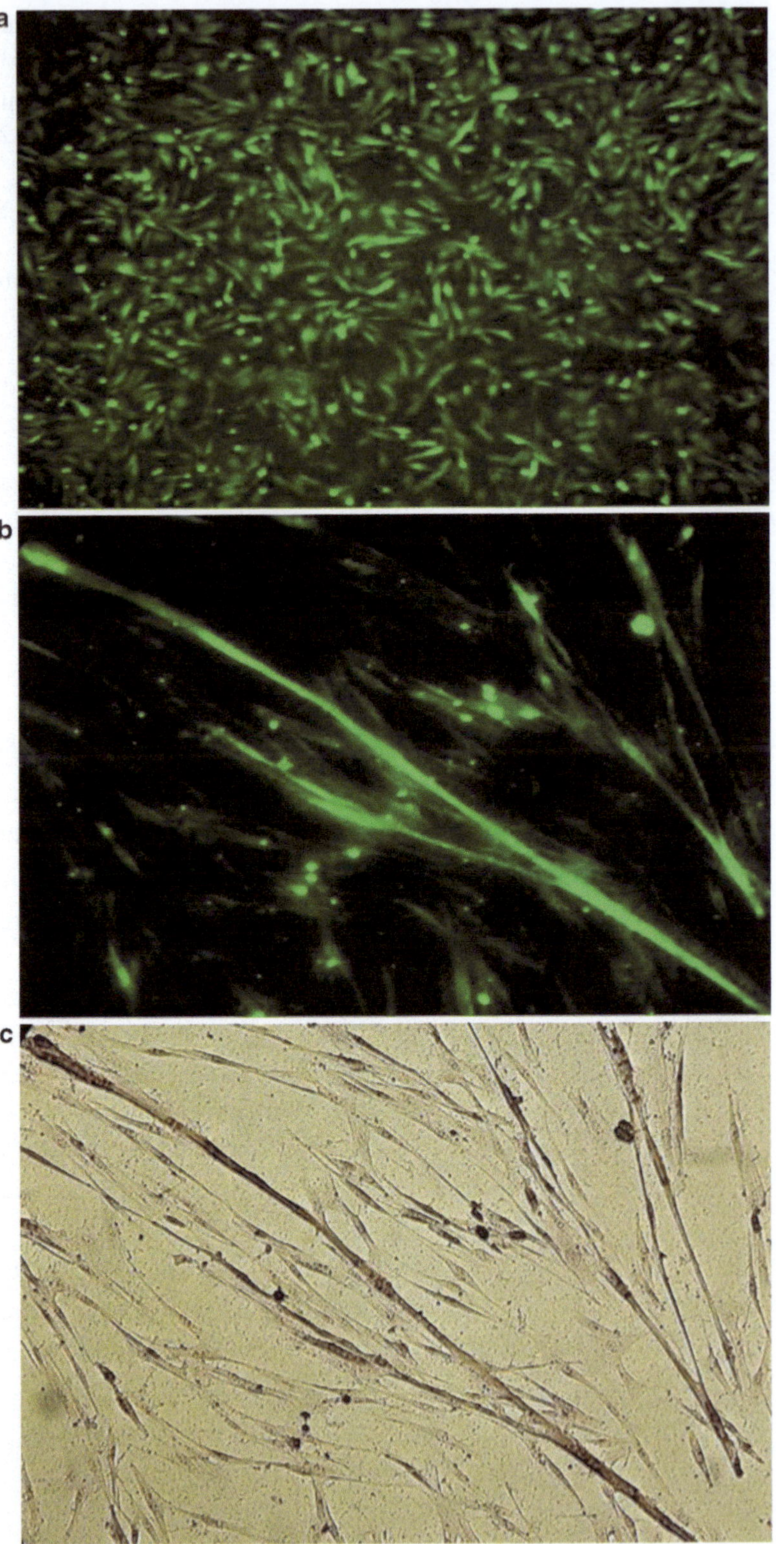

Fig. 3 Satellite cells (**a**) labeled with green fluorescence protein (GFP). The formation of myotube from GFP-labeled satellite cells under fluorescent microscope (**b**) and the same field under light microscope (**c**)

21. Denature cellular DNA by immersing in 2× SSC with 70 % formamide (15 mL 2× SSC + 35 mL formamide) at 70 °C for 2 min.
22. After denaturation, place slides in ice-cold 70 % ethanol for 2 min.
23. Dehydrate through ethanol series for 2 min each.
24. Air-dry slides.
25. Apply 12.5 μL of biotin-labeled probes on to the slide (this is for 22 × 22 mm coverslip, adjust amount base on area).
26. Seal the slide with coverslip using rubber cement.
27. Incubate at 85 °C for 10 min.
28. Hybridize for approximately 16 h at 37 °C in a humidified chamber.
29. Remove rubber cement and place in 1× SSC to remove coverslip (do not allow slide to dry).
30. Wash twice in 1× SSC with 50 % formamide at 45 °C for 5 min each.
31. Wash again in 1× SSC twice for 5 min each time at 45 °C.
32. Incubate in detergent wash solution at 45 °C for 4 min.
33. Apply 100 μL of working reagent onto the slide and cover the slide with Parafilm immediately.
34. Incubate slide in a humidified chamber at 37 °C for 15–20 min.
35. Remove Parafilm from slide and wash three times in the detergent wash solution for 4 min each time.
36. Drain slide well, stain with DAPI if desired, and mount with a glass coverslip.
37. Store slide in dark at 4 °C or observed under confocal microscope for Cy3 (Fig. 4).

4 Notes

1. For animals, young adults are preferred over than the aged animals for higher yield of satellite cells and less non-myogenic cells [20, 21]. For small animals (rat, mouse), inbred animals can be used to avoid rejection. For human or large animals, autologous samples are used.
2. Highly purified collagenase offer no advantage as compared to crude collagenase for satellite cell isolation other than higher cost. Same units of collagenase will have same function for cell isolation. The endotoxin contamination in collagenase is a major concern; low or undetectable endotoxin is preferred. Most collagenase products were obtained through acid precipitation, and the acid residue can alter the pH of the

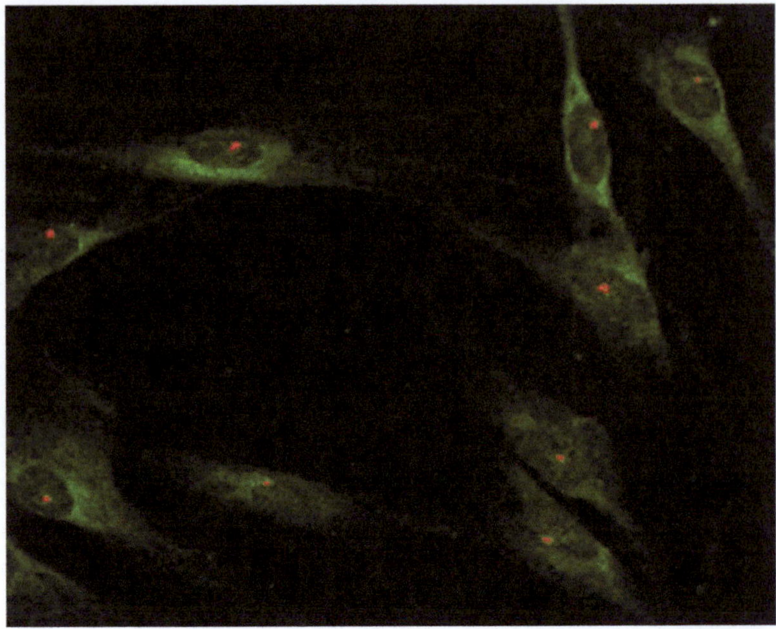

Fig. 4 Cultured satellite cells from male mouse that have been labeled with GFP and also subjected to Y chromosome FISH and revealed with Cy3 streptavidin

enzyme solution. Proper amount of sodium bicarbonate solution can be added to overcome this. For each lot of collagenase, the amount of sodium bicarbonate required is quite consistent for a fixed amount of the enzyme; therefore, the calculated volume can be applied for the complete lot of collagenase.

3. Different lots of fetal bovine serum will support the growth and multiplication of satellite cells differently. The supplier will give free samples from different lots of fetal bovine serum for evaluation. Once a good lot is identified, it will be wise to purchase sufficient amount to last for many experiments.

4. Sterile filtration is necessary to prevent pathogen growth in satellite cell culture. The enzymes (collagenase, hyaluronidase, protease) after dissolved in medium must be sterile filtered using the vacuum filter system (Corning or Nalgene all work well). Due to the high particulate content of collagenase, it will be wise to do step by step filtration using decreasing pore size filters (0.45 μ then 0.2 μ) to prevent membrane becomes blockage. Alternatively high capacity mini capsule filter of 0.2 μ (Gelman Sciences, Ann Arbor, MI) can be used.

5. The sterile filtered Polybrene stock solution can be divided into small aliquots (1 mL per tube) and stored at −20 °C for long duration. Freezing/thawing the stock solution will lose its activity. Polybrene is a polycation that reduces charge

repulsion between the virus and the cellular membrane to enhance transfection efficiency. The contact of virus with cell membrane is necessary for successful transfection. Excessive exposure to Polybrene can be toxic to cells, and the optimal dose (usually 2–12 μg/mL), viral concentration (usually $>1 \times 10^7$ multiplicity of infection), as well as transfection duration (usually 8–24 h) needs to be worked out for different laboratories. Repetitive freezing and thawing of the viral stock solution is not recommended because it may result in loss of viral titer. Divide the stock solution into small aliquots and store in −80 °C freezer.

6. For small animals, it is important to carefully stay away from the anal area to avoid contamination. For large animals, other skeletal muscle can be selected for satellite cell isolation. There is a neurovascular bundle passing through the middle deep portion of the tibialis anterior muscle; salvaging this neurovascular bundle is recommended. Muscle sample size less than 5 g will make satellite cells isolation difficult.
7. If muscle has been teased into thin bundles, mincing will not be necessary.
8. Washing out the Ca^{++} and Mg^{++} is necessary to loosen the intercellular cement and allow the enzymes to digest it.
9. Despite the inclusion of safety features for the virus, they still pose some biohazardous risk of transducing primary human cells. The person should be familiar with the handling of virus [22–24] and the "Biosafety in Microbiological and Biomedical Laboratories" (www.cdc.gov/biosaftey/publications/bmbl5/index.htm).
10. For all the procedures, if temperature is not specified, it is performed at room temperature. For washes performed in Coplin jars, it is the temperature of the solution in the jars not just the water bath temperature.

Acknowledgement

This work was supported by NIH grants HL072138, GM093878 and AHA grants 09GRNT2020111, 02555009B to RLK.

References

1. Mauro A (1978) Muscle regeneration. Raven, New York
2. Brack AS, Rando TA (2012) Tissue-specific stem cells: lessons from the skeletal muscle satellite cell. Cell Stem Cell 10:504–514
3. Carlson BM, Faulkner JA (1983) The generation of skeletal muscle fibers following injury: a review. Med Sci Sports Exerc 15:187–198
4. Snow MH (1978) An autoradiographic study of satellite cells differentiation into regenerating myotubes following transplantation of muscle in young rat. Cell Tissue Res 186:535–540
5. Wang YX, Rudnicki MA (2011) Satellite cells, the engines of muscle repair. Nat Rev Mol Cell Biol 13:127–133

6. Pallafacchina G, Blaauw B, Schiaffino S (2012) Role of satellite cells in muscle growth and maintenance of muscle mass. Nutr Metab Cardiovasc Dis. [Epub ahead of print]
7. Kao RL, Chiu RCJ (1997) Satellite cell implantation. In: Kao RL, Chiu RCJ (eds) Cellular cardiomyoplasty: myocardial repair with cell implantation. Chapman & Hall, New York, pp 129–162
8. Campion DR (1984) The muscle satellite cell: a review. Int Rev Cytol 87:225–251
9. Zhang M, McLennan IS (1994) Use of antibodies to identify satellite cells with a light microscope. Muscle Nerve 17:987–994
10. Kao RL (2001) Autologous satellite cell for myocardial regeneration. E-biomed: J Regen Med 2:1–8
11. Mauro A (1961) Satellite cells of skeletal muscle fibers. J Biophys Biochem Cytol 9: 493–495
12. Usas A, Mačiulaitis J, Mačiulaitis R et al (2011) Skeletal muscle-derived stem cells: implications for cell-mediated therapies. Medicina (Kaunas) 47:469–479
13. Aziz A, Sebastian S, Dilworth FJ (2012) The origin and fate of muscle satellite cells. Stem Cell Rev 8:609–622
14. Kao RL, Browder W, Li C (2009) Cellular cardiomyoplasty: what have we learned? Asian Cardiovasc Thorac Ann 17:89–101
15. Huu AL, Prakash S, Shum-Tim D (2012) Cellular cardiomyoplasty: current state of the field. Regen Med 7:571–582
16. Zhao R, Kao RL (2000) Comparison of labeling procedures for myogenic cells. Cardiac Vasc Regen 1:85–91
17. Al-Khaldi A, Lachapelle K, Galipeau J (2000) Endogenous β-galactosidase enzyme activities in normal tissue and ischemic myocardium. Cardiac Vasc Regen 1:283–290
18. Grajales L, García J, Geenen DL (2012) Induction of cardiac myogenic lineage development differs between mesenchymal and satellite cells and is accelerated by bone morphogenetic protein-4. J Mol Cell Cardiol 53:382–391
19. Danoviz ME, Yablonka-Reuveni Z (2012) Skeletal muscle satellite cells: background and methods for isolation and analysis in a primary culture system. Methods Mol Biol 798:21–52
20. Neal A, Boldrin L, Morgan JE (2012) The satellite cell in male and female, developing and adult mouse muscle: distinct stem cells for growth and regeneration. PLoS One 7(e37950):1–11
21. Di Foggia V, Robson L (2012) Isolation of satellite cells from single muscle fibers from young, aged, or dystrophic muscles. Methods Mol Biol 916:3–14
22. Yi Y, Noh MJ, Lee KH (2011) Current advances in retroviral gene therapy. Curr Gene Ther 11:218–228
23. Durand S, Cimarelli A (2011) The inside out of lentiviral vectors. Viruses 3:132–159
24. Sakuma T, Barry MA, Ikeda Y (2012) Lentiviral vectors: basic to translational. Biochem J 443:603–618

Chapter 3

Bone Marrow Stem Cells

Minh Ngoc Duong, Yu-Ting Ma, and Ray C.J. Chiu

Abstract

The "mesenchymal stem cells (MSCs)" are cells adherent in the bone marrow, which can be isolated to induce differentiation. In contrast to the "embryonic stem cells" whose goal is to develop a new organism, the "MSC adult stem cells" can participate in tissue growth and repair throughout postnatal life. Addition of 5-*azacytidine* to MSCs in vitro induces the gradual increase in cellular size and begins spontaneous beatings, thereafter differentiating into cardiomyocytes. The "Methods" and "Protocols" to induce structural and functional maturations of MSCs, thus to achieve "Cellular Cardiomyoplasty," are described. With appropriate media, differentiations of MSCs to various kinds of cells such as chondrocytes, osteocytes, and adipocytes are also achievable.

Key words Cellular cardiomyoplasty, Bone marrow stem cells (BMSC), Mesenchymal stem cell (MSC), MSC isolation and culture, MSC differentiation, 5-Azacytidine, Connexin 43, Troponin I-c, Transfection, LacZ, DAPI, Echocardiography

1 Introduction: Bone Marrow Stromal Cells for Cellular Cardiomyoplasty

In bone marrow, there are two types of stem cells, hematopoietic stem cells and bone marrow stromal cells (MSCs). Bone marrow stromal cells are fibroblast-like cells and were thought to play only supportive roles in hematopoiesis by expressing various cytokines, growth factors, and adhesion molecules [1]. In the 1970s, Friedenstein and his colleagues demonstrate that these cells can differentiate into fibroblasts as well as other mesenchymal cells [2]. When they cultured whole bone marrow tissue in vitro, there was a certain population of cells adhered to the bottom of the culture dish. Then the supernatants were discarded which contain the hematopoietic stem cells. The adherent cells which are the "marrow stromal cells" can be differentiated into cells such as osteoblasts, chondrocytes, adipocytes, and muscle cells both in vitro and in vivo; thus they are also called "mesenchymal stem cells" to indicate their ability to differentiate into cells of mesenchymal lineage [3].

Race L. Kao (ed.), *Cellular Cardiomyoplasty: Methods and Protocols*, Methods in Molecular Biology, vol. 1036,
DOI 10.1007/978-1-62703-511-8_3, © Springer Science+Business Media New York 2013

Since Friedenstein's initial observation, more evidences have shown the existence and the property of mesenchymal stem cells. Moreover, many investigators show that such cells could also differentiate into cells of other lineage, such as endoderm-derived hepatocytes [4] and ectodermal neuron cells [5, 6]. Hence, they are given the name "adult stem cells" which indicate they are capable of differentiating into virtually all somatic cell types in adult animals.

In contrast to the embryonic stem cells, whose goal is to develop a new organism, the adult stem cells participate in tissue growth and repair throughout postnatal life. In fact, there is currently ample evidence suggesting that mesenchymal stem cells (MSCs) can be recruited from the bone marrow to various tissues to participate in tissue repair and regeneration in response to either apoptosis or tissue injury. For example, MSCs differentiated into endothelial cells, hepatocytes, and myoblasts in the cases of ischemia, cirrhosis, and muscular dystrophy [7–9].

In 1995, Wakitani et al. [10] was the first group to demonstrate that MSCs can differentiate into beating myotubules and stained positive for skeletal muscle-specific myosin when treated with 5-azacytidine, a hypomethylating agent, in vitro. This finding is further confirmed by Makino et al. [11]. By adding 5-azacytidine to the medium, MSCs can be differentiated into cardiomyocytes with the characteristics of cardiomyocyte-specific genes including ANP, BNP, GATA4, and Nkx2.5/Csx. Using the phase-contrast photography, the morphology of MSCs changed from fibroblast-like to myotube-like and connected to adjoining cells and beat spontaneously 3 weeks after adding 5-azacytidine (Fig. 1). Furthermore, electrophysiological study shows that they have sinus node-like potentials and ventricular myocyte-like potentials (Fig. 2).

To confirm the in vitro studies mentioned above, many laboratories, including ours, have demonstrated a series of studies showing MSCs could differentiate into cardiomyocytes without adding 5-azacytidine when injected directly into a viable myocardium. Furthermore, they can improve ventricular function in a coronary artery ligation model. In the first study, our team isolated and cultured MSCs from femoral and tibial bones of donor rats; then the cells were labeled and injected into left ventricular wall of the recipient rats, near the peri-infarct area [12]. The rats were sacrificed from 4 days to 12 weeks later, and the phenotype of the labeled cells was examined. By week 4, DAPI-labeled cells were found to have morphology similar to the cardiomyocytes (Fig. 3) and were stained positive for sarcomeric myosin heavy-chain molecules (Fig. 4a). These labeled cells aligned in parallel with host cardiomyocytes and were incorporated into the host myocardial fibers. They were connected to each other or with the host

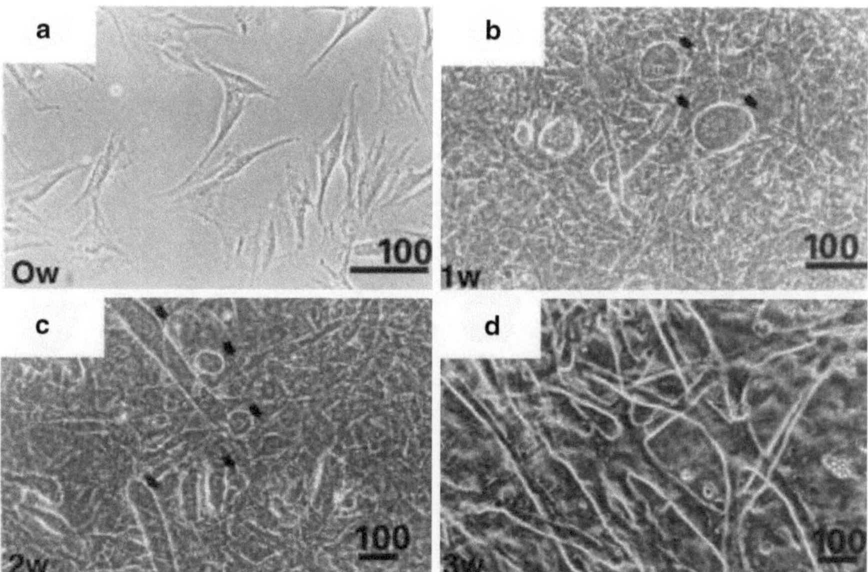

Fig. 1 Phase-contrast photographs of MSCs before and after adding 5-azacytidine. (**a**) At 0 week, MSCs show fibroblast-like morphology before adding 5-azacytidine. (**b**) One week after adding 5-azacytidine, some cells gradually increased in size and formed a ball-like appearance. Moreover, these cells began spontaneously beating thereafter. (**c**) Two weeks after adding 5-azacytidine, ball-like cells connected to adjacent cells and began to form myotube-like structure. (**d**) Three weeks after adding 5-azacytidine, most of the beating cells were connected together and formed myotube-like structure (scale bars: 100 μm)

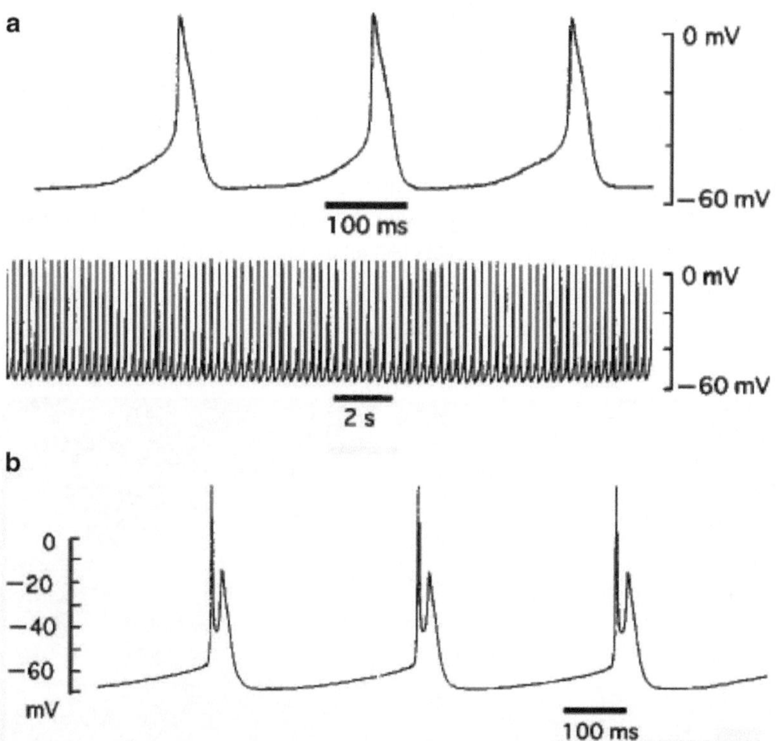

Fig. 2 Action potential was recorded from the spontaneously beating MSCs-differentiated cardiomyocytes at day 28 after 5-azacytidine treatment. Makino et al. categorized these action potentials into two groups: (**a**) sinus node-like action potential and (**b**) ventricular cardiomyocyte-like action potential

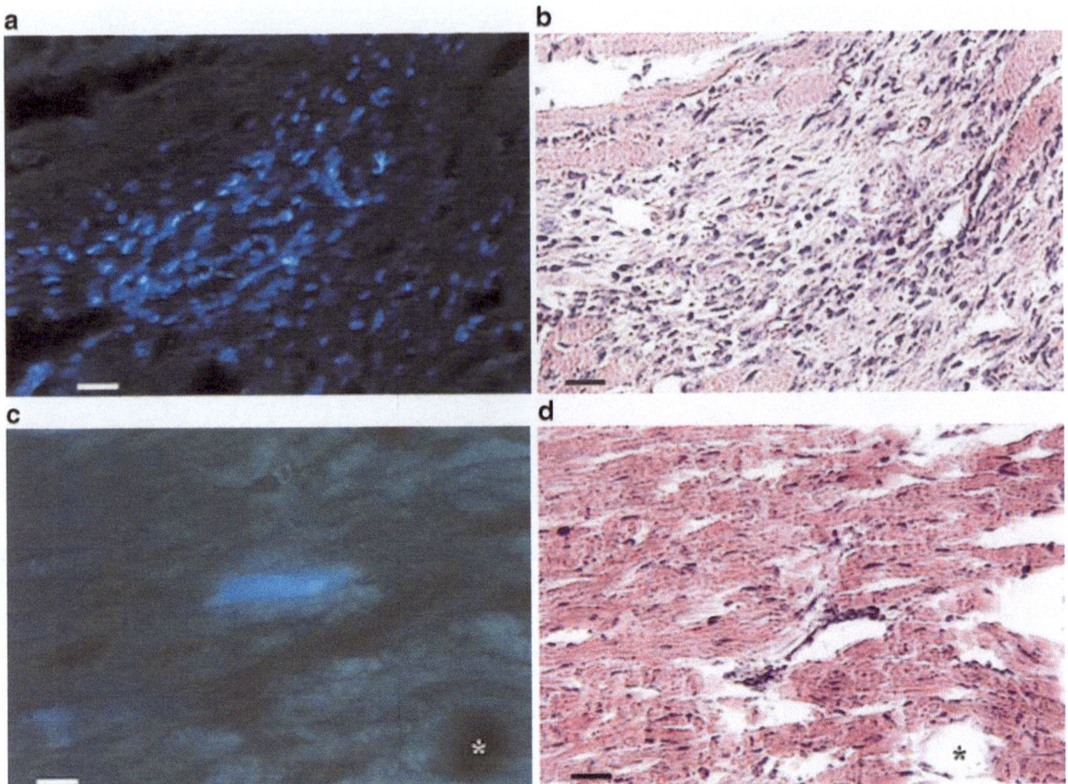

Fig. 3 (**a**) and (**b**) MSCs grafts in isogenic rat recipient hearts 4 days after implantation. (**a**) Numerous DAPI-labeled cells (*blue* fluorescent) scattered in the field. (**b**) Hematoxylin and eosin stain. Note that the concordance between dense hematoxylin staining and presence of DAPI epifluorescence. In addition, the labeled MSC-derived donor cells show immature appearance with large nucleus-to-cytoplasm ratio (**c**) and (**d**) MSCs grafts in isogenic rat recipient hearts 4 weeks after implantation. (**c**) DAPI-labeled cells were incorporate with the host myocardium. (**d**) Hematoxylin and eosin stain. Note the labeled MSC-derived cells have the same structure with the surrounding host cardiomyocytes (scale: 30 μm) (Wang et al.)

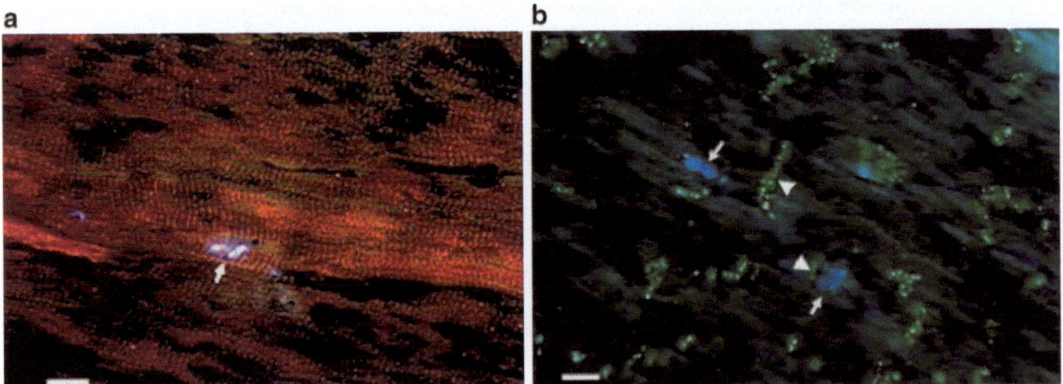

Fig. 4 (**a**) The *arrow* shows that DAPI-labeled cell is stained positively with sarcomeric myosin heavy-chain immunofluorescence (with the use of MF20 primary antibody and Texas Red conjugated secondary antibody). The clear striation can also be observed here. (**b**) Positive connexin 43 staining (*arrowheads*) is found at the interfaces between one DAPI-labeled cells (*arrow*) and neighboring non-labeled host cardiomyocytes and between non-labeled host cardiomyocytes (scale: 15 μm)

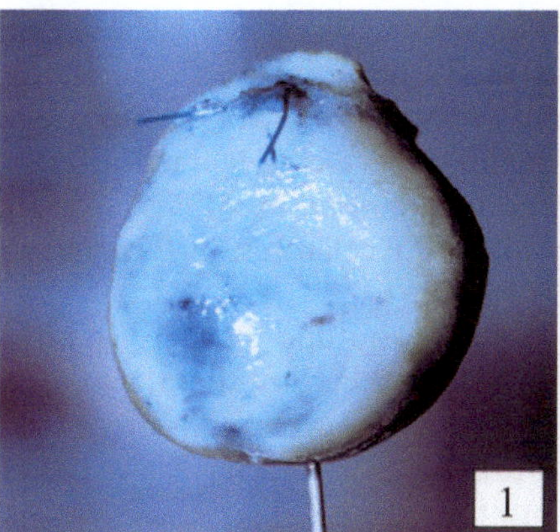

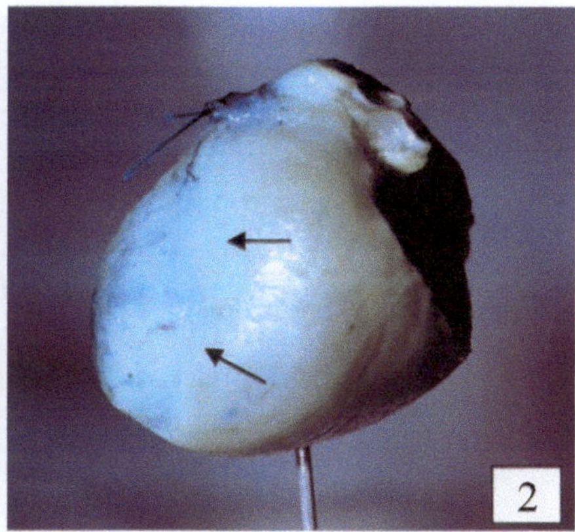

Fig. 5 The hearts were stained with X-gal solution to reveal the implant cells at 4 weeks after coronary ligation. *View "2"*: Note the *blue* discoloration localized in the area of scarred myocardium. *View "3"*: In the oblique view of the same gross heart specimen, the adjacent normal myocardium remained unstained, which indicates the labeled MSCs only presence in the territory of the infarcted myocardium. The *arrows* denote the border zone between scar and normal myocardium (Bittira et al.)

cardiomyocytes through gap junction, which stained positive for connexin 43, a major gap junction protein in cardiomyocyte junctions (Fig. 4b). This result appeared consistent with the subsequent study by Wang et al. in which MSCs were injected into the coronary artery of a heart, which had previously undergone coronary artery ligation to produce an infarct scar [13]. These MSCs were found to migrate out of the coronary microvasculature and differentiated into phenotypes similar to those found in the surrounding. The MSCs migrated to scar tissue differentiated into fibroblast-like morphology and those migrated to myocardium differentiated into cardiomyocytes. Our lab called this phenomenon "milieu dependent differentiation" which means that the microenvironment in vivo supplied the signals required for the differentiation of these MSCs.

To further verify that MSCs are recruited to the heart upon myocardial infarction and played pathophysiological roles in healing and adaption process, Bittira et al. [14] injected labeled donor MSCs intravenously into recipient rats, and after 1 week, ten rats were killed, and they examined the distribution of the labeled MSCs. Other rats underwent coronary artery ligation ($n=14$). The rats that did not undergo coronary artery ligation have their labeled MSCs found in bone marrow, and none were found in the hearts. In coronary ligated hearts, labeled cells were found in the region of the scar (Fig. 5). Moreover, the labeled cells were stained positive for cardiac specific connexin 43 and troponin I-c, which indicated their cardiomyogenic differentiation. In the aspect of cardiac function, Saito et al. [15] from our lab used echocardiogram to measure ejection fraction and fractional shortening and compare the difference between control group (medium was injected) and MSCs group. The ejection fraction and fractional shortening were significantly higher in MSCs group compared with the control group following cell infusion. This indicates MSCs can improve cardiac function.

In this chapter, we will first outline the steps of how to isolate bone marrow MSCs from the rat, culture them, and then differentiate them into chondrocytes, adipocytes, and osteocytes. Then we will describe how to label the MSCs with LacZ and DAPI transfection before injecting into the rats.

Myocardial infarction remains an important leading cause of morbidity and mortality worldwide. Deficiency of cardiomyocytes results from necrosis or apoptosis, combined with limited endogenous repair mechanism eventually leading to ventricular remodeling which ultimately leads to progressive heart failure caused by various etiologies. In addition to the current medical therapy for heart failure such as surgical techniques, mechanical ventricular assist device, and heart transplant, MSCs cellular transplantation maybe a novel approach to directly solve the problem of loss of cardiomyocytes. Moreover, MSCs are reasonable stem cell source which does not encounter ethical, biologic, or technical limitations. They are easy to grow in vitro, they do not have oncogenicity potential, and they are "universal donor cells."

2 Materials

2.1 MSC Isolation and Culture

1. Pentobarbital sodium injection, 50 mg/mL (pentobarbital).
2. 70 % Ethanol.
3. Phosphate buffer saline (PBS): containing 137 mM NaCl, 2.7 mM KCl, 10 mM Na_2HPO_4, and 2 mM KH_2PO_4 at pH 7.4.
4. Dulbecco's Modified Eagle's Medium (DMEM), low glucose (catalogue number 11885) (Gibco company).
5. Fetal bovine serum (FBS).
6. Penicillin/streptomycin (P/S), 100× solution (catalogue number 15070063) (Invitrogen company).
7. Trypsin. 2.5 %, 10× solution (catalogue number 15090046) (Invitrogen company).
8. 5 % CO_2 incubator.
9. Sterile forceps, scissors, and gauze.

2.2 MSC Differentiation

1. StemPro Chondrogenesis Differentiation Kit.
2. StemPro Adipogenesis Differentiation Kit.
3. StemPro Osteogenesis Differentiation Kit.

All differentiation kits are from Invitrogen company.

2.3 Freezing of MSC

1. Freezing medium: 80 mL DMEM medium, 10 mL FBS, and 10 mL dimethyl sulfoxide (DMSO).
2. DMEM.
3. FBS.
4. Dimethyl sulfoxide (DMSO).
5. Hanks balance salt solution (HBSS).
6. PBS.
7. Centrifuge.

2.4 LacZ Transfection

1. 1 T-75 flask of cultured BM stem cells, around 80 % confluent.
2. 1 T-75 flask of cultured GP + E86 cells which produce a retrovirus contain beta-galactosidase gene.
3. 0.8 μm filter.
4. Growth medium: DMEM media with 10 % FBS and P/S antibiotic.
5. Polybrene stock solution is 4 mg/mL in PBS (Sigma Chemical Co., St. Louis, MO, USA).

2.5 Labeling with DAPI

1. 4′,6-Diamidino-2-phenylindole (DAPI) (Sigma Chemical Co., St. Louis, MO, USA).
2. DMEM growth medium with P/S, FBS.

3 Methods

3.1 MSC Isolation and Culture

1. The procedure must be done under aseptic condition.
2. Sacrifice the rat with an overdose of pentobarbital (100 mg/kg given intraperitoneally).
3. Collect the femoral and tibial bones, cleanse the tissue with the scissor, and place them in a Petri dish.
4. In the laminar hood, wash the bones briefly with 70 % ethanol and then PBS.
5. With the help of sterile forceps and gauze, separate the two bones from each other.
6. Cut the two edges of each bone by sterile scissors.

7. With 10 mL of 10 % DMEM complete medium in a sterile syringe, flush the cells from the bone marrow into a test tube several times.
8. Pipet the cells into T-75 tissue culture flask and place in 5 % CO_2 incubator for 48 h to allow the stem cells to attach to the bottom of the flask (*see* **Note 1**).
9. After 2 days, replace the medium and discard the nonadherent cells.
10. Change the medium twice a week and observe the cultured MSC under the microscope every day to assess the level of expansion as well as verify the cells' morphology. After three to four times of changing medium, most of the adherent cells are pure BM stem cells.
11. When the cells are around 70–80 % confluent, divide them into two flasks as the following steps:
    (a) Discard the medium from the flask.
    (b) Wash with PBS.
    (c) Add 2 mL trypsin and leave on 2–3 min to detach the cells from the bottom. Add another 2 mL of complete medium to stop trypsin reaction.
    (d) Divide 4 mL into 2 flasks, 2 mL each, plus another 10 mL complete medium, so the cells can grow again.

3.2 MSC Differentiation

1. One of an important character of stem cells is the ability to differentiate into other kind of cells like chondrocytes, adipocytes, and osteocytes. To make sure the cells we isolated are real stem cells, we did the differentiation experiment (*see* **Note 2**).
2. All of the kits come from Invitrogen company. This experiment is easy and straightforward, so all you have to do is to follow the manual. In general, we seed around 10–15 thousand cells in a well of 12-well plate. When the cells are around 60–80 % confluent, then you feed the cells with the differentiation medium and keep them for 14–21 days. At the end, stain the plates to see the result (Figs. 6, 7, and 8).

3.3 Freezing of MSC

1. First, we have to prepare the freezing medium and keep at 4 °C.
2. Bone marrow stem cells are grown in CO_2 incubator at 37 °C until around 80 % confluent.
3. Take out the flasks and discard the medium, and wash briefly with 5 mL HBSS or PBS.
4. Add 2 mL trypsin to each flask and leave it on for 2 min. Trypsin will lift the cells attached on the bottom of the flask up. Add another 2 mL of medium to each flask; the FBS in

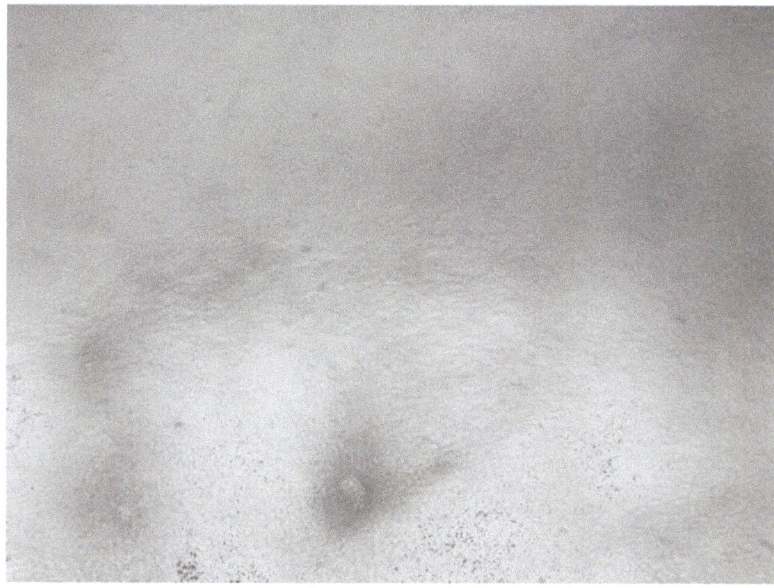

Fig. 6 This is an example of chondrocyte differentiation

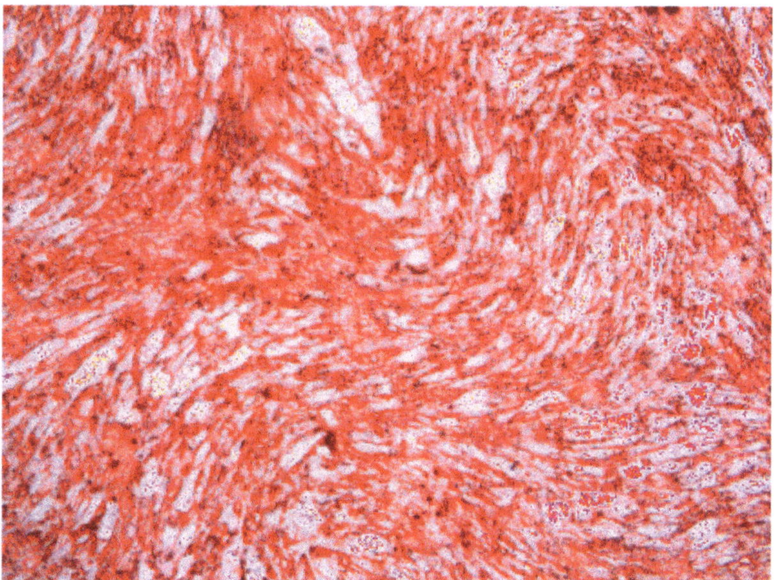

Fig. 7 This is osteocyte differentiation

medium solution will stop trypsin reaction. Pipet all cell solution to a new, sterile tube and centrifuge at $580 \times g$ for 5 min.

5. Discard the supernatant and count the cell pellet.
6. Mix one million cells in 1 mL of freezing medium in a cryotube.
7. Immediately store the cryotubes at −80 freezer and the cells can be saved for many years.

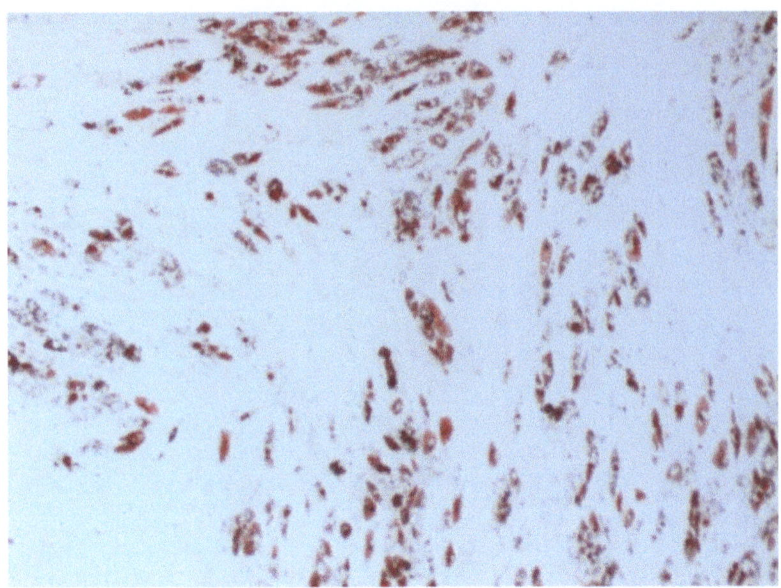

Fig. 8 This is adipocyte differentiation

8. When the cells are needed for experiment, get a cryotube out and thaw it in 37° water bath for 1 min. Pipet the cells and freezing medium of each cryotube into a new 10 mL tube containing 5 mL of growth medium.
9. Centrifuge the tube at 580×*g* for 3 min. Discard the supernatant and mix the cells pellet with 3 mL growth medium. Transfer this solution to a T-25 tissue culture flask and keep it in CO_2 incubator.
10. Change into new growth medium after 24 h and wait for the cells to multiply.

3.4 LacZ Transfection

In order to follow the cells injected in the rat's heart, we usually transfected the cells with either (a) retrovirus containing LacZ plasmid or (b) DAPI.

DAPI is a fluorescent chemical. It gets in the nucleus of the cells and gives a blue nucleus, so it is very easy to recognize when the cells are implanted. In our lab, DAPI is used for a short-term follow-up (2–4 weeks) because DAPI is not very stable in vivo; when the cells divide, only one nucleus has DAPI, not two, so the real number of cells survived is less recognized. For a long-term experiment (4–12 weeks), we transfect bone marrow MSCs with LacZ-containing retrovirus (*see* **Note 3**). The cells will give an *aqua* (blue greenish) color when stain with beta-galactosidase solution (Fig. 9).

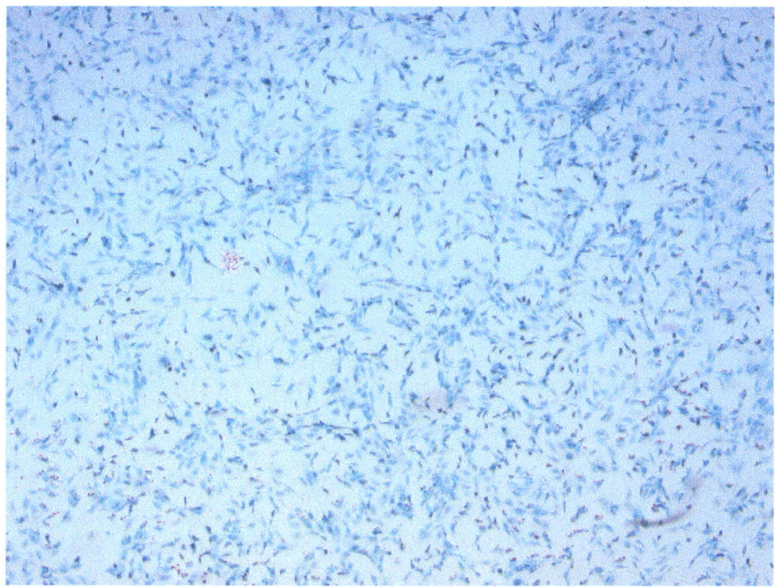

Fig. 9 The *blue* cells are LacZ-transfected bone marrow cells

1. In the laminar hood, filter the supernatant of GP+E86 cells culture by 0.8 μm filter to get rid of dead floating cells. This supernatant contains retrovirus required for transfection.
2. Pipet 40 μl of stock Polybrene solution into 10 mL retrovirus supernatant. Mix well. Polybrene is used to facilitate the transfer of virus into stem cells.
3. Discard the media in cultured stem cells flask.
4. Pipet the mixture of Polybrene and retrovirus supernatant into stem cells flask.
5. After 24 h, change back to normal growth medium.
6. Repeat this experiment three to four times to increase the number of cells transfected.

3.5 Labeling with DAPI

1. Two hours before we use the cells for implantation, replace the medium in one flask with new DMEM growth medium containing 25 microgram of DAPI/1 mL of medium.
2. Put the flask back in the CO_2 incubator for 2 h.
3. Take the flask out and rinse the flask with sterile PBS several times until all of the extra, unabsorbing DAPI particles are removed. This is very important because we don't want the free DAPI particles in the injection.
4. Trypsinize the flask, collect the cells, and implant the cells in the heart as usual.

3.6 Prepare BMSC for Injection

In order to mimic the heart problem of patient, the myocardial infarction is done in the rat. In this model, ultrasound is done on rat before experiment as a baseline. After that, an artery ligation is done to create a sick condition. Then, three million bone marrow stem cells are injected either directly to the heart or through penile vein. After 24 h or 2, 4, 8, or 12 weeks later, another ultrasound will be done to see the heart's function improvement.

3.6.1 Harvesting BMSC

1. Discard the growth medium in the flasks and wash the flask with 5 mL of HBSS. This step is important because the salt solution will remove all dead cells and some leftover of FBS in growth medium. In the presence of FBS, trypsin solution can't work.
2. Add 2 mL of trypsin to each flask and leave it on for 2–3 min.
3. Collect all cells solution in a new sterile tube containing 5 mL growth medium and centrifuge at 580 × *g* for 2 min. Discard supernatant and count the cells.
4. Mix three million cells to150 μl of DMEM and inject to a rat.

3.6.2 LAD Ligation

1. Insert 18-gauge intravenous catheter into rat's trachea, then connect the catheter to a ventilator. The ventilator is set at 85 breaths/min.
2. Turn on the isoflurane to 2.5 which is connected properly to the ventilator. The anesthesia is maintained until the surgery is over.
3. Place the animal in lateral position with its left chest facing the surgeon.
4. Under sterile condition, a transverse incision is made on the chest, from the midaxillary line to the midsternal line through the skin. The muscles are transected to expose ribs and intercostal spaces.
5. Made an incision between 4th and 5th intercostal space.
6. Use a retractor to open the chest to expose the heart.
7. The left coronary artery is identified, and a suture is made approximately 1–2 mm from its origin with a 7-0 Prolene suture. You will see a segment of the anterior wall become pale.
8. Use a 28-gauge insulin syringe to inject MSCs (3×10^6 cells suspended in 150 μl DMEM) directly into the peri-ischemic region of the myocardium.
9. Close the incision with 3-0, 4-5 sutures passing around the two adjacent ribs.
10. Close the skin incision with 3-0.

3.6.3 Echocardiography

1. The transthoracic echocardiography should be performed on all animals preoperation (baseline) and postoperation (3 days, 1, 2, and 3 weeks).
2. Shave the left chest of the rat and place the animal in lateral position with its left chest facing the surgeon.
3. Put rat under anesthesia and keep the isoflurane at 2.5.
4. Put quarter amount of gel on the shaved chest.
5. Image the left ventricle in parasternal long-axis view in 2-dimensional mode.
6. At the level of papillary muscles of the mitral valves, M-mode images were obtained.
7. Measure the end-diastolic diameter of left ventricle (LVEDD) and end-systolic diameter of the left ventricle (LVESD).
8. Then calculate the ejection fraction (EF) and fractional shortening (FS) by the following equation:

$$\left[\frac{\text{LVEDD}-\text{LVESD}}{\text{LVEDD}}\right]\times 100\% = \text{Fractional shortening}$$

$$\left[\frac{\text{LVEDV}-\text{LVESV}}{\text{LVEDV}}\right]\times 100\% = \text{Ejection fraction}$$

$$\text{where LVEDV} = \frac{7.0\times \text{LVEDD}^3}{2.4+\text{LVEDD}}$$

$$\text{where LVESV} = \frac{7.0\times \text{LVESD}^3}{2.4+\text{LVESD}}$$

4 Notes

1. Bone marrow MSC is an easy cell type to grow; however, the number of cells put in a flask initially is very important. Too little cells can make the growth sluggish, and the cells will need more time to be confluent. Sometimes they die because there is no cell-to-cell contact. Normally, for a T-75 flask, at 80 % confluent, we have around three million cells; this amount should be divided into two or three flasks only. This high seeding will make the cells grow quicker and healthier.
2. This differentiation experiment is simple, but there is only one thing we should pay attention which is the number of passages we use. The cells we use for this experiment undergo passage number 3 or 4, not more than that because we suspect that continuously passaged stem cells might lose their multipotency.

3. The technique for retrovirus transfection is quite simple, but this experiment is very difficult to achieve a high yield of cells transfected number. We usually have to repeat the experiment 2–3 times to get around 70–80 % cell transfected. In order to have a good yield, the following points should be kept in mind.

The cell culture of BM stem cells and GP + E86 should be fresh. We usually plate the cells the day before the experiment.

The medium used to grow GP + E86 has no P/S; FBS has to be heat inactivated. These changes in medium composition help the transfected cells to survive more.

After 24 h, change back to normal medium for 1–2 days and then perform the X-gal staining to see how much cells are transfected. If the percentage is low, we can repeat the experiment 1–2 times to have a good transfection. The final transfected BM then will be spread to have a lot of cells for freezing and implanting later.

References

1. Cohnheim J (1867) Ueber Entzündung und Eitenung. Virchows Arch Path Anat 40:1
2. Friedenstein AJ (1976) Precursor cells of mechanocytes. Int Rev Cytol 47:327–359
3. Caplan AI (1991) Mesenchymal stem cells. J Orthop Res 9:641–650
4. Peterson BE, Bowen WC, Patrene KD et al (1999) Bone marrow as a potential source of hepatic oval cells. Science 284:1168–1170
5. Woodbury D, Schwarz EJ, Prockop DJ, Black IB (2000) Adult rat and human bone marrow stromal cells differentiate into neurons. J Neurosci Res 61:364–370
6. Sanchez-Ramos J, Song S, Cardozo-Pelaez F et al (2000) Adult bone marrow stromal cells differentiate into neural cells in vitro. Exp Neurol 164:247–256
7. Gussoni E, Soneoka Y, Strickland CD et al (1999) Dystrophin expression in the MDX mouse restored by stem cell transplantation. Nature 1401:390–394
8. Lagasse E, Connors H, Al-Dhalimy M et al (2000) Purified hematopoietic stem cells can differentiate into hepatocytes in vivo. Nat Med 6:1229–1234
9. Thesise ND, Nimmakayalu M, Gardner R et al (2000) Liver from bone marrow in humans. Hepatology 32:11–16
10. Wakitani S, Saito T, Caplan A (1995) Myogenic cells derived from rat bone marrow mesenchymal stem cells exposed to 5-Azacytidine. Muscle Nerve 18:1417–1426
11. Makino S, Fukudi K, Miyoshi S et al (1999) Cardiomyocytes can be generated from marrow stromal cells in vitro. J Clin Invest 103:697–705
12. Wang JS, Shum-Tim D, Galipeau J et al (2000) Marrow stromal cells for cellular cardiomyoplasty: feasibility and potential clinical advantages. J Thorac Cardiovasc Surg 20:999–1006
13. Wang JS, Shum-Tim D, Chedrawy E, Chiu RCJ (2001) The coronary delivery of marrow stromal cells for myocardial regeneration: pathophysiologic and therapeutic implications. J Thorac Cardiovasc Surg 122:699–705
14. Bittira B, Kuang JQ, Al-Khaldi A, Shum-Tim D, Chiu RCJ (2003) Mobilization and homing of bone marrow stromal cells in myocardial infarction. Eur J Cardiothorac Surg 24:393–398
15. Saito T, Kuang J-Q, Bittira B, Al-Khaldi A, Chiu RCJ (2002) Xenotransplant cardiac chimera: Immune tolerance of adult stem cells. Ann Thorac Surg 74:19–24

Chapter 4

Adipose Tissue-Derived Mesenchymal Stem Cells: Isolation, Expansion, and Characterization

Miriam Araña, Manuel Mazo, Pablo Aranda, Beatriz Pelacho, and Felipe Prosper

Abstract

Over the last decade, cell therapy has emerged as a potentially new approach for the treatment of cardiovascular diseases. Among the wide range of cell types and sources, adipose-derived mesenchymal stem cells have shown promise, mainly due to its plasticity and remarkable paracrine-secretion capacity, largely demonstrated at the in vitro and in vivo levels. Furthermore, its accessibility and abundance, the low morbidity of the surgical procedure, its easy isolation, culture, and long-term passaging capacity added to its immunomodulatory properties that could allow its allogeneic transplantation, making it one of the most attractive candidates for clinical application. In this chapter, we will focus on the methodology for the isolation, expansion, phenotypical characterization, differentiation, and storage of the adipose-derived stem cells.

Key words Adipose tissue, Stem cells, Stromal vascular fraction, ADSC, Isolation, Expansion, Characterization, Storage

1 Introduction

The adipose tissue (AT) has traditionally been regarded as an energy-storing organ, composed of mature adipocytes, nurtured by an intermingling vasculature and containing fibroblasts and immune/hematopoietic cells. It was Zuk and coworkers however who first described the isolation of a population with multilineage differentiation capacity from human lipoaspirates [1], named as stromal vascular fraction (SVF) and composed by a mixture of phenotypes, including endothelial, smooth muscle, cardiac, immune, and stromal cells [1–4]. Furthermore, if cultured under concrete conditions, SVF was homogenized, giving rise to the adipose-derived stem cells (ADSC), a pure mesenchymal cell population (*see* Fig. 1) able to give rise to mesodermal phenotypes such as osteoblasts, chondrocytes, adipocytes, and myogenic cells [5–8]. Both SVF and ADSC differ in their phenotypic profile, their capacity

Race L. Kao (ed.), *Cellular Cardiomyoplasty: Methods and Protocols*, Methods in Molecular Biology, vol. 1036,
DOI 10.1007/978-1-62703-511-8_4, © Springer Science+Business Media New York 2013

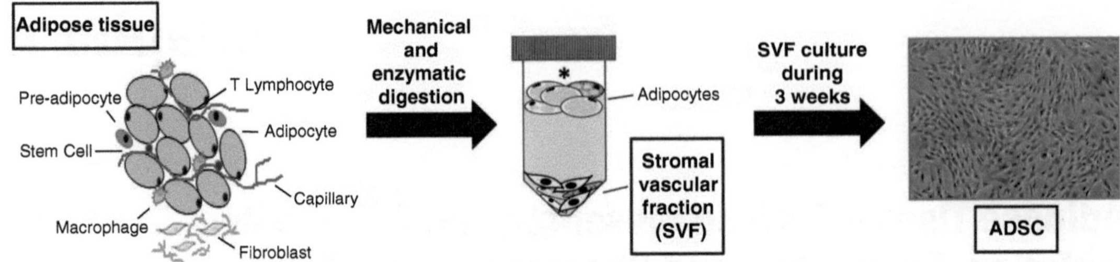

Fig. 1 Adipose-derived stem cells (ADSC) isolation from adipose tissue. After mechanical and enzymatic digestion of an adipose tissue biopsy and following centrifugation to eliminate mature adipocytes [top layer (*)], the adipose stromal vascular fraction (SVF) (pellet) is plated and kept in culture during 3 weeks, deriving into a homogeneous mesenchymal cell population, the ADSC

of differentiation, and their secretome [9–12], although both cases have shown, at the experimental level, a positive effect for the treatment of different pathologies at the experimental level (reviewed in [13]). Importantly, together with their therapeutic potential, adipose-derived stem cells present a number of advantages over other cell types. First, AT is easily accessible, requiring a minimally invasive and conventional surgery for its harvesting. Second, progenitor cells are present in a greater number [14] than in other tissues (e.g., bone marrow) and have a larger expansion potential [5, 15], making high-dosage treatments readily available. Third, the isolation process is relatively simple and does not require specific equipment, and fourth, cell culture and characterization do not imply the use of expensive reagents, making any prospective therapy more affordable. Thus, clinical application has been pursued, focusing not only on ADSC mesenchymal differentiation potential for bone or cartilage reconstruction surgery [16] but also on their implication on the healing process (*see* www.clinicalTrials.gov, Identifier NCT00475410) and their immunomodulatory effects in pathologies like Crohn's [17] and graft-versus-host disease (Identifier NCT01222039). Also, the putative beneficial effect of the ADSC at the paracrine level, stimulating different mechanisms such as cell survival, tissue revascularization, and tissue remodeling (reviewed in [18]), is being evaluated on heart and limb ischemia clinical trials (Identifier NCT00426868 and NCT01211028) and also in brain disease (Identifier NCT01453829).

In order to elucidate the real beneficial potential of the ADSC and compare the results of different clinical trials, it is indeed of capital importance a standardized isolation and expansion protocol together with an adequate ADSC characterization, since their phenotypic profile is not completely specific of ADSC and is shared by commonly contaminating cells as fibroblasts. Along this chapter we will describe the procedures for the isolation, expansion, storage, and characterization of mouse, rat, pig, and human AT-derived cells.

2 Materials

2.1 ADSC Isolation and Culture

1. Sterile dishes.
2. Sterilized scissors or blades.
3. Collagenase type I.
4. 0.2 μm filters.
5. ADSC basal medium: Dulbecco's Modified Eagle's Medium (DMEM) supplemented with 10 % fetal bovine serum (FBS) and 1 % penicillin/streptomycin.
6. 100 and 40 μm filters.
7. Erythrocyte lysis buffer: 155 mM NH_4Cl, 10 mM $KHCO_3$, 0.1 mM EDTA.
8. Phosphate Buffer Saline (PBS).
9. Trypan blue.
10. Culture flasks 175 cm^2.
11. 0.05 % trypsin and 200 mg/l EDTA.
12. Freezing medium: DMEM, 50 % FBS, and 10 % dimethyl sulfoxide (DMSO).
13. Cryogenic vials.
14. Isopropanol.
15. Freezing container.
16. Conical tubes (50 and 15 ml).

2.2 Flow Cytometry

1. PBS.
2. Cytometry tubes.
3. Antibodies (*see* Table 1).
4. 0.4 % paraformaldehyde (PFA).

2.3 Osteogenic Differentiation

1. Osteogenic differentiation medium: alpha-MEM supplemented with 0.2 mM ascorbic acid, 0.1 μM dexamethasone, 10 mM β-glycerophosphate, 10 % FBS, and 1 % penicillin/streptomycin.
2. 6-well cell culture plates.
3. 10 % neutral buffered formalin solution.
4. Alizarin Red S solution.
5. Acetone.
6. Sodium citrate.
7. Alkaline staining: mix 6 mg of Fast Blue BB Salt with 1 ml of Naphtol AS-MX and 24 ml of distilled water.

Table 1
Antibody list. Antibodies used for ADSC characterization by flow cytometry

Antibody	Specificity (species)	Commercial reference
CD29	Pig	BD 552369
	Human	Immunotech 0791
CD31	Rat/pig Mouse Human	BD 555027 BD 551262 BD 555446
CD34	Mouse Human	BD 551387 BD 345802
CD44	Rat Human Mouse	BD 554869 BD 555478 BD 553134
CD45	Mouse Rat Human	BD 557235 BD 554881 BD 557059
CD73	Rat Human	BD 551124 BD 550257
CD90	Human/pig Rat Mouse	BD 555596 BD 554898 eBioscience 17090082
CD105	Human	Ancell 326-050
CD117	Mouse Human	BD 553356 BD 332785
HLA-A, HLA-B, HLA-C	Human	BD 555553
HLA-DR, HLA-DP, HLA-DQ	Human	BD 555558
MHC-I	Mouse	BD 553573
MHC-II	Mouse	BD 553623
RT1A	Rat	BD 559993
RT1B	Rat	BD 554929

2.4 Adipogenic Differentiation

1. Adipogenic differentiation medium: alpha-MEM supplemented with 50 μM indomethacin, 1 μM dexamethasone, 0.5 mM isobutyl-methylxanthine (IBMX), 10 % FBS, and 1 % penicillin/streptomycin.
2. 6-well cell culture plates.
3. 10 % neutral buffered formalin solution.
4. 0.5 % Oil Red O in isopropanol.
5. Harris' hematoxylin.

2.5 Chondrogenic Differentiation

1. Chondrogenic differentiation medium: Dulbecco's Modified Eagle's Medium High Glucose (4.5 g/l) (DMEM-HG) supplemented with 0.1 μM dexamethasone, 100 μg/ml sodium pyruvate, 50 μg/ml ascorbic acid, 1 % ITS + Premix Tissue Culture Supplement, 1 % penicillin/streptomycin, 500 ng/ml bone morphogenetic protein-6 (BMP-6), and 10 ng/ml transforming growth factor beta-1 (TGFβ-1).
2. Conical tubes (15 ml).
3. 10 % neutral buffered formalin solution.
4. Toluidine blue.
5. Acetic acid.
6. Ethanol.
7. Xylene.
8. DPX (BDH).

3 Methods

3.1 Ex Vivo Expansion of ADSC

Mammalian AT can be classified in three types, brown, beige, and white, of whom the last is the most abundant. In humans, white AT represents on average 16 % of body weight, distributed throughout the body but especially in the abdomen, buttocks, and abdominal zone. It appears however that not all of the fat accumulations are equivalent, and at least in mice, the potential of the cells can be different according to their location [19].

3.1.1 Cell Isolation

1. Place the AT sample (*see* **Note 1**) in a sterile dish and mince thoroughly (around 15 min) with scissors and blades until a mush is obtained (*see* **Note 2**).
2. Collect the minced tissue in a 50 ml tube and weigh it. Prepare 10 ml of collagenase I solution per 3 g tissue (for the collagenase I solution, dissolve 2 mg/ml collagenase type I in DMEM and filter through a 0.2 μm filter).
3. Incubate the minced tissue with the collagenase I solution during 1 h at 37 °C, gently shaking on a water bath (*see* **Note 3**).
4. After digestion, dilute the sample 1:1 in DMEM and 10 % FBS and sequentially filter through 100 and 40 μm filters.
5. Centrifuge the filtered sample at 600 × *g* for 7 min and discard the formed lipid layer on the top and the supernatant by collecting them with a pipette. Resuspend the pellet in 1 ml of basal medium and add 3 ml of erythrocyte lysis buffer (155 mM NH_4Cl, 10 mM $KHCO_3$, 0.1 mM EDTA) for 5 min at room temperature (RT).
6. Add 10 ml of PBS and centrifuge at 600 × *g* for 7 min.

7. Discard the supernatant and resuspend the pellet in 1 ml of basal medium.
8. Pick a small aliquot and count cells, checking viability through trypan blue dye exclusion (*see* **Note 4**).
9. Plate isolated cells (SVF) at a density of 15–30 × 10^3 cells/cm^2 in basal medium (DMEM supplemented with 10 % FBS and 1 % antibiotics) (*see* **Notes 5** and **6**).
10. Incubate at 37 °C with 5.5 % CO_2 (*see* **Note 7**).

3.1.2 Subculture of Cells

1. Remove the medium from the flasks and wash the cells with PBS. Add the appropriate volume of trypsin/EDTA (0.05 % trypsin; 200 mg/l EDTA) and incubate the flasks during 5 min at 37 °C to detach the cells (*see* **Note 8**).
2. Check complete detachment by gently tapping the side of the flask and observing cells under the microscope.
3. Inactivate trypsin adding pre-warmed basal medium (*see* **Note 8**).
4. Collect the cells with basal medium and plate them at 4 × 10^3 cells/cm^2 (*see* **Note 5**).
5. Incubate the cells at 37 °C with 5.5 % CO_2, 90–95 % humidity.

3.2 Long-Term Preservation

SVF or ADSC can be cryopreserved for later use. Optimal preservation is crucial for ensuring cell survival and proliferation after thawing. Cells can be aliquot and stored in liquid nitrogen at recommended density [20, 21].

3.2.1 Cryopreservation

1. Remove medium from flasks and wash cells with PBS. Add the appropriate volume of trypsin/EDTA (0.05 % trypsin; 200 mg/l EDTA) and incubate flasks during 5 min at 37 °C to detach cells (*see* **Note 8**).
2. Check cell detachment under the microscope and inactivate trypsin, adding basal medium (*see* **Note 8**).
3. Collect and centrifuge cells at 600 × *g* for 5 min.
4. Discard the supernatant and resuspend the cells at 1–10 × 10^6 cells/1 ml in freezing medium (40 % DMEM, 50 % FBS, 10 % DMSO).
5. Aliquot cells into previously labeled cryogenic vials (*see* **Note 9**).
6. Place the cryogenic vials in a freezing container and transfer to a −80 °C freezer.
7. For long-term storage, after overnight freezing at −80 °C, move vials to a liquid nitrogen container.

3.2.2 Recovery of Cryopreserved Cells

1. Rapidly thaw the frozen vial in a pre-warm water bath. Maximum cell viability depends on the rapid thawing of frozen cells.
2. As soon as the cells are completely thawed, disinfect the outside of the vial with 70 % ethanol.

3. Transfer the cell suspension with a 1 ml pipette to a 15 ml conical tube containing approximately 10 ml of basal medium.
4. Mix the cell suspension by gently pipetting up and down.
5. Centrifuge the tubes at 600 × *g* for 5 min to pellet the cells and remove DMSO.
6. Discard the supernatant and resuspend the cell pellet in a suitable volume of basal medium (*see* **Note 5**).
7. Plate the resuspended cells at a density of 12×10^3 cells/cm^2.

3.3 Cell Characterization

As stated above, the characterization of ADSC requires fulfilling both the phenotype and differentiation capacity criteria (*see* Fig. 3). As a heterogeneous population, freshly isolated SVF expresses hematopoietic markers (CD34 and CD45), mesenchymal markers (CD29, CD44, CD73, CD90, and CD105), endothelial cell markers (CD34 and CD31), and other stem cell markers (CD117). The subsequent culture and homogenization (taking usually 2–3 weeks) that gives rise to ADSC is reflected in their phenotypic profile, showing that stem cell, endothelial, or hematopoietic markers progressively disappear, obtaining a homogeneous population which only expresses mesenchymal cell markers [2, 6].

On the differentiation side, ADSC, similarly to bone marrow-derived mesenchymal stem cells (BM-MSC), have a multilineage differentiation capacity, giving rise to mesodermal lineages, including bone, fat, and cartilage [1]. However, although ADSC can be easily differentiated into the adipose lineage, it has been reported that they are less committed towards the osteogenic and chondrogenic lineages than BM-MSC [22, 23].

3.3.1 Flow Cytometry Analysis

The phenotypic analysis performed by flow cytometry with specific antibodies (*see* Table 1) must confirm the mentioned heterogeneity of the freshly isolated SVF and the homogeneity of the in vitro cultured ADSC (*see* Table 2) (*see* **Note 10**):

1. Remove medium from flasks, wash cells with PBS, and add the appropriate volume of trypsin/EDTA (0.05 trypsin; 200 mg/l EDTA). Incubate flasks during 5 min at 37 °C to detach cells (*see* **Note 8**).
2. Check cell detachment under the microscope and inactivate trypsin, adding basal medium (*see* **Note 8**).
3. Collect cells and centrifuge at 600 × *g* for 5 min.
4. Discard the supernatant. Add 1 ml of basal medium and count cells.
5. Resuspend $0.1–1 \times 10^6$ cells in 100 μl of PBS in a cytometry tube.
6. Add 10 μl of each antibody (*see* Table 1) and incubate during 15 min at RT. The incubation must be done in the dark.
7. Add 2 ml of PBS and vortex the sample.

Table 2
Flow cytometry analysis

	Mouse		Rat		Pig		Human	
	SVF (d0)	ADSC (d15)	SVF (d0)	ADSC (d21)	SVF (d0)	ADSC (d21)	SVF (d0)	ADSC (d21)
MHC-I	+++	++	+++	+++	n.d.	n.d.	++	+++
MHC-II	++	+	–	–	n.d.	n.d.	+	±
CD29	n.d.	n.d.	n.d.	n.d.	++	+++	++	+++
CD31	++	±	++	–	±	–	+	–
CD34	+	+	n.d.	n.d.	n.d.	n.d.	++	–
CD44	++	+++	++	+++	n.d.	n.d.	++	+++
CD45	++	+	+	–	n.d.	n.d.	+	–
CD73	n.d.	n.d.	+	+++	n.d.	n.d.	++	+++
CD90	+	++	+	+++	++	+++	++	+++
CD105	n.d.	n.d.	n.d.	n.d.	n.d.	n.d.	++	+++
CD117	–	–	n.d.	n.d.	n.d.	n.d.	+/–	–

Results of ADSC phenotype are shown as +++: ≥90 %, ++: 50–90 %, +: 5–50 %, ±: ≤5 %, –: 0 % positive cells. Data obtained from the average of 3–6 independent samples (*d* days in culture, *n.d.* not determined)

8. Centrifuge at 600 × *g* for 5 min.
9. Remove the supernatant and resuspend the pellet in 400 μl of 0.4 % PFA.
10. Store the cell suspensions immediately at 4 °C in the dark until analysis (*see* **Note 11**).

3.3.2 ADSC Differentiation

Aside from marker expression, ADSC must meet the differentiation criteria for a proper characterization (*see* **Note 12**).

Osteogenic Differentiation (See Note 13)

1. Trypsinize cells and plate 5×10^3 cells/cm^2 in ADSC medium.
2. One day after, change medium to osteogenic differentiation medium.
3. Change medium every 3 days.
4. Maintain cells for 3 weeks in culture with the osteogenic differentiation medium.
5. After 3 weeks of differentiation, cells can be fixed and stained with Alizarin Red S or alkaline phosphatase.

Alizarin Red S Staining

1. Aspirate the medium from each well.
2. Fix cells with 10 % formalin during 30 min at RT.

3. Carefully aspirate the formalin and rinse first with PBS and distilled water.
4. Stain with 2 % Alizarin Red S solution pH 4.5 in distilled water for 5 min.
5. Wash three times with distilled water to remove remaining staining solution.
6. Visualize stained samples using a microscope.

Alkaline Phosphatase Test

1. Wash cells with PBS and then fix cells with 60 % acetone in 3 mM sodium citrate during 30 s, then wash with distilled water.
2. Stain samples with alkaline staining (*see* Subheading 2.3) for 30 min at RT and dark.
3. Wash three times with distilled water to remove remaining staining solution.
4. Visualize stained samples using a microscope.

Adipogenic Differentiation (See Note 14)

1. Culture ADSC cells in basal medium until 95–100 % confluence is reached.
2. Wash cells with PBS and add the adipogenic differentiation medium.
3. Change medium every 3 days.
4. Maintain for 3 weeks in culture in differentiation medium.
5. After 3 weeks of differentiation, cells can be fixed and stained with Oil Red O.

Oil Red O Staining

1. Aspirate the medium from each well.
2. Fix cells with 10 % formalin during 30 min, then wash with PBS and distilled water.
3. Stain with 60 % Oil Red O solution in distilled water (from a stock solution of 0.5 % Oil Red O in isopropanol) 20 min.
4. Wash three times with PBS to remove remaining Oil Red O solution.
5. Counterstain samples with Harris' hematoxylin diluted 1:2 in distilled water.
6. Visualize stained samples using a microscope.

Chondrogenic Differentiation (See Note 15)

1. Trypsinize and count cells.
2. Centrifuge ADSC cells (2×10^5 cells) at $450 \times g$ for 5 min to form a pelleted micromass. Discard the supernatant.
3. Culture pellets in 15 ml conical tubes with chondrogenic medium.
4. Change medium every 3 days, avoiding removing pellets.

5. Maintain for 3 weeks in culture in chondrogenic differentiation medium.
6. Collect pellets and use them for toluidine blue staining.

Toluidine Blue Staining

1. Fix pellets with 10 % formalin during 30 min.
2. Transfer the pellets to 70 % ethanol in H_2O.
3. Dehydrate the samples and embed the pellets with paraffin, following the routine histological procedures (see elsewhere).
4. Cut the samples in 5 μm sections using a microtome.
5. Deparaffinize the sections 15 min at 60 °C and immerse twice on xylene (for 5 and 15 min).
6. Rehydrate the sections using decreasing alcohol series (100, 96, 80, 70 %, 2 min each), followed by a rinse with tap water for 5 min.
7. Rinse the sections with deionized water for 1 min.
8. Stain samples with 1 % toluidine blue reagent and 1 % acetic acid (1:4) for 10 min.
9. Rinse the stained sections with distilled water.
10. Dehydrate in graded ethanol (96 and 100 %, 2 min each) followed by two steps in xylene for 15 min, and mount with DPX.
11. Visualize samples using a microscope.

4 Notes

1. It is important to collect samples in a sterile container and process them maintaining sterile conditions and within the first 24 h to obtain the highest cell yield. The AT samples are processed in a Class II biological laminar flow hood, and the personnel processing the samples must wear a lab coat, gloves, and surgical mask.
2. Lipoaspirate samples are directly incubated with the collagenase solution; mincing is not required. Nevertheless, an appropriate mincing of the sample is mandatory for a proper enzymatic digestion. In our experience, a careful and thorough mincing facilitates filtration and renders a higher cell yield.
3. For rat or mouse adipose tissue processing, incubate the samples with the collagenase solution during 30 min.
4. Approximately, 0.5–1 million cells per gram of processed adipose tissue are obtained.
5. For a 175 cm^2 culture flask, add 18–20 ml of basal medium.
6. As shown in Table 3 there are several similar media formulations available for the cultivation of ADSC, with the most frequent basic components being DMEM or alpha-MEM

Table 3
Different cell medias used for ADSC expansion

Basic medium	Serum	Supplements	References
DMEM	10 % FBS	–	[6, 7]
DMEM-LG	10 % FBS	–	[29]
DMEM F12	10 % FBS	–	[22, 30]
α-MEM	10 % FBS	–	[26]
α-MEM	10 % FBS	1 ng/ml bFGF	[24]

supplemented with 10 % FBS. Also, bFGF is used to enhance the proliferation rate [24]. Animal serum is also added to support optimal cell growth as it provides crucial cues for the adequate cell growth. For clinical application, however, animal components must be avoided. As a consequence, a very low human serum expansion medium and a completely serum-free medium have been developed [25]. Another option is the replacement of bovine serum by autologous serum [26] in order to prevent undesirable animal-derived viral transmissions or immunologic reactions. A recently used serum substitute for culture of ADSC is platelet lysate obtained by subjecting platelets to several cycles of freezing-thawing and collecting the supernatants. Recent studies have compared the ADSC and bone marrow MSC yield obtained with platelet lysate in comparison with other serum-containing media [27, 28].

7. ADSC are cultured in plastic flasks at 37 °C with a 95 % humidified atmosphere of 5.5 % CO_2. ADSC form fibroblast-like loose colonies composed of spindle-shaped cells which are visible under microscope 1–2 days after their isolation. The colonies grow and cells proliferate, reaching confluence in approximately 3–4 days. ADSC proliferate at high density and are subcultured when they reach 80–90 % confluence (*see* Fig. 2); it is important to note that the ADSC growth is not inhibited by cell-to-cell contact. For subculturing, cells are washed to eliminate old medium and serum and detached with trypsin/EDTA. ADSC are replated at 4×10^3 cells/cm^2, requiring 3 weeks for proper homogenization. Media must be changed every 3 days.
8. For a 175 cm^2 culture flask, wash with 10 ml of PBS, trypsinize with 2 ml trypsin/EDTA, and inactivate the trypsin with 6 ml of basal medium (DMEM supplemented with 10 % FBS and 1 % antibiotics).

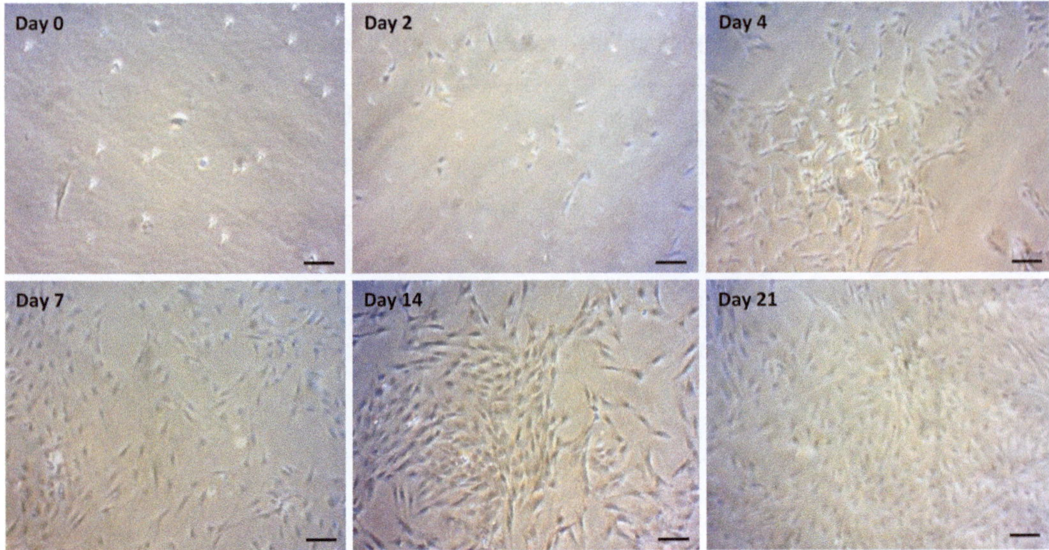

Fig. 2 Adipose-derived stem cell (ADSC) culture. Representative photographs of rat adipose tissue-derived cells at d0, d2, d4, d7, d14, and d21 of cell culture. Scale bars: 50 μm

9. It is recommended to label the cryogenic vials with the number of the experiment, cryopreserved cells, and cell passage; also, it is important to add the cryopreservation date.

10. Although some of the markers depicted on Table 1 are different among species, this does not reflect differences among those populations but lack of specific antibodies. Researcher is highly encouraged to try cross-reactivity of existing antibodies or newly developed ones. However, it is important to keep in mind the above requirements for each population, which must be met for a proper characterization.

11. For best results, analyze the cells on the flow cytometer as soon as possible.

12. As multipotent progenitors, ADSC give rise to osteoblasts, chondrocytes, and adipocytes. At least two of these lineages must be achieved for a proven multipotency. Cell differentiation is triggered by culturing ADSC for 3 weeks with specific induction media, as specified below. As depicted on Table 4, media supplements may vary slightly depending on the chosen protocol.

13. This assay is performed in 6-well cell culture plates. Add 3 ml medium/each well. After 3 weeks of culture with the osteogenic medium, verify the differentiation towards osteoblasts by Alizarin Red S staining and alkaline phosphatase tests. Alizarin Red S stains calcified depositions characteristic of osteogenic differentiation, whereas alkaline phosphatase tests the activity of this enzyme (*see* Fig. 3b).

Table 4
Factors for ADSC differentiation

Differentiation	Differentiation factors	References
Osteogenic	1,25-Dihydroxycholecalciferol, β-glycerophosphate, ascorbic acid, dexamethasone	[22, 23, 29, 31]
Adipogenic	Insulin, IBMX, dexamethasone, indomethacin	[23, 32, 33]
Chondrogenic	TGF-β2, TGF-β3, dexamethasone, insulin, transferrin, ITS, sodium-l-ascorbate, sodium pyruvate, ascorbate-2-phosphate	[22, 23, 29, 33]

BMP bone morphogenetic protein, *IBMX* 3-isobutyl-1-methylxanthine, *TGF-β* transforming growth factor-β

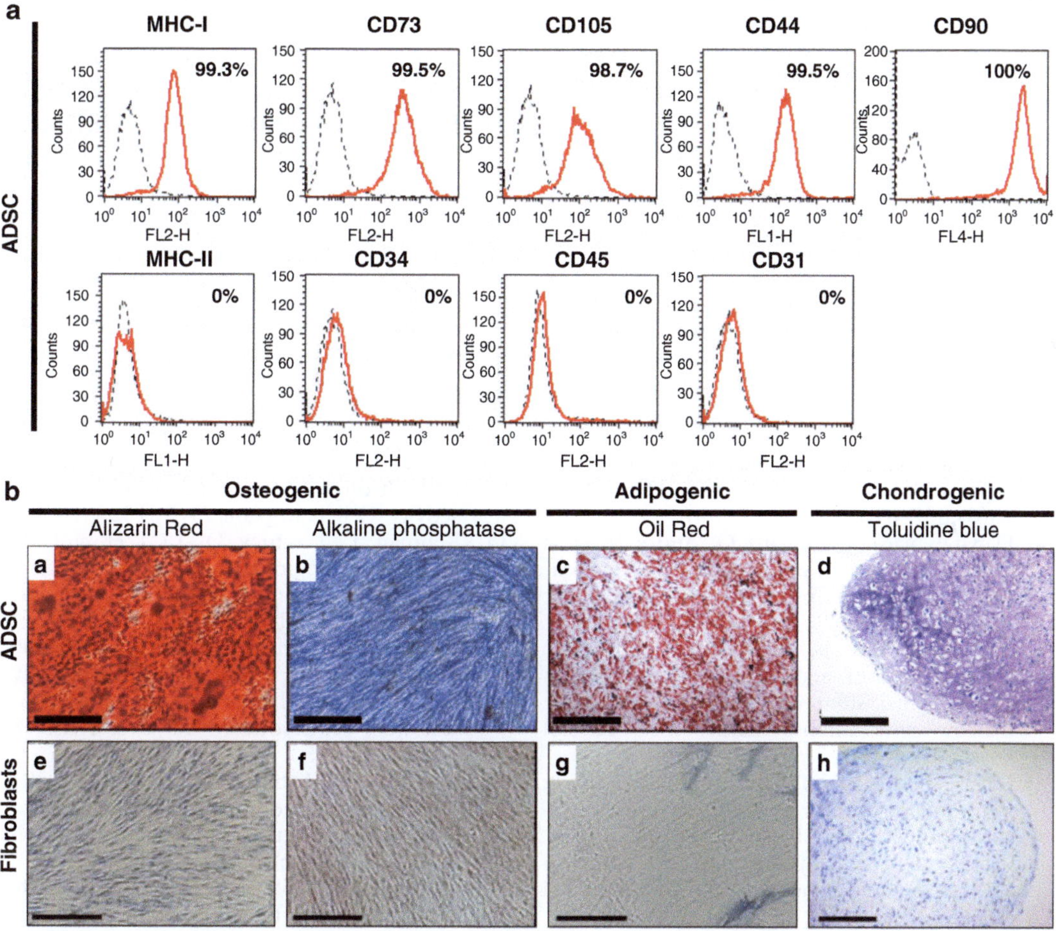

Fig. 3 ADSC characterization. (**a**) ADSC phenotype characterization. Representative example of antigen expression of human ADSC by flow cytometry analysis. The dotted line corresponds to isotype control IgG and the red line to the specific antibody. Expression of each antigen is also indicated as percentage. (**b**) ADSC differentiation potential. ADSC differentiates in vitro towards osteocytes (Alizarin Red and alkaline phosphatase stainings), adipocytes (Oil Red O staining), and chondrocytes (toluidine blue staining). Fibroblasts' staining is shown as negative control. Scale bars: 250 μm (*A–C, E–H*), 100 μm (*d*)

14. This assay is performed in 6-well cell culture plates. Add 3 ml medium/each well. After the differentiation is completed (3 weeks), Oil Red O staining can be performed to visualize lipid deposit and ascertain if lineage conversion has been successful (*see* Fig. 3b).
15. This assay is performed in 15 ml polypropylene centrifuge tubes to obtain cell aggregates. Cartilage produces an extracellular matrix rich in collagen type II, type X, or aggrecans. The chondrogenic differentiation can thus be assessed by staining the samples with toluidine blue, whereby cartilaginous extracellular matrix stains purple and undifferentiated tissue stains blue (*see* Fig. 3b).

Acknowledgement

This work was supported in part by funds from the ISCIII (RD06/0014, PI10/01621, CP09/00333), MINECO (PLE2009-0116), FP7 Program (INELPY), and the "UTE project CIMA."

References

1. Zuk PA, Zhu0000onnenberg VS, Pfeifer ME et al (2010) Stromal vascular progenitors in adult human adipose tissue. Cytometry A 77(1):22–30
3. Lin CS, Xin ZC, Deng CH et al (2010) Defining adipose tissue-derived stem cells in tissue and in culture. Histol Histopathol 25(6):807–815
4. Planat-Benard V, Menard C, Andre M et al (2004) Spontaneous cardiomyocyte differentiation from adipose tissue stroma cells. Circ Res 94(2):223–229
5. Lee RH, Kim B, Choi I et al (2004) Characterization and expression analysis of mesenchymal stem cells from human bone marrow and adipose tissue. Cell Physiol Biochem 14(4–6):311–324
6. Lin G, Garcia M, Ning H et al (2008) Defining stem and progenitor cells within adipose tissue. Stem Cells Dev 17(6):1053–1063
7. Zuk PA, Zhu M, Ashjian P et al (2002) Human adipose tissue is a source of multipotent stem cells. Mol Biol Cell 13(12):4279–4295
8. Guilak F, Awad HA, Fermor B, Leddy HA, Gimble JM (2004) Adipose-derived adult stem cells for cartilage tissue engineering. Biorheology 41(3–4):389–399
9. Yoshimura K, Shigeura T, Matsumoto D et al (2006) Characterization of freshly isolated and cultured cells derived from the fatty and fluid portions of liposuction aspirates. J Cell Physiol 208(1):64–76
10. Mazo M, Cemborain A, Gavira JJ et al (2012) Adipose stromal vascular fraction improves cardiac function in chronic myocardial infarction through differentiation and paracrine activity. Cell Transplant 21(5):1023–1037
11. Rehman J, Traktuev D, Li J et al (2004) Secretion of angiogenic and antiapoptotic factors by human adipose stromal cells. Circulation 109(10):1292–1298
12. Mitchell JB, McIntosh K, Zvonic S et al (2006) Immunophenotype of human adipose-derived cells: temporal changes in stromal-associated and stem cell-associated markers. Stem Cells 24(2):376–385
13. Mizuno H, Tobita M, Uysal AC (2012) Concise review: adipose-derived stem cells as a novel tool for future regenerative medicine. Stem Cells 30(5):804–810
14. Strem BM, Hicok KC, Zhu M et al (2005) Multipotential differentiation of adipose tissue-derived stem cells. Keio J Med 54(3):132–141
15. Kern S, Eichler H, Stoeve J, Kluter H, Bieback K (2006) Comparative analysis of mesenchymal stem cells from bone marrow, umbilical cord blood, or adipose tissue. Stem Cells 24(5):1294–1301

16. Mesimaki K, Lindroos B, Tornwall J et al (2009) Novel maxillary reconstruction with ectopic bone formation by GMP adipose stem cells. Int J Oral Maxillofac Surg 38(3): 201–209
17. Herreros MD, Garcia-Arranz M, Guadalajara H, De-La-Quintana P, Garcia-Olmo D (2012) Autologous expanded adipose-derived stem cells for the treatment of complex cryptoglandular perianal fistulas: a phase III randomized clinical trial (FATT 1: fistula Advanced Therapy Trial 1) and long-term evaluation. Dis Colon Rectum 55(7):762–772
18. Mirotsou M, Jayawardena TM, Schmeckpeper J, Gnecchi M, Dzau VJ (2011) Paracrine mechanisms of stem cell reparative and regenerative actions in the heart. J Mol Cell Cardiol 50(2):280–289
19. Prunet-Marcassus B, Cousin B, Caton D et al (2006) From heterogeneity to plasticity in adipose tissues: site-specific differences. Exp Cell Res 312(6):727–736
20. Goh BC, Thirumala S, Kilroy G, Devireddy RV, Gimble JM (2007) Cryopreservation characteristics of adipose-derived stem cells: maintenance of differentiation potential and viability. J Tissue Eng Regen Med 1(4):322–324
21. Gonda K, Shigeura T, Sato T et al (2008) Preserved proliferative capacity and multipotency of human adipose-derived stem cells after long-term cryopreservation. Plast Reconstr Surg 121(2):401–410
22. Im GI, Shin YW, Lee KB (2005) Do adipose tissue-derived mesenchymal stem cells have the same osteogenic and chondrogenic potential as bone marrow-derived cells? Osteoarthritis Cartilage 13(10):845–853
23. Noel D, Caton D, Roche S et al (2008) Cell specific differences between human adipose-derived and mesenchymal-stromal cells despite similar differentiation potentials. Exp Cell Res 314(7):1575–1584
24. Zaragosi LE, Ailhaud G, Dani C (2006) Autocrine fibroblast growth factor 2 signaling is critical for self-renewal of human multipotent adipose-derived stem cells. Stem Cells 24(11): 2412–2419
25. Parker AM, Shang H, Khurgel M, Katz AJ (2007) Low serum and serum-free culture of multipotential human adipose stem cells. Cytotherapy 9(7):637–646
26. Mazo M, Hernandez S, Gavira JJ et al (2012) Treatment of reperfused ischemia with adipose-derived stem cells in a preclinical swine model of myocardial infarction. Cell Transplant 21(12):2723–2733
27. Perez-Ilzarbe M, Diez-Campelo M, Aranda P et al (2009) Comparison of ex vivo expansion culture conditions of mesenchymal stem cells for human cell therapy. Transfusion 49(9): 1901–1910
28. Shih DT, Chen JC, Chen WY et al (2011) Expansion of adipose tissue mesenchymal stromal progenitors in serum-free medium supplemented with virally inactivated allogeneic human platelet lysate. Transfusion 51(4): 770–778
29. Rada T, Reis RL, Gomes ME (2011) Distinct stem cells subpopulations isolated from human adipose tissue exhibit different chondrogenic and osteogenic differentiation potential. Stem Cell Rev 7(1):64–76
30. Szoke K, Beckstrom KJ, Brinchmann JE (2012) Human adipose tissue as a source of cells with angiogenic potential. Cell Transplant 21(1):235–250
31. Leong DT, Abraham MC, Gupta A et al (2012) ATF5, a possible regulator of osteogenic differentiation in human adipose-derived stem cells. J Cell Biochem 113(8):2744–2753
32. Pittenger MF, Mackay AM, Beck SC et al (1999) Multilineage potential of adult human mesenchymal stem cells. Science 284(5411): 143–147
33. Liu TM, Martina M, Hutmacher DW et al (2007) Identification of common pathways mediating differentiation of bone marrow- and adipose tissue-derived human mesenchymal stem cells into three mesenchymal lineages. Stem Cells 25(3):750–760

Chapter 5

Cardiac Side Population Cells and Sca-1-Positive Cells

Toshio Nagai, Katsuhisa Matsuura, and Issei Komuro

Abstract

Since the resident cardiac stem/progenitor cells were discovered, their ability to maintain the architecture and functional integrity of adult heart has been broadly explored. The methods for isolation and purification of the cardiac stem cells are crucial for the precise analysis of their developmental origin and intrinsic potential as tissue stem cells. Stem cell antigen-1 (Sca-1) is one of the useful cell surface markers to purify the cardiac progenitor cells. Another purification strategy is based on the high efflux ability of the dye, which is a common feature of tissue stem cells. These dye-extruding cells have been called side population cells because they locate in the side of dye-retaining cells after fluorescent cell sorting. In this chapter, we describe the methodology for the isolation of cardiac SP cells and Sca-1 positive cells.

Key words Cardiac progenitor cells, Cardiac stem cells, Side population (SP), Hoechst 33342, Stem cell antigen-1 (Sca-1)

1 Introduction

The recent discovery of resident cardiac stem cells in postnatal heart has opened the new era of cardiac regenerative medicine. Several laboratories have identified distinct population of cardiac stem cells including side population (SP) cells [1, 2], stem cell antigen-1-positive (Sca-1^+) cells [3, 4], c-kit-positive (c-kit^+) cells [5], Isl-1-positive cells [6], and Wilms' tumor 1-positive epicardial progenitor cells [7]. In addition it has been reported that cardiospheres, which are grown from the heart specimens after multistep culture, contain Sca-1^+ and c-kit^+ cardiac stem cells [8]. The methods for isolation and purification of the cardiac stem cells are crucial for the precise analysis of their developmental origin and intrinsic potential as tissue stem cells. Isl-1 and Wilms' tumor-1 are transcription factors, and therefore, the transgenic animals are necessary to genetically mark the transcription factors to isolate the live cells [6, 7]. In contrast, Sca-1^+ and c-kit^+ cells are detected by the specific cell surface markers, and SP cells are identified based on the efflux ability of the dye, thus being simply isolated by the fluorescent-activating sorting system. It is important to note that these

Race L. Kao (ed.), *Cellular Cardiomyoplasty: Methods and Protocols*, Methods in Molecular Biology, vol. 1036,
DOI 10.1007/978-1-62703-511-8_5,

cell surface marker- and dye-based methods enable us to obtain fresh cells without transgenic animals and long-term culture, which may affect the intrinsic profiles of stem cells.

SP cells were first identified as mouse hematopoietic stem cells with long-term multi-lineage reconstitution abilities based on their unique ability to efflux the DNA-binding dye Hoechst 33342 [9]. SP cells have been reported to exist in a variety of organs, such as bone marrow, skeletal muscle, mammary gland, liver, lung, skin, and heart, and play an important role as tissue-specific stem cells [10]. Zhou et al. have reported that the ATP-binding cassette transporter subfamily G member 2 (Abcg2), also known as breast cancer-resistant protein 1 (BCRP-1), is a molecular determinant of this SP phenotype in hematopoietic stem cells [11]. In cardiac SP cells, Abcg2 controls dye efflux in early postnatal period, whereas multidrug resistance 1 (Mdr1) is required for the dye efflux phenotype in adulthood [12]. Abcg2 supports long-term survival of stem cells via the enhancement of ability to export cytotoxic compounds [10]. Recently, Abcg2 has been reported to reduce intracellular heme/porphyrin accumulation and provide the tolerance to hypoxic condition [13]. Mdr1 transports cytotoxic drugs delivered as chemotherapy out of the cells, thereby reducing drug-mediated cell death. In addition, a recent report has shown that Mdr1 inhibits the apoptosis induced by a various kind of cell stimuli, suggesting that the mechanisms other than a simple excretion of cytotoxic substrates exist [14]. The cardiomyogenic potential of cardiac SP cells has been reported in vitro and in vivo. Adult cardiac SP cells spontaneously express cardiac proteins when cultured on laminin-coated dishes; however, coculture with cardiomyocytes is necessary to develop organized sarcomere and contractile capacity [1]. Our group has reported that cardiac SP cells from postnatal rat hearts differentiate into spontaneously beating cardiomyocytes when cultured and stimulated with oxytocin or trichostatin A [2]. When cardiac SP cells were intravenously transplanted into the cryoinjured heart, the transplanted SP cells differentiated into cardiomyocytes in the infarct area [2]. The molecular mechanisms, which regulate the differentiation and proliferation of cardiac SP cells, are still elusive. Recently, Oikonomopoulos et al. have reported that canonical Wnt signaling and its downstream mediator, insulin-like growth factor-binding protein 3, negatively regulate the proliferation of adult cardiac SP cells [15].

Sca-1 is a member of the Ly-6 family and has first reported as one of the cell surface markers of hematopoietic stem cells [16]. Our and another group have reported that adult cardiac Sca-1^+ cells differentiate into cardiomyocytes in vitro under the treatment with 5-azacytidine [3] and oxytocin [4]. Intravenously injected cardiac Sca-1^+ cells home, migrate, and differentiate into cardiomyocyte in the infarct area [3]. Furthermore the report from our group has demonstrated that transplantation of cardiac Sca-1$^+$ cells improves cardiac function after myocardial infarction through cardiomyocyte differentiation and paracrine factors, including soluble vascular cell adhesion molecule-1 [17]. The biological hierarchy and correlation between cardiac SP cells and Sca1$^+$ cells is still unclear. Interestingly, it has been reported that a high percentage (~80 %) of adult cardiac SP cells express Sca1; however, only a very small percentage (1 ~ 3.5 %) of cardiac Sca-1$^+$ cells is included in SP fraction [1, 3]. Pfister et al. have identified that Sca1$^+$ CD31$^-$ subpopulations within cardiac SP cells were enriched for cardiomyogenic potential [1]. These reports suggest that there is a substantial heterogeneity in each of the primary isolated cardiac SP and Sca-1$^+$ cells. The purification of cardiac SP and Sca-1$^+$ cells in combination with more specific markers may allow us to examine the more precise dynamics of proliferation and differentiation of cardiac stem cells.

2 Materials

In this section, subheadings from 2.1 to 2.3 list the materials for isolation of cardiac SP cells and subheadings from 2.4 to 2.6 list the materials for isolation of cardiac Sca-1$^+$ cells.

2.1 Enzymatic Digestion of Adult Murine Hearts for Isolation of Cardiac SP Cells

1. Collagenase type 2 (26.5 U/ml), lyophilizate. The final concentration for the digestion is 1 %. Store dry at 4 °C and protected from light.
2. Dispase II, lyophilizate. The final concentration for the digestion is 4.6 U/ml.
3. $CaCl_2$. The final concentration for the digestion is 2.4 mM.
4. 0.01 M Phosphate Buffered Saline (PBS): one pouch of Phosphate Buffered Saline is dissolved in distilled water to make up a total volume of 1 l.
5. PBS supplemented with 3 % fetal bovine serum.
6. 70 μm cell strainer.

2.2 Hoechst 33342 Incubation for Isolation of Cardiac SP Cells

1. Hoechst 33342 dissolved in PBS at a final concentration of 5 mg/ml.
2. PBS supplemented with 3 % fetal bovine serum.
3. Verapamil 50 mM stock solution in distilled water.

2.3 Flow Cytometry and Sorting for Isolation of Cardiac SP Cells

1. Flow cytometer and cell sorter: EPICS ALTRA HyperSort.
2. Test tubes.

2.4 Enzymatic Digestion of Adult Murine Hearts for Isolation of Cardiac Sca-1+ Cells

1. Collagenase type 2, lyophilized. The final concentration for the digestion is 0.1 %.
2. Type XIV protease. The final concentration for the digestion is 0.01 %.
3. 2,3-Butanedione monoxime. The final concentration for the digestion is 30 mM.
4. NaCl. The final concentration for the digestion is 63 mM.
5. D-glucose. The final concentration for the digestion is 5.6 mM.
6. HEPES. The final concentration for the digestion is 12 mM.
7. Taurine. The final concentration for the digestion is 10 mM.
8. Creatine monohydrate. The final concentration for the digestion is 2.2 mM.
9. Sodium pyruvate. The final concentration for the digestion is 2.5 mM.
10. $NaH_2PO_4 \cdot 2H_2O$. The final concentration for the digestion is 0.5 mM.
11. $CaCl_2$. The final concentration for the digestion is 100 μM.
12. KCl. The final concentration for the digestion is 4.4 mM.
13. $MgCl_2 \cdot 6H_2O$. The final concentration for the digestion is 1 mM.
14. NaOH (1 N).
15. Masterflex perfusion system.
16. Tube (size 13).
17. Water bath.
18. 24GA Autoguard Winged (0.75I N 0.7 × 19 mm).
19. 5-0 nylon suture.
20. 0.22 and 0.45 μm filters.
21. 10 ml syringe.
22. Stereomicroscope.
23. 70 μm strainer.

2.5 Immunostaining for Isolation of Cardiac Sca-1+ Cells

1. Phycoerythrin (PE)-conjugated anti-Sca-1 (anti-Ly6A/E) antibody. The final concentration is 0.5 %.
2. Anti-PE MicroBeads. The final concentration is 20 %.
3. 0.01 M Phosphate Buffered Saline (PBS): one pouch of Phosphate Buffered Saline is dissolved in distilled water to make up a total volume of 1 l.
4. PBS supplemented with 3 % fetal bovine serum.

2.6 Flow Cytometer and Cell Sorting for Isolation of Cardiac Sca-1+ Cells

1. Flow cytometer: EPICS ALTRA HyperSort.
2. Cell separation column.
3. MiniMACS separator.

3 Methods

In this section, we explain the protocol for the isolation of adult murine cardiac SP cells (Subheadings 3.1–3.3) and that for the isolation of cardiac Sca-1$^+$ cells (Subheadings 3.4–3.6) from C57Bl/6JJ mice.

An average of the total cardiac SP cell yield was 0.2 ± 0.08 % in mice 10–12 weeks of age according to our experience. Approximately 40 and 1.8 % of cardiac SP cells express Sca-1 and CD31, respectively. Pfister et al. have reported that 84 and 75 % of cardiac SP cells express Sca-1 and CD31, respectively [1]. An average of the total cardiac Sca-1$^+$ cells yield was 3 % in mice 8 weeks of age according to our experiences. Approximately 40, 10, and 9 % of cardiac Sca-1$^+$ cells express CD45, CD34, and CD117 (c-kit). It is important to note that the yield and composition of cardiac SP and Sca-1$^+$ cells depend on the protocols, including digestion of the hearts, cell staining, and sorting procedure. In order to obtain cardiac SP and Sca-1$^+$ cells of good quality, reproducibility of the total yield and components of the cells must be examined in each laboratory under correct techniques.

3.1 Enzymatic Digestion of Adult Murine Hearts for Isolation of Cardiac SP Cells

1. Make fresh digestion buffer containing 1 % collagenase type 2, 4.6 U/ml dispase II, and 2.4 mM $CaCl_2$. Prewarm 5 ml of this digestion buffer in a 50 ml conical tube in 37 °C water bath prior to use. Utilize 5 ml digestion buffer per one mouse heart and 10 ml for two hearts. We recommend digesting no more than two hearts. Prepare one 59 × 15 mm culture dishes with PBS and one watch glass on ice.
2. A mouse is killed by cervical dislocation. Note that alternative methods of anesthesia can be used in accordance with the individual Institutional Animal Care and Use Committee's guidelines and approval. Spray 70 % ethanol on the chest region. Cut the rib in bilateral sides of sternum to expose the thoracic cavity. Open the thorax, and lift and cut the heart out by forceps. Put the heart immediately in the one 59 × 15 mm culture dishes containing cold PBS to wash away any residual blood.
3. After washing, place the heart on a precooled watch glass. Cut the heart with ophthalmologic iris scissors into small pieces until the heart tissue become slurry. Transfer the minced cardiac tissue in 5 ml prewarmed digestion buffer per one heart. Thoroughly homogenate the tissue in digestion buffer by a water bath shaker at 37 °C for 20 min with shaking speed at 160 return/min and shaking width at 40 mm. After digestion, ensure that the tissue is entirely dispersed in the digestion buffer.
4. Following 20 min of incubation, stop the enzymatic reaction by adding 5 ml of cold PBS with 3 % FBS. Centrifuge at 440 × g for 5 min at 4 °C, discard the supernatant, and suspend the

pellet with 11 ml of cold PBS with 3 % FBS. The cell suspension was filtered through a 70 μm cell strainer. Take 10–20 μl of this cell suspension and count the mononucleated cells with a hemocytometer. We check the existence of the rod-shaped cardiomyocytes at this step to ensure the cell damage through digestion was held to a minimum. The total number of cardiomyocyte-depleted mononucleated cells is approximately 1.6×10^6 per heart from a ~10-week-old C57Bl/6J mouse.

3.2 Hoechst Incubation for Isolation of Cardiac SP Cells

1. Take 1 ml from filtered 11 ml of cell suspension and put in a 15 ml conical tube for a negative control sample. As the Hoechst staining procedure is light sensitive, turn off the light in the clean bench after this step if possible. Add 5 μl of Hoechst 33342 to 10 ml of cell suspension, which contains approximately 1.5×10^6 of mononuclear cells (*see* **Note 1**). To prepare a negative control sample, add 2 μl of verapamil to 1 ml of cell suspension and incubate for 10 min in a 37 °C water bath before adding 0.5 μl of Hoechst 33342. Gently invert the tube several times to mix the cells and Hoechst dye, and then leave for 90 min in a 37 °C water bath. Since verapamil inhibits the ABC transporter, the SP cells treated with verapamil retain Hoechst dye and disappear from the SP fraction, thus making easy to distinguish SP cells from non-SP cells and to determine the SP gate precisely. It is crucial to analyze the verapamil-treated SP cells as a negative control in each staining protocol.
2. After the 90-min incubation time, spin the cells down at $440 \times g$ for 5 min at 4 °C. Remove the supernatant and resuspend the cells in 10 and 1 ml of cold PBS with 3 % FBS for non-treated and verapamil-treated SP cells, respectively. Repeat the spin and resuspension one more time in the same way. Keep the cell suspension on ice and protect from light until flow cytometry and sorting analysis.

3.3 Flow Cytometry and Sorting Analysis for Isolation of Cardiac SP Cells

We are used to use EPICS ALTRA equipped with two argon lasers (Innova 70 and Innova 90c, Coherent). Hoechst 33342 dye is excited at 350 nm (UV range). Fluorescent emission is detected through 450 nm BP (Hoechst blue) and 675 nm LP (Hoechst red) filters, respectively. It is important to note that stable excitation of Hoechst dye and a correct detection of the emission are necessary to perform Hoechst dye efflux analysis. To set up an optimal condition, we recommend asking a technical assistance from the manufacture of your own flow cytometer. For those first starting to isolate cardiac SP cells, it is recommended to establish the optimal incubation time or concentration of Hoechst 3342 dye. Figure 1 showed a relationship between the percentage of SP cells and the incubation time with Hoechst dye. The percentage of Hoechst low or negative cells decreases as the Hoechst incubation time is getting longer from 5 to 75 min (Fig. 1a–d) and then does

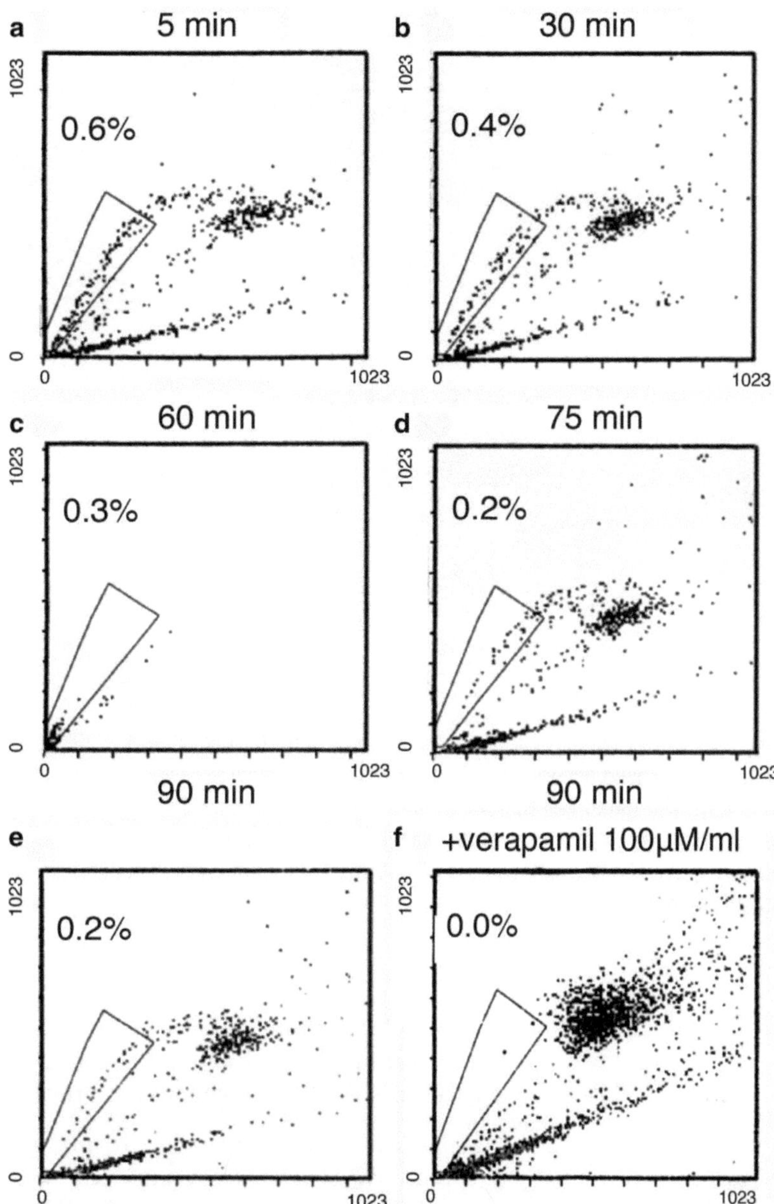

Fig. 1 (**a**)–(**f**) Determination of optimal Hoechst incubation time. Representable results of flow cytometry are displayed according to the emission profile against the Hoechst blue (*vertical axis*) versus red (*horizontal axis*). The isolated cardiac mononuclear cells were incubated with 2.5 μg/ml of Hoechst 33342 for various periods (**a**, 5 min; **b**, 30 min; **c**, 60 min; **d**, 75 min; **e**, 90 min). The percentage of SP cells in the boxed area was shown in each graph. The profile of SP cells was confirmed by the disappearance of SP cells in the boxed area after the treatment with verapamil (**f**)

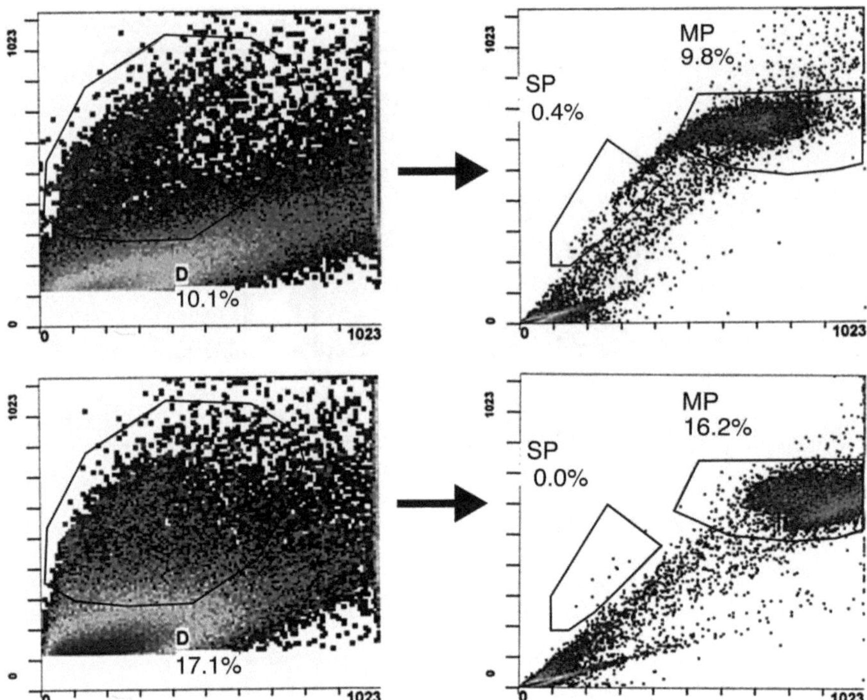

Fig. 2 (**a**)–(**d**) Representable process of gating and display of cardiac SP cells. Isolated cardiac mononuclear cells are displayed according to forward scatter (*vertical axis*) versus side scatter parameters (*horizontal axis*) (**a** and **c**). The gated cell population in the *boxed area* was displayed according to the Hoechst blue (*vertical axis*) versus red profile (*horizontal axis*) (b and d). The *boxed areas* in (**b** and **d**) indicate the population of cardiac SP cells. The treatment with 100 μM/ml of verapamil removes the cells in the boxed area, confirming the specificity of the SP profile (**d**)

not change between 75 and 90 min (Fig. 1d, e). The treatment with verapamil completely eliminated the SP fraction (Fig. 1f). Finally we determined that the incubation for 90 min with 2.5 μg/ml of Hoechst is the best to obtain a SP profile.

1. Nonviable or dead cells are excluded by displaying forward scatter (vertical axis) versus side scatter parameters (horizontal axis) (Fig. 2a, c) (*see* **Note 2**). The gated cell population was displayed according to the Hoechst blue versus red profile, with blue on the vertical axis (450 nm BP filter) and red (675 nm LP filter) on the horizontal axis on linear scale. The cardiac SP cells are in the boxed are represented as SP in Fig. 2b.
2. The specificity of the SP profile is confirmed using the sample treated with verapamil and Hoechst. Almost no cells exist in the boxed area (Fig. 2d).
3. Once the SP gate was fixed properly, sort and collect SP cells in desired media. We confirm the profile of SP cells by immunostaining with Mdr1 antibodies. As shown in Fig. 3, SP cells are small round cells with high nuclear cytoplasm ratio and expression of Mdr1 on their cell surface.

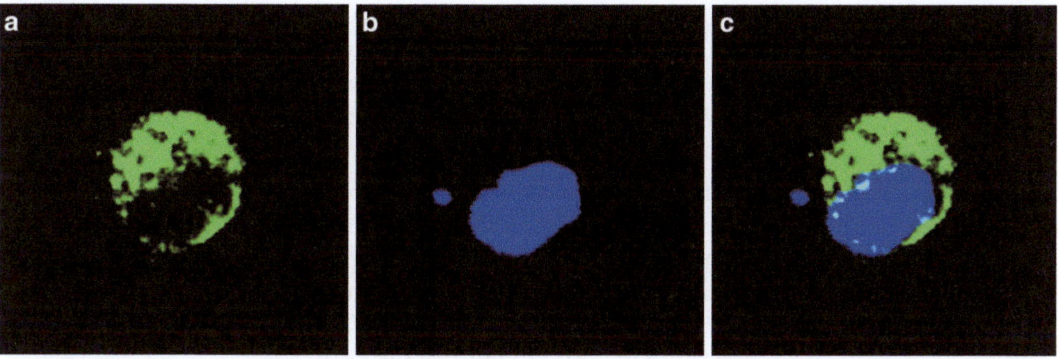

Fig. 3 (**a**)–(**c**) Cardiac SP cells expressing Mdr1. Freshly isolated cardiac SP cells were corrected by using cytospin and immunostained for Mdr1 (**a**, *green*) and DAPI (**b**, *blue*). A merged image was represented as in (**c**)

3.4 Enzymatic Digestion of Adult Murine Heart for Isolation of Cardiac Sca-1⁺ Cells

1. Make the buffer (0 mM Ca^{2+} solution) containing 63 mM NaCl, 5.6 mM D-glucose, 12 mM HEPES, 10 mM taurine, 2.2 mM creatine monohydrate, 2.5 mM sodium pyruvate, 0.5 mM $NaH_2PO_4 \cdot 2H_2O$, 4.4 mM KCl, and 1 mM $MgCl_2 \cdot 6H_2O$ in distilled water. By adjusting the pH of the buffer around 7.52–7.6 with 1 N NaOH (26 ml for 2 l buffer), the pH in 37 °C should be 7.4. This buffer is sterilized with 0.22 μm filter (Millipore). Prewarm 50 ml of this buffer in a 50 ml conical tube in 37 °C water bath prior to use. Prepare two 10 cm culture dishes with 10 ml of 0 mM Ca^{2+} solution. Prepare a 10 ml syringe with 10 ml of 0 mM Ca^{2+} solution and fit the syringe with external cylinder of intravenous cannula through 0.45 μm filter.
2. Make the buffer (100 μM Ca^{2+} solution) containing 63 mM NaCl, 5.6 mM D-glucose, 12 mM HEPES, 10 mM taurine, 2.2 mM creatine monohydrate, 2.5 mM sodium pyruvate, 0.5 mM $NaH_2PO_4 \cdot 2H_2O$, and 100 μM $CaCl_2$ in distilled water. This buffer is sterilized with 0.22 μm filter (Millipore). Prewarm 50 ml of this buffer in a 50 ml conical tube in 37 °C water bath prior to use.
3. Make fresh digestion buffer containing 0.1 % collagenase type 2, 0.01 % protease, and 30 mM BDM in 100 μM Ca^{2+} solution. This digestion buffer is sterilized with 0.22 μm filter. Prewarm 50 ml of this digestion buffer in a 50 ml conical tube in 37 °C water bath prior to use. Utilize 50 ml digestion buffer per one mouse heart.
4. Wash the line with sterilized distilled water for 3 min using perfusion system (2 ml/min).
5. Wash the line with sterilized 0 mM Ca^{2+} solution for 3 min using perfusion system (2 ml/min).
6. A mouse is killed by cervical dislocation. Note that alternative methods of anesthesia can be used in accordance with the individual Institutional Animal Care and Use Committee's

guidelines and approval. Spray 70 % ethanol on the chest region. Cut the rib in bilateral sides of sternum to expose the thoracic cavity. Open the thorax, and lift and cut the heart out by forceps. Put the heart immediately in the one 10 cm dish containing 0 mM Ca^{2+} solution to wash away residual blood.

7. After washing, pass the external cylinder of intravenous cannula through ascending aorta and lash the external cylinder and aorta with 5-0 nylon suture using a stereomicroscope. Take care not to pass the external cylinder over the aortic valve. Wash the heart with 10 ml of 0 mM Ca^{2+} solution using a syringe in a 10 cm culture dish.
8. Remove the syringe and fix the heart with the cylinder and 0.45 μm filter to the tube.
9. Perfuse the heart with 0 mM Ca^{2+} solution for 5 min using the perfusion system (2 ml/min).
10. Perfuse the heart with the digestion buffer for 12 min using the perfusion system (2 ml/min). When the perfusion solution is changed to the digestion buffer from 0 mM Ca^{2+} solution, stop the perfusion system to avoid the air incorporation in the perfusion tube.
11. Perfuse the heart with 100 μM Ca^{2+} solution for 5 min the perfusion system (2 ml/min). When the perfusion solution is changed to 100 mM Ca^{2+} solution from the digestion buffer, stop the perfusion system to avoid the air incorporation in the perfusion tube.
12. Collect the heart by cutting the ascending aorta with a sterilized scissor in 10 cm culture dish. Add 5 ml of 100 μM Ca^{2+} solution and cut the heart with a scissor into small pieces until the heart tissue become slurry. Transfer the minced cardiac tissue to a 50 ml conical tube through 70 μm strainer.

3.5 Immunostaining for Isolation of Cardiac Sca-1⁺ Cells

1. Centrifuge the tube at 300 × *g* for 5 min at 4 °C and aspirate the supernatant.
2. Resuspend the cells in 2 ml of cold PBS with 3 % FBS and add 10 μl of biotin or PE-conjugated anti-Sca-1 antibody.
3. Mix well and incubate for 10 min on ice.
4. Wash cells by adding 10 ml of cold PBS with 3 % FBS and centrifuge the tube at 300 × *g* for 5 min at 4 °C and aspirate the supernatant.
5. Repeat **step 4** further two times.
6. Resuspend the cells in 160 μl of cold PBS with 3 % FBS and add 40 μl of anti-biotin or PE MicroBeads. Mix well and incubate for 15 min at the refrigerator (4 °C).
7. Wash cells by adding 10 ml of cold PBS with 3 % FBS and centrifuge the tube at 300 × *g* for 5 min at 4 °C and aspirate the supernatant.

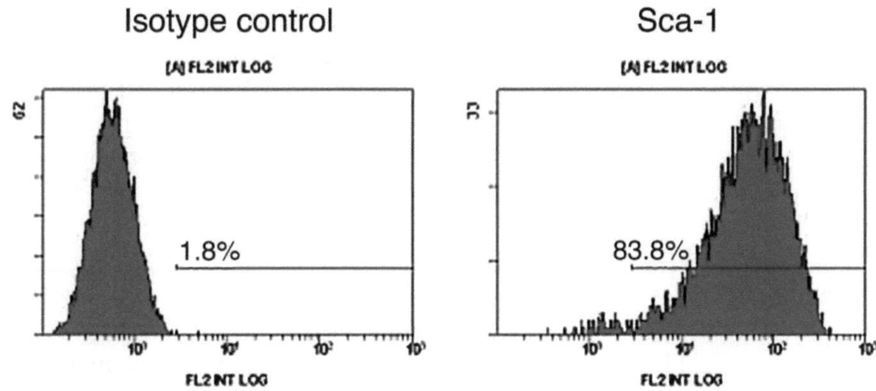

Fig. 4 FACS analysis of Sca-1 expression of cells after MACS sorting

8. Repeat **step 7** further two times.
9. Resuspend the cells in 5 ml of cold PBS with 3 % FBS.

3.6 Cell Sorting for Isolation of Cardiac Sca-1⁺ Cells

1. Place column in the magnetic field of a MACS separator.
2. Rinse the column with 3 ml of cold PBS with 3 % FBS.
3. Apply cell suspension onto the column. Discard the flow-through containing unlabeled cells.
4. Wash column with 3 ml of cold PBS with 3 % FBS. Discard the unlabeled cells that pass through and combine with the effluent from **step 12**. Repeat this step further two times.
5. Remove column from the separator and place it on a 50 ml conical tube.
6. Pipette 5 ml of cold PBS with 3 % FBS onto the column. Immediately flush out the magnetically labeled cells by firmly pushing the plunger into the column.
7. Repeat **steps 1–6** one more time.
8. After 2-time sorting, about 95 % purity of Sca-1 positive cells are obtained (Fig. 4).

4 Notes

1. Once the digestion protocol is established, relatively a constant number of the cells are obtained. For those who have just started SP cell isolation, we recommend checking the cell number in this step and adjusting the cell density to 1.5×10^5/ml by cold PBS with 3 % FBS, because the ratio of Hoechst dye to the cell number affects the yield and quality of SP cells.
2. To exclude the dead cells, we used to use propidium iodide (PI). PI is dissolved in PBS at 5 mg/ml and used at a final concentration of 2 μg/ml. Before flow cytometry and sorting

analysis, add 4 μl of PI to 10 ml of cell suspension, respectively. PI in cells is excited at 488 nm and fluorescence emission is detected through a 610 nm BP filter. PI-positive cells are excluded as the dead cells. After many times of PI staining experiences, we empirically determine the gate according to the forward and side scatter parameters.

Acknowledgements

The authors thank A. Furuyama for the excellent technical assistance. This work was supported by a Grant-in-Aid for Scientific Research, Developmental Scientific Research, and Scientific Research on Priority Areas from the Ministry of Education, Science, Sports, and Culture.

References

1. Pfister OF, Mouquet M, Jain R et al (2005) CD31- but Not CD31+ cardiac side population cells exhibit functional cardiomyogenic differentiation. Circ Res 97:52–61
2. Oyama T, Nagai T, Wada H et al (2007) Cardiac side population cells have a potential to migrate and differentiate into cardiomyocytes in vitro and in vivo. J Cell Biol 176:329–341
3. Oh H, Bradfute SB, Gallardo TD et al (2003) Cardiac progenitor cells from adult myocardium: homing, differentiation, and fusion after infarction. Proc Natl Acad Sci U S A 100:12313–12318
4. Matsuura K, Nagai T, Nishigaki N et al (2004) Adult cardiac Sca-1-positive cells differentiate into beating cardiomyocytes. J Biol Chem 279:11384–11391
5. Beltrami AP, Barlucchi L, Torella D et al (2003) Adult cardiac stem cells are multipotent and support myocardial regeneration. Cell 114:763–776
6. Laugwitz KL, Moretti A, Lam J et al (2005) Postnatal isl1+ cardioblasts enter fully differentiated cardiomyocyte lineages. Nature 433:647–653
7. Smart N, Bollini S, Dubé KN et al (2011) De novo cardiomyocytes from within the activated adult heart after injury. Nature 474:640–644
8. Messina E, De Angelis L, Frati G et al (2004) Isolation and expansion of adult cardiac stem cells from human and murine heart. Circ Res 95:911–921
9. Goodell MA, Brose K, Paradis G et al (1996) Isolation and functional properties of murine hematopoietic stem cells that are replicating in vivo. J Exp Med 183:1797–1806
10. Challen GA, Little MH (2006) A side order of stem cells: the SP phenotype. Stem Cells 24:3–12
11. Zhou S, Schuetz JD, Bunting KD et al (2001) The ABC transporter Bcrp1/ABCG2 is expressed in a wide variety of stem cells and is a molecular determinant of the side-population phenotype. Nat Med 7:1028–1034
12. Pfister O, Oikonomopoulos A, Sereti KI et al (2008) Role of the ATP-binding cassette transporter Abcg2 in the phenotype and function of cardiac side population cells. Circ Res 103:825–835
13. Krishnamurthy P, Ross DD, Nakanishi T et al (2004) The stem cell marker Bcrp/ABCG2 enhances hypoxic cell survival through interactions with heme. J Biol Chem 279: 24218–24225
14. Smyth MJ, Krasovskis E, Sutton VR et al (1998) The drug efflux protein, P-glycoprotein, additionally protects drug-resistant tumor cells from multiple forms of caspase-dependent apoptosis. Proc Natl Acad Sci U S A 95: 7024–7029
15. Oikonomopoulos A, Sereti KI, Conyers F et al (2011) Wnt signaling exerts an antiproliferative effect on adult cardiac progenitor cells through IGFBP3. Circ Res 109:1363–1374
16. van der Rijn M, Heimfeld S, Spangruade GJ et al (1989) Mouse hematopoietic stem-cell antigen Sca-1 is a member of the Ly-6 antigen family. Proc Natl Acad Sci U S A 86: 4634–4638
17. Matsuura K, Honda A, Nagai T et al (2009) Transplantation of cardiac progenitor cells ameliorates cardiac dysfunction after myocardial infarction in mice. J Clin Invest 119:2204–2217

Chapter 6

Two-Step Protocol for Isolation and Culture of Cardiospheres

Lijuan Chen, Yaohua Pan, Lan Zhang, Yingjie Wang, Neal Weintraub, and Yaoliang Tang

Abstract

Cardiac progenitor cells (CPC) are a unique pool of progenitor cells residing in the heart that play an important role in cardiac homeostasis and physiological cardiovascular cell turnover during acute myocardial infarction (MI). Transplanting CPC into the heart has shown promise in two recent clinical trials of cardiac repair (SCIPIO & CADUCEUS). CSCs were originally isolated directly from enzymatically digested hearts followed by cell sorting using stem cell markers. However, long exposure to enzymatic digestion can affect the integrity of stem cell markers on the cell surface and also compromise stem cell function. Here, we describe a two-step procedure in which a large number of intact cardiac progenitor cells can be purified from small amount of heart tissue.

Key words Cardiac progenitor cells, Cardiosphere, Magnetic-activated cell sorting (MACS)

1 Introduction

The mammalian heart has long been considered a postmitotic organ, with little regenerative capacity following ischemic necrosis, thereby leading to scarring. Recent evidence indicates that the adult mammalian heart (including the human heart) possesses a pool of intermediate cardiac progenitors which can differentiate into cells that phenotypically resemble cardiomyocytes, endothelial cells, and vascular smooth muscle cells, the major components of myocardial tissue [1, 2]. Unfortunately, resident mammalian CPC cell populations become acutely depleted following MI [3], which limits their endogenous regenerative capacity. A recent clinical trial from Cedars-Sinai Heart Institute and Johns Hopkins University demonstrated that transplanting autologous CPC can increase cardiac muscle mass and reduce scar size [4]. Conventional methods use enzymatic digestion to isolate resident cardiac progenitor cells (c-kit+, Sca-1+) from heart in one step. However, enzymatic digestion of myocardium compromises the integrity of important surface antigens of resident

Race L. Kao (ed.), *Cellular Cardiomyoplasty: Methods and Protocols*, Methods in Molecular Biology, vol. 1036,
DOI 10.1007/978-1-62703-511-8_6, © Springer Science+Business Media New York 2013

cardiac stem cells and leads to dysfunctional sorted cells, which makes the method hard to be reproduced.

To avoid these problems, we have developed a two-step procedure to isolate and expand pure population of cardiac progenitor cells from heart tissue. First, we use primary heart tissue explanting technology to expand endogenous cardiac progenitor cells for about 2 to 3 weeks depending on age; second, we use magnetic-activated cell sorting (MACS) or fluorescence-activated cell sorting (FACS) to isolate pure population of progenitor cells from cardiac explant tissue and cloning. We use a cardiac fibroblast conditional medium to maintain the proliferation of cardiac progenitor cells at first three generations. We demonstrated that Sca-1+ cells isolated by this method keep their self-renewal and clonogenic character in vitro and can directly differentiate into normal cells in myocardium, including cardiomyocytes, endothelial cells, and smooth muscle cells, after transplantation in ischemic hearts of mice.

In this protocol, we describe a two-step procedure in which a large number of Sca-1+ cardiac progenitor cells can be purified from small amount of heart tissue. The cultured cardiac progenitor cells can keep their capacity for self-renewal and clonogenic in vitro with fibroblast-free conditional medium.

2 Materials

2.1 Cell Isolation and Expansion

1. Heart tissue.
2. Dulbecco's PBS (D-PBS, without calcium chloride and magnesium chloride).
3. Bovine serum albumin (BSA, Fraction V, 7.5 % (wt/vol)) solution.
4. Collagenase IV.
5. 24-well plate, with lid, flat bottom, ultralow attachment surface.
6. Dulbecco's Modified Eagle Medium (DMEM)/Ham's F-12 nutrient broth (1:1, vol/vol) with 15 mM HEPES buffer, L-glutamine, and pyridoxine hydrochloride.
7. Fetal bovine serum (FBS).
8. Human fibroblastic growth factor, basic (rh-bFGF).
9. Trypsin/EDTA [0.05 % (wt/vol)].
10. Penicillin/streptomycin/amphotericin B.
11. Cryogenic vials.
12. Dimethylsulfoxide Hybri-Max.
13. Freezing container (1 °C)

14. 40-μm cell strainer.
15. Fibronectin-coated dish.
16. Poly-D-lysine-coated dish.

2.2 MACS Sorting

1. Anti-Sca-1 microbeads.
2. Magnetic cell sorter device.

2.3 Equipment

1. Centrifuge water bath shaker.

2.4 Reagent Setup

1. Enzyme mix: prepare fresh a solution of 0.2 % (wt/vol) trypsin and 0.1 % (wt/vol) collagenase IV in D-PBS, usually 30–50 ml for each mouse heart.
2. Explant medium: Iscove's Modified Dulbecco's IMDM with 10 % fetal calf serum (FBS), 100 U/mL penicillin G, 100 μg/ml streptomycin, 2 mmol/L L-glutamine, and 0.1 mmol/L 2-mercaptoethanol.
3. Cell growth medium (CGM): [DMEM/F12, 10 % FBS, 200 mmol/L L-glutamine, 0.1 mmol/L β-mercaptoethanol, 1 % nonessential amino acids, 1,000 U/ml LIF, 0.1 U/ml thrombin, and 5 ng/ml basic fibroblast growth factor (bFGF)].
4. Cardiac fibroblast conditional medium (CFCM): CGM was conditioned by exposing it for 48 h to cardiac fibroblast in 10-cm dish to dissolve paracrine factors from cardiac fibroblasts. The conditional medium will be mixed with fresh CGM medium at a 3:1 ratio, sterilized by filtration, and supplemented with additional bFGF at 5 ng/ml.

3 Methods

3.1 Step One: Dissociating and the Primary Tissue Explant

1. Mince mouse heart tissues into small 1×1 mm^3 pieces in a 10-cm dish.
2. Transfer the minced heart tissues to 10 ml enzyme mix in 50-ml centrifuge tube for enzymatic dissociation.
3. Place the tube in the 37 °C shaker water bath and gently shake (80 rpm/min) for 5 min. Aspirate off the supernatants; leave pellets of minced heart tissues. Add 10 ml new enzyme mix, and repeat Subheading 3.1 **steps 2–4** for another two times.
4. Aspirate the supernatants, and resuspend each remaining tissue fragments in 3 ml explant medium and pool the suspensions into 10-cm fibronectin-coated dish at 37 °C and 5 % CO_2.
5. Add 7 ml explant medium 2 days after tissue explanting, change medium every 3 days, and note the date of a layer of fibroblasts covering the culture dish, and note the date of round, phase-bright cells with different sizes migrating from

the adherent explants. These migrated cardiac cells are loosely attached to the fibroblast layer and could be collected periodically by simply washing and centrifuging (*see* **Note 1**).

3.2 Step Two: The Cell Enrichment

1. Collect small, phase-bright cells migrated from heart explants by washing with D-PBS at 2–3 weeks after tissue explanting (*see* **Note 2**).
2. Filter the cell suspension through a 40-μm cell strainer, wash the filter with 10 ml of D-PBS, centrifuge the filtered cells at 300 × *g* for 10 min at RT, and count the cell numbers.
3. Deplete mature hematopoietic cells and their committed precursors from the migrated cardiac cells using Lineage Cell Depletion Kit (mouse).
   (a) Resuspend cell pellet in 40 μL of buffer, add 10 μL of Biotin-Antibody Cocktail, mix well and incubate for 10 min at 4–8 °C, and add 30 μL of buffer to cells.
   (b) Add 20 μL of Anti-Biotin MicroBeads to cells. Mix well and incubate for additional 15 min at 4–8 °C. Wash cells by adding 1 mL of buffer and centrifuge at 300 × *g* for 10 min. Pipette off supernatant completely. Resuspend cells in 500 μL of buffer.
   (c) Magnetic separation with MS Columns, apply cell suspension onto the column, allow the cells to pass through, and collect effluent as fraction with unlabeled cells, representing the enriched lineage negative cell fraction.
4. Purify the Sca-1+ cardiac progenitor cells from lineage negative cells using anti-Sca-1-microbead kit from Miltenyi Biotec.
   (d) Resuspend cell pellet in 90 μL of buffer, add 10 μL of Biotinylated Anti-Sca-1 antibody, mix well, and incubate for 10 min at 4–8 °C. Wash cells by adding 1 mL of buffer. Centrifuge at 300 × *g* for 10 min. Aspirate supernatant completely.
   (e) Resuspend cell pellet in 80 μL of buffer; add 20 μL Anti-Biotin MicroBeads. Mix well and incubate for 10 min at 4–8 °C. Wash cells by adding 1 mL of buffer. Resuspend cells in 500 μL of buffer.
   (f) Apply cell suspension onto MS column, wash three times, and remove column from the separator and place it on a suitable collection tube; pipette 1 ml of CFCM medium onto the column. Immediately flush out fraction with the magnetically labeled cardiac cells by firmly applying the plunger supplied with the column.
5. Seed newly isolated cardiac Sca-1+ cells at 6 well plates precoated with Matrigel using CFCM medium for first three passages (*see* **Note 3** and **4**).

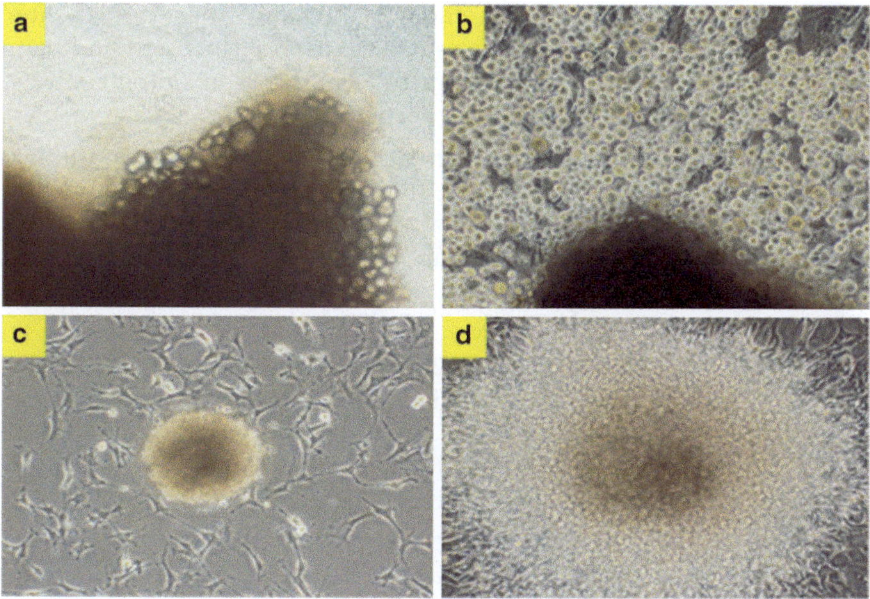

Fig. 1 Isolation, expansion of cardiosphere-derived cells (CDCs). (**a**) Explanted minced heart tissue. (**b**) *Round*, phase-bright cells migrating from the primary culture of mouse ventricular explants, (**c**) cardiosphere formation from purified Sca-1 positive cardiac progenitors in poly-D-lysine-coated dish, (**d**) monolayer expansion of cardiosphere-derived cells in fibronectin-coated dish

6. After cell sorting via MACS, purified Sca-1+ cells were cultured in CFCM (*see* **Note 5**) in poly-D-lysine-coated dishes. Cardiospheres form after 4–7 days on poly-D-lysine-coated dishes (Fig. 1c).
7. Formed cardiospheres can be plated on fibronectin-coated dishes to become a monolayer (cardiosphere-derived cells) (Fig. 1d) for cell transplantation.

4 Notes

1. During **step 1** preparation, a layer of fibroblasts will cover the culture dish at about 7 days, and then the round, phase-bright cells with different size will migrate from the adherent explants.
2. The round, phase-bright cells migrated from cardiac explants are loosely attached to the fibroblast layer and could be collected periodically by simply washing and centrifuging without using trypsin.
3. Cardiac fibroblasts provide a feeder layer for cardiac progenitor cell proliferation and migration from explants. The paracrine factors released from cardiac fibroblasts are important for CPC maintenance and self-renewal. We use CFGM medium which

includes conditioned medium from cardiac fibroblast to support cardiac stem cell maintenance and find that CFCM is sufficient to maintain Sca-1+ cells in a proliferative state without the need for fibroblasts.

4. Extracellular matrix (ECM) is also important for purified CPC maintenance. We found the Matrigel can provide the required ECM for survival and proliferation of purified CPC since it contains laminin, collagen IV, and heparin sulfate proteoglycan.
5. Sca-1+ cells were bright, round without fibroblast contamination. Some of them proliferated and became 2- to 3-cell aggregates in suspension after 3–5 days. These aggregates slowly increased in size and gradually attached to the plate. After 2 weeks in poly-D-lysine-coated dish, the Sca-1+ cells form three-dimensional spheres (Fig. 1c).

Acknowledgement

This work was supported by the American Heart Association Beginning Grant-in-Aid 0765094Y (to Y.T.), NIH grant HL086555 (to Y.T.), and NIH grants HL076684 and HL62984 (to N.L.W.).

References

1. Urbanek K, Torella D, Sheikh F et al (2005) Myocardial regeneration by activation of multipotent cardiac stem cells in ischemic heart failure. Proc Natl Acad Sci USA 102:8692–8697
2. Kajstura J, Gurusamy N, Ogorek B et al (2010) Myocyte turnover in the aging human heart. Circ Res 107:1374–1386
3. Mouquet F, Pfister O, Jain M et al (2005) Restoration of cardiac progenitor cells after myocardial infarction by self-proliferation and selective homing of bone marrow-derived stem cells. Circ Res 97:1090–1092
4. Makkar RR, Smith RR, Cheng K et al (2012) Intracoronary cardiosphere-derived cells for heart regeneration after myocardial infarction (CADUCEUS): a prospective, randomised phase 1 trial. Lancet 379:895–904

Chapter 7

Generation of Human iPSCs from Human Peripheral Blood Mononuclear Cells Using Non-integrative Sendai Virus in Chemically Defined Conditions

Jared M. Churko, Paul W. Burridge, and Joseph C. Wu

Abstract

Human-induced pluripotent stem cells (hiPSCs) have received enormous attention because of their ability to differentiate into multiple cell types that demonstrate the patient's original phenotype. The use of hiPSCs is particularly valuable to the study of cardiac biology, as human cardiomyocytes are difficult to isolate and culture and have a limited proliferative potential. By deriving iPSCs from patients with heart disease and subsequently differentiating these hiPSCs to cardiomyocytes, it is feasible to study cardiac biology in vitro and model cardiac diseases. While there are many different methods for deriving hiPSCs, clinical use of these hiPSCs will require derivation by methods that do not involve modification of the original genome (non-integrative) or incorporate xeno-derived products (such as bovine serum albumin) which may contain xeno-agents. Ideally, this derivation would be carried out under chemically defined conditions to prevent lot-to-lot variability and enhance reproducibility. Additionally, derivation from cell types such as fibroblasts requires extended culture (4–6 weeks), greatly increasing the time required to progress from biopsy to hiPSC. Herein, we outline a method of culturing peripheral blood mononuclear cells (PBMCs) and reprogramming PBMCs into hiPSCs using a non-integrative Sendai virus.

Key words hiPSC, Cardiac disease modeling, Sendai virus, Cardiomyocytes, Blood reprogramming

1 Introduction

Pluripotent stem cells have the ability to differentiate into many different cellular lineages. The use of pluripotent stem cells is particularly important in regenerative medicine because these cells can be induced to differentiate into most cell types and can further be used to repair damaged tissue. While there are ethical concerns regarding the use of human embryonic stem cells (hESCs) [1], human-induced pluripotent stem cells (hiPSCs) can be created from differentiated adult and mature cell types. Initially, mouse iPSCs were created by exogenously expressing only four genes *POU5F1* (*OCT4*), *SOX2*, *KLF4*, and *MYC* (*c-MYC*) in mouse embryonic fibroblasts (MEF) [2]. Since this discovery, hiPSCs have been successfully derived by

Race L. Kao (ed.), *Cellular Cardiomyoplasty: Methods and Protocols*, Methods in Molecular Biology, vol. 1036, DOI 10.1007/978-1-62703-511-8_7, © Springer Science+Business Media New York 2013

expressing these four genes, and other similar combinations, in human adult fibroblasts [3, 4], keratinocytes [5, 6], blood [7, 8], adipose stromal cells [9], and multiple other cell types.

For hiPSCs to be efficiently created, reprogramming factors must be expressed in the proper stoichiometry [10]. In addition, for clinical use of hiPSCs, any exogenous genes should not be carried over and expressed within the hiPSCs after creation. Viral delivery of *OCT4*, *SOX2*, *KLF4*, and *MYC* reprogramming factors is commonly used to create hiPSCs. Lentiviral and retroviral methods of delivery require integration of exogenous genes within the host genome and subsequent epigenetic downregulation of expression; however, leaky expression of *OCT4*, *SOX2*, *KLF4*, and *MYC* can be found in hiPSCs even after prolonged culture [11]. Therefore, it is important to deliver *OCT4*, *SOX2*, *KLF4*, and *MYC* by a non-integrating method such as episomal plasmid [12], minicircle plasmid [13], mRNA [14], miRNA [15], or more recently Sendai virus [16]. It will also be important to develop chemically defined culture conditions because they are more cost-effective and elimination of xeno-proteins can prevent activation of the host immune response [17].

Acquiring patient cells may be difficult because some patients are reluctant to donate biological material, such as punch biopsies. It is therefore imperative to derive strategies to create hiPSCs by noninvasive procedures. A mildly, noninvasive procedure is drawing blood from a patient. hiPSCs can be created by isolating the nucleated cells contained in blood (peripheral blood mononuclear cells (PBMCs)) and expressing *OCT4*, *SOX2*, KLF4, and *MYC* into these cells.

In the following text, we have outlined a method of isolating PBMCs from patient blood by Percoll centrifugation and described the culture conditions necessary for PBMC expansion and survival. In addition, we have provided a protocol for reprogramming PBMCs into hiPSCs using non-integrative Sendai virus expressing the reprogramming factors *OCT4*, *SOX2*, *KLF4*, and *MYC*. Cardiomyocytes derived in this manner will be a valuable resource in studying various cardiac diseases and conditions.

2 Materials

2.1 Media

1. *Blood media* [7] [modified to be xeno-free]: *1:1* IMDM with glutamine/F12, 5 mg/mL Human serum albumin, 1× lipid concentrate, 10 μg/mL insulin, 100 μg/mL transferrin, 14 ng/mL sodium selenite, 64 μg/mL L-ascorbic acid 2-phosphate, 450 μM 1-thioglycerol, 50 ng/mL SCF, 10 ng/mL IL3, 2 U/mL EPO, 40 ng/mL IGF1, 1 μM dexamethasone.
2. *iPSC Media*: Essential 8 (combine supplement with base media) and Essential 6 supplemented with 100 ng/mL FGF2 (combine supplement with base media).

2.2 Reagents

1. Matrigel—Growth factor reduced, hESC-qualified.
2. DMEM/F12.
3. TrypLE Express, store at RT, there is no need to warm to 37 °C before use.
4. Y27632 (ROCK inhibitor): 10 mM stocks in Ultrapure water, store at −20 °C.
5. Ultrapure water.
6. Sodium butyrate (NaB).
7. Ficoll-Paque PLUS at room temperature (GE Healthcare).
8. PBS.
9. EDTA.
10. Patient blood: At least 10 mL in EDTA preservatives (lavender tubes).
11. CytoTune®-iPS Sendai Reprogramming Kit (Life Technologies).

2.3 Equipment

1. 6-well cell culture plates (surface area = 9.8 cm^2) coated with 2 mL Matrigel.
2. 12-well cell culture plates (surface area = 3.8 cm^2) coated with 1 mL Matrigel.
3. 10 cm tissue culture plates (surface area = 58.95 cm^2) coated with 12 mL Matrigel.
4. 15 and 50 mL polypropylene conical tubes.
5. 2 mL plastic aspiration pipettes.
6. 5, 10, 25, and 50 mL plastic pipettes.
7. 250 and 500 mL PES media filters.
8. Countess Cell Counter, slides, and trypan blue.
9. Tissue culture incubator capable of 37 °C, 5 % CO_2, and 85 % relative humidity (such as New Brunswick Galaxy 170R).
10. Dual gas tissue culture incubator capable of 37 °C, 5 % CO_2, 5 % O_2, and 85 % relative humidity with split inner door.
11. Centrifuge.
12. Inverted tissue culture microscope (such as Nikon Ti) with heated stage.

3 Methods

3.1 PBMC Isolation from Blood by Percoll Separation

1. Prepare the blood media by combining each component and filter sterilize.
2. Prepare a PBS buffer mix solution containing phosphate-buffered saline (PBS), pH 7.2, and 2 mM EDTA. Filter sterilize and keep buffer cold (2–8 °C).

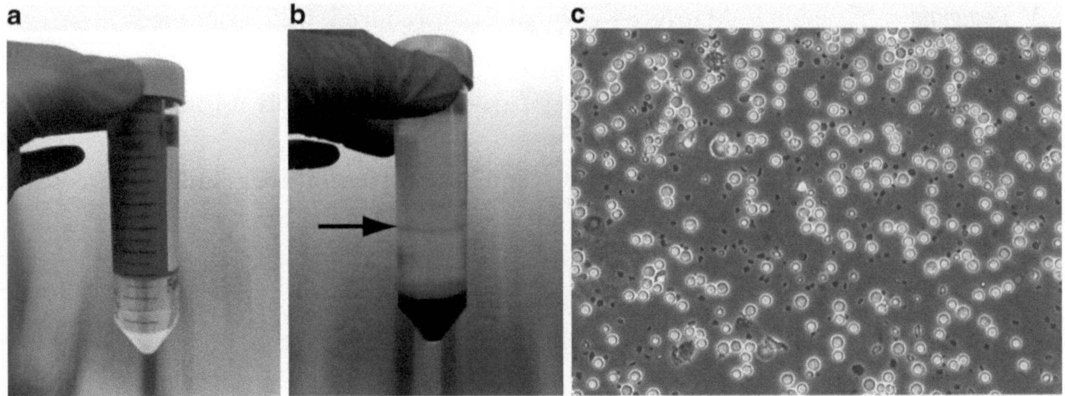

Fig. 1 Purification of PBMCs. (**a**) Slowly layer 35 mL of blood onto 15 mL of Percoll. (**b**) After centrifugation, remove the thin layer of PBMCs (*arrow* denotes layer of PBMCs). (**c**) After multiple rounds of washing, PMBCs will appear as rounded spheres in suspension

3. Dilute blood cells in 2–4× the volume of buffer (the more dilute the blood sample, the better the purity of the mononuclear cells).
4. Carefully layer 35 mL of diluted cell suspension over 15 mL of Ficoll-Paque 15 mL ($\rho = 1.077$ g/mL at room temperature) in a 50 mL conical tube (*see* **Note 1**) (Fig. 1a).
5. Centrifuge at 400 × *g* for 30–40 min at 20 °C in a swinging-bucket rotor *without* brake.
6. Aspirate the upper layer leaving the mononuclear cell layer (lymphocytes, monocytes, and thrombocytes) (Fig. 1b) undisturbed at the interphase.
7. Carefully transfer the mononuclear cell layer to a new 50 mL conical tube.
8. Fill the conical tube with PBS buffer, mix, and centrifuge at 300 × *g* for 10 min at 20 °C. Carefully remove the supernatant completely to remove the Percoll.
9. Resuspend PBMC in 50 mL of PBS buffer mix and centrifuge at 300 × *g* for 10 min at 20 °C (*see* **Note 2**).
10. Aspirate PBS buffer mix and resuspend PBMC in blood medium to two to three million cells per mL.
11. Plate out PBMC in a standard TC-coated 24-well plate; change media by removal, centrifugation, and resuspension every 2–3 days (*see* **Note 3**) for 6–8 days (Fig. 1c).

3.2 Infect PBMCs with Sendai Virus Reprogramming Factors

1. Prepare Sendai virus cocktail: 10 μL each of *OCT4*, *SOX2*, *KLF4*, and *MYC* as per the manufacturer's instructions. Keep on ice.
2. Plate 1×10^5—5×10^5 PBMCs into 200 μL of blood media in a 24-well plate.

3. Add combined Sendai virus reprogramming cocktail (40 μL) to PBMCs.
4. The following day, remove the virus by centrifugation (300 × *g* for 6 min). Note: Some PBMCs may be left behind so additional washes of the well may be required. Resuspend the PBMCs into 500 μL of blood media and add to 1 well of a 12-well plate.
5. Allow PBMCs to grow for 3 days in suspension in the blood media + 0.5 mM NaB.

3.3 Prepare Matrigel Plates

1. Thaw stock bottle of Matrigel at 4 °C overnight.
2. Add one 300 μL of Matrigel to 50 mL of cold DMEM/F12 media. Add 2 mL to each well of a 6-well plate.
3. Place the 6-well plates in the incubator and allow the Matrigel to set overnight (*see* **Note 4**).

3.4 PBMC Reprogramming

1. Three days after Sendai virus infection, remove the blood media by centrifugation and resuspend the cells in 2 mL of E7 media + 0.5 mM NaB.
2. Add the PBMCs to one well of a 6-well plate coated with Matrigel.
3. Monitor the cells over the next 3 days. Suspended cells should settle and adhere to the bottom of the Matrigel-coated wells (Fig. 2a). Once cells have become adherent, aspirate Essential 6+FGF2 media and feed cells daily with 2 mL of Essential 6+FGF2.
4. Continue to monitor the cells for proliferation and morphology change.
5. At day 15 after Sendai virus infection, replace Essential 6+FGF2 media with Essential 8 media.
6. Colonies will appear around day 20 (Fig. 2b) and should be picked (using a stem cell knife or p20 pipette tip) onto 1 well of a fresh Matrigel-coated 6-well plate into Essential 8 + 10 μM Y27632 (*see* **Note 5**) [passage 1 (=p1)]. Total protocol time from isolating PBMCs to hiPSC colonies being picked should be approximately one month (Fig. 3).

3.5 Colony Purification and Expansion

1. After 7–10 days, colonies will have grown out and become dense. Cut up colonies into 10–20 pieces with a p10 pipette tip and transfer using a p200 pipette into 1 well of a Matrigel-coated 6-well plate into Essential 8 + 10 μM Y27632 (=p2) (*see* **Note 6**).
2. After 7–10 days, colonies will have grown out and become dense; add 1 mL TrypLE and passage into 1 well of a Matrigel-coated 6-well plate into Essential 8 + 10 μM Y27632 (=p3).

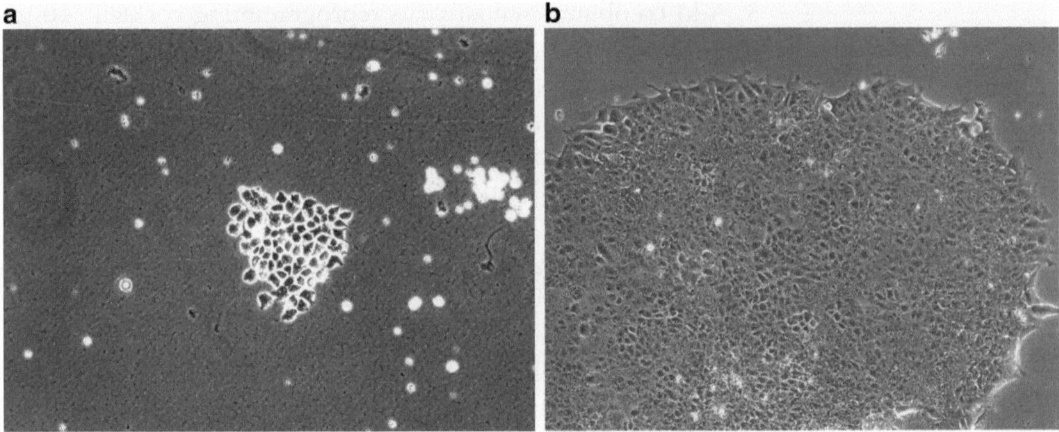

Fig. 2 Reprogramming of PBMCs. (**a**) After Sendai virus infection, PMBCs will be adherent to Matrigel-coated plates. (**b**) Twenty days after Sendai virus infection, hiPSC colonies can be seen

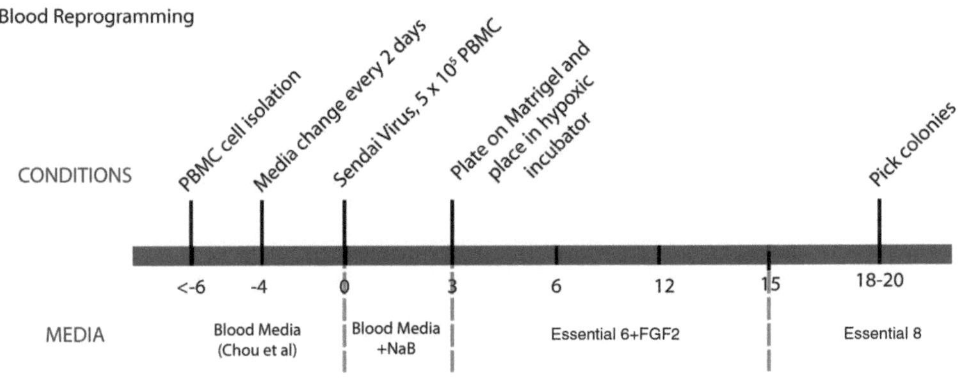

Fig. 3 Timeline of blood reprogramming. The timeline outlines cell culture conditions and media requirements for the different stages of reprogramming PBMCs to hiPSC

3. After 4–5 days, colonies will have grown out and become dense; add 1 mL TrypLE and passage into 3 wells of a Matrigel-coated 6-well plate into Essential 8 + 10 μM Y27632 (=p4).
4. Freeze down 5 vials from the 3 wells and continue to grow at a 1:6 split ratio, freezing vials every 5–10 passages.
5. Grow cells to at least passage 20 for efficient differentiation.

4 Notes

1. This step is critical to get a clear distinct band of mononuclear cells. Place the pipet-aid on gravity setting to slowly pour the blood onto the Ficoll layer.

2. Additional washes may be performed to lower platelet levels.
3. In the first 24 h of plating, some cells will adhere to the bottom of the well. However, after 3 days, refresh the media and replate at a high density (one to two million cells/mL of media); proliferation difference should become obvious at 6 to 9 days after Sendai virus infection.
4. Matrigel-coated plates are essential for the adherence and reprogramming stage. Keep everything cold. After the diluted Matrigel is added to each plate, these plates can also be wrapped in parafilm and stored at 4 °C for 1 week.
5. Manually cutting and picking the optimal size of colony will help in the expansion of the next passage. Picked colonies that are too large will stick down easier but will differentiate earlier. Picked colonies that are too small however may not survive.
6. Early colonies may need to be manually picked a few times to prevent the passage of unwanted differentiated cell types.

Acknowledgement

This work was supported by NIH R01 HL113006, NIH U01 HL099776, CIRM TR3-05556, CIRM DR2-05394 (to JCW) and AHA Postdoctoral Fellowship Grant (PWB).

References

1. Lebacqz K (2012) Stumbling on status: abortion, stem cells, and faulty reasoning. Theor Med Bioeth 33(1):75–82
2. Takahashi K, Yamanaka S (2006) Induction of pluripotent stem cells from mouse embryonic and adult fibroblast cultures by defined factors. Cell 126(4):663–676
3. Itzhaki I, Maizels L, Huber I et al (2011) Modelling the long QT syndrome with induced pluripotent stem cells. Nature 471(7337):225–229
4. Lai WH, Ho JC, Lee YK et al (2010) ROCK inhibition facilitates the generation of human-induced pluripotent stem cells in a defined, feeder-, and serum-free system. Cell Reprogram 12(6):641–653
5. Itoh M, Kiuru M, Cairo MS, Christiano AM (2011) Generation of keratinocytes from normal and recessive dystrophic epidermolysis bullosa-induced pluripotent stem cells. Proc Natl Acad Sci USA 108(21):8797–8802
6. Raya A, Rodriguez-Piza I, Navarro S et al (2010) A protocol describing the genetic correction of somatic human cells and subsequent generation of iPS cells. Nat Protoc 5(4):647–660
7. Chou BK, Mali P, Huang X et al (2011) Efficient human iPS cell derivation by a non-integrating plasmid from blood cells with unique epigenetic and gene expression signatures. Cell Res 21(3):518–529
8. Burridge PW, Thompson S, Millrod MA et al (2011) A universal system for highly efficient cardiac differentiation of human induced pluripotent stem cells that eliminates interline variability. PLoS One 6(4):e18293
9. Sun N, Panetta NJ, Gupta DM et al (2009) Feeder-free derivation of induced pluripotent stem cells from adult human adipose stem cells. Proc Natl Acad Sci USA 106(37): 15720–15725
10. Tiemann U, Sgodda M, Warlich E et al (2011) Optimal reprogramming factor stoichiometry increases colony numbers and affects molecular characteristics of murine induced pluripotent stem cells. Cytometry A 79(6):426–435
11. Hanley J, Rastegarlari G, Nathwani AC (2010) An introduction to induced pluripotent stem cells. Br J Haematol 151(1):16–24
12. Chen G, Gulbranson DR, Hou Z et al (2011) Chemically defined conditions for human

iPSC derivation and culture. Nat Methods 8(5):424–429

13. Jia F, Wilson KD, Sun N et al (2010) A nonviral minicircle vector for deriving human iPS cells. Nat Methods 7(3):197–199
14. Warren L, Manos PD, Ahfeldt T et al (2010) Highly efficient reprogramming to pluripotency and directed differentiation of human cells with synthetic modified mRNA. Cell Stem Cell 7(5):618–630
15. Anokye-Danso F, Trivedi CM, Juhr D, Gupta M, Cui Z, Tian Y, Zhang Y, Yang W, Gruber PJ, Epstein JA, Morrisey EE (2011) Highly efficient miRNA-mediated reprogramming of mouse and human somatic cells to pluripotency. Cell Stem Cell 8(4): 376–388
16. Fusaki N, Ban H, Nishiyama A, Saeki K, Hasegawa M (2009) Efficient induction of transgene-free human pluripotent stem cells using a vector based on Sendai virus, an RNA virus that does not integrate into the host genome. Proc Jpn Acad Ser B Phys Biol Sci 85(8):348–362
17. Martin MJ, Muotri A, Gage F, Varki A (2005) Human embryonic stem cells express an immunogenic nonhuman sialic acid. Nat Med 11(2):228–232

Chapter 8

Identification of Stem Cells After Transplantation

Yingjie Wang, Lan Zhang, Yaohua Pan, Lijuan Chen, Neal Weintraub, and Yaoliang Tang

Abstract

The ability to identify the donor stem cells following transplantation into injured hearts is critical. This is particularly important in evaluating stem cell survival and lineage differentiation into mature cardiovascular cells. Several approaches have been employed for tracking the donor stem cells, including fluorescent dyes and fluorescent protein gene transfer. Here, we will induce a protocol using lentivirus-mediated green fluorescent protein (GFP) to monitor the fate of donor stem cells following transplantation.

Key words Green fluorescent protein (GFP), Lentivirus, Stem cells, Myocardial infarction (MI)

1 Introduction

Ischemic heart disease is the leading cause of morbidity and mortality in the western world. Endogenous cardiac stem cells are rapidly exhausted after myocardial ischemia [1]; therefore, transplantation with ex vivo expansion stem cells may replenish the pool of stem cells in injured heart and lead to heart regeneration. Identifying the engrafted cells will help us to compare the efficacy of different source of cells and identify the relative mechanisms for heart repair. A number of approaches have been employed to tracking the engrafted stem cells in vivo, for example, (1) fluorescent dye labeling, like PKH26 [2] and DAPI [3]—the limitation of dye labeling is that the observed signal may not come from donor cells but from host cells which have acquired free dye released from dead donor cells; in addition, this approach is transient and suffered from signal dilution—and (2) reporter gene transfer, like GFP [4], *beta-galactosidase* (β-gal) [5, 6], and luciferase [7]. Lentiviral vector can infect divided and nondivided cells [8]; it allows monitoring of the fate of donor cells for long term since the reporter genes can be integrated into chromosome [9, 10]. Stem cells from genetically modified animals, for example, GFP mice, provide an alternative strategy to identify donor cells following cell

Race L. Kao (ed.), *Cellular Cardiomyoplasty: Methods and Protocols*, Methods in Molecular Biology, vol. 1036,
DOI 10.1007/978-1-62703-511-8_8, © Springer Science+Business Media New York 2013

transplantation. In this chapter, we will introduce a detailed protocol to use lentiviral GFP vector to label donor stem cells and identify engrafted cells in ischemic myocardium.

2 Materials

2.1 Plasmids for Lentivirus Packaging

1. pRRLSIN.cPPT.PGK-GFP.WPRE.
2. psPAX2.
3. pMD2.G.
4. 293FT cells.
5. FuGENE® HD Transfection Reagent.
6. 0.45 μm syringe filter.
7. Ultracentrifuge and rotor.
8. Ultra-Clear ultracentrifuge tubes.
9. OPTI-MEM® Reduced Serum Medium.
10. Dulbecco's Modified Eagle Medium (DMEM).
11. Fetal bovine serum (FBS).
12. Hexadimethrine bromide (polybrene).
13. Prepare a 1 mg/mL solution of polybrene in 0.9 % NaCl, and then filter-sterilize through 0.2 μm filter. Stock solution stored at 4 °C.
14. Small animal ventilator.
15. Accutase cell detachment solution.
16. Abbocath-T I.V. 18 G catheter.
17. BD 3/10 ml SafetyGlide Insulin Syringe with 31G needle.
18. 12. Vectashield Hardset mounting medium with DAPI vector.
19. Leica TCS confocal microscope.

3 Methods

3.1 Lentiviral-GFP-Vector Packaging (See Note 1)

Viral vectors encoding GFP were produced by transfection of 293FT cells with the lentiviral backbone plasmid (pRRLSIN.cPPT.PGK-GFP.WPRE plasmid), an envelope plasmid (pMD2.G), and a packaging plasmid (psPAX2).

This protocol is for transfection in a 15-cm dish.

Day 1: Plate 1.2×10^7 293 FT cells in 20 mL of media in a 10-cm tissue culture dish. Incubate cells at 37 °C, 5 % CO_2 overnight.

Day 2:

1. In tube 1, create a mix of plasmids.

   6.3 μg pRRLSIN.cPPT.PGK-GFP plasmid.

   4.7 μg psPAX2 packaging plasmid.

   1.6 μg pMD2.G envelope plasmid to 125 μl OPTI-MEM.

2. In tube 2, create a master mix of FuGENE® HD transfection reagent in OPTI-MEM. Mix 38 μL FuGENE HD + 462 μL OPTI-MEM for each 15 dish transfection (*see* **Note 2**).
3. Pipette 500 μL of FuGENE HD master mix to tube 1. Mix by gently flicking the tube. Incubate for 30 min at room temperature.
4. Gently add DNA:FuGENE® mix dropwise to 293FT. Swirl to disperse mixture evenly (*see* **Note 3**).
5. Incubate cells at 37 °C, 5 % CO_2 overnight.

Day 3: In the morning, change the media (*see* **Note 4**). Incubate cells at 37 °C, 5 % CO_2 for 24 h.

Day 4 and Day 5: Harvest supernatant containing lentiviral vector and transfer to 50 ml polypropylene storage tube. Filter the media through a 0.45-μm filter to remove 293FT cells (*see* **Note 5**). Add ~37 ml of viral supernatant to each ultracentrifuge tube and balance, and then spin at ~82,000 × g for 90 min at 4 °C in SW28 rotor; resuspend viral pellet in 400 μl of PBS. Virus should be frozen at −80 °C for long-term storage (*see* **Note 6**).

3.2 Stem Cell GFP Labeling

Lentivirus can efficiently transduct a broad range of cell types, including both dividing and nondividing cells.

Day 1: Plate 0.3×10^6 stem cells to 6-well plate and incubate at 37 °C, 5 % CO_2 overnight.

Day 2: Stem cells should be approximately 70 % confluent before infection. Change to fresh culture media containing 8 μg/mL polybrene. Add 100 μl lentiviral solution (*see* **Note 7**). Incubate cells at 37 °C, 5 % CO_2 for 3 days.

Day 5: Change to fresh media, and determine the transduction efficacy using florescent microscopy (Fig. 1).

3.3 Myocardial Infarction Model and Cell Transplantation

1. Remove hair from chest region using hair clippers. After anesthesia, surgical preparation, and preemptive analgesics, mice will be intubated with an 18-gauge catheter and mechanically ventilated at 120 breaths per minute with a stroke volume of 150 μl on a positive pressure ventilator with room air. Body temperature will be maintained with a heated water blanket.
2. Make lateral incision to open the chest under the dissecting microscope; cut the intercostals muscle between left 3rd and

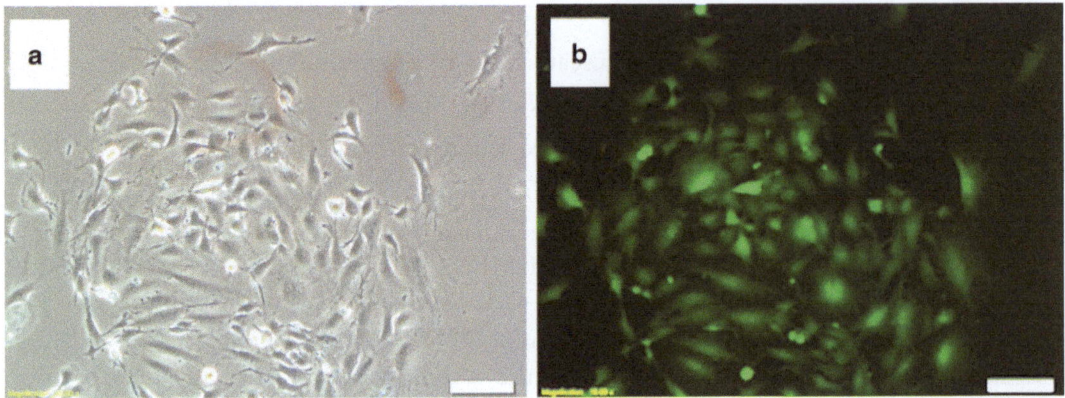

Fig. 1 Transduced cardiac stem cells with GFP lentivirus. (**a**) Phase contrast picture of stem cell clone; (**b**) GFP expression in transuded stem cells

4th ribs with a cautery pen. Tear the pericardium to make a small opening, identify the left anterior descending coronary artery (LAD), and pass 8-0 suture under 2–3 mm from the tip of the left auricle. Permanently occlude the LAD by ligation (*see* **Note 8**).

3. Harvest the GFP-labeled stem cells using Accutase; inactivate Accutase with MEM complete medium. Count cells using a hemacytometer; centrifuge at 300 × g for 5 min. Carefully aspirate supernatant and resuspend pellet at a concentration of 5×10^5 cells/30 μl of PBS for cell transplantation; keep cells in ice prior to injection.
4. Intramyocardial injection: identify the border zone of the heart; make two 15 μL injections of GFP cell suspension using a 31-gauge needle (*see* **Note 9**).
5. Following injection, use 6-0 absorbable sutures to close the ribs and muscle layers. Suture skin closed using 6-0 nylon suture also. Allow mouse to recover from anesthesia and extubate.

3.4 Identify Donor Stem Cells in Infarct Heart

1. Five days after surgically induced MI and intramyocardial injection of GFP stem cells, harvest mouse hearts, embed it in OCT compound, snap frozen, and cut into 5-μm sections.
2. Identify the donor cells, and analyze stem cell differentiation by immunostaining:
   (a) Fix with 4 % formaldehyde for 10 min at room temperature.
   (b) Wash slides twice in PBS for 5 min ×2.
   (c) Mount slides in DAPI mounting medium.
   (d) Examine the sections under confocal microscope; identify the GFP-positive cells (Fig. 2).

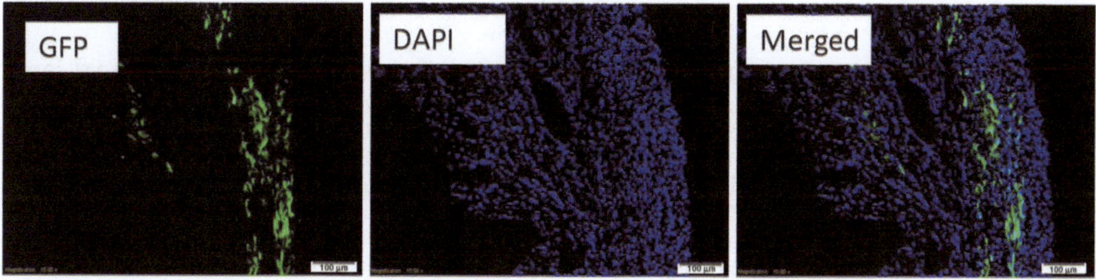

Fig. 2 Confocal imaging of donor cells in infarcted mouse heart 5 days after surgical MI and cell injection

4 Notes

1. Before this step, you must contact your institution's biosafety office to receive permission and institution-specific instructions. You must follow safety procedures and work in a BL2+ environment suitable for handling HIV-derivative viruses.
2. Directly add FuGENE HD into the OPTI-MEM; avoid FuGENE HD in contact with the walls of the polypropylene tube before it has been diluted.
3. 293FT cells should be 70 % confluent and in DMEM in 10 % FBS without antibiotics.
4. Be cautious not to disturb the transfected cells when pipetting the medium.
5. Do not use a 0.2-µm filter since it may shear the envelope of lentiviral particles.
6. Avoid repeated freeze/thaw cycles since they will decrease the efficiency of the virus.
7. Polybrene can significantly increase the efficiency of viral infection; however, it is toxic to cell. To sensitive stem cells, substitute protamine sulfate for polybrene. It is recommended using high MOI (multiplicity of infection) for stem cell infection to reach high transduction efficiency and bright GFP signal.
8. Successful coronary occlusion will be verified by the development of a pale color in the distal myocardium after ligation.
9. Bending the needle head ~45° can avoid the injection of cells into left ventricular chamber.

Acknowledgement

This work was supported by the American Heart Association Beginning Grant-in-Aid 0765094Y (to Y.T.), NIH grant HL086555 (to Y.T.), and NIH grants HL076684 and HL62984 (to N.L.W.).

References

1. Mouquet F, Pfister O, Jain M et al (2005) Restoration of cardiac progenitor cells after myocardial infarction by self-proliferation and selective homing of bone marrow-derived stem cells. Circ Res 97:1090–1092
2. Shao-Fang Z, Hong-Tian Z, Zhi-Nian Z, Yuan-Li H (2011) PKH26 as a fluorescent label for live human umbilical mesenchymal stem cells. In Vitro Cell Dev Biol Anim 47:516–520
3. Tang YL, Zhao Q, Zhang YC et al (2004) Autologous mesenchymal stem cell transplantation induce VEGF and neovascularization in ischemic myocardium. Regul Pept 117:3–10
4. Chen L, Ashraf M, Wang Y et al (2012) The role of notch 1 activation in cardiosphere derived cell differentiation. Stem Cells Dev 21:2122–2129
5. Tang YL, Zhu W, Cheng M et al (2009) Hypoxic preconditioning enhances the benefit of cardiac progenitor cell therapy for treatment of myocardial infarction by inducing CXCR4 expression. Circ Res 104:1209–1216
6. Tang YL, Shen L, Qian K, Phillips MI (2007) A novel two-step procedure to expand cardiac Sca-1+ cells clonally. Biochem Biophys Res Commun 359:877–883
7. Hu S, Huang M, Nguyen PK et al (2011) Novel microRNA prosurvival cocktail for improving engraftment and function of cardiac progenitor cell transplantation. Circulation 124:S27–S34
8. Lewis P, Hensel M, Emerman M (1992) Human immunodeficiency virus infection of cells arrested in the cell cycle. EMBO J 11:3053–3058
9. Naldini L, Blomer U, Gage FH, Trono D, Verma IM (1996) Efficient transfer, integration, and sustained long-term expression of the transgene in adult rat brains injected with a lentiviral vector. Proc Natl Acad Sci USA 93:11382–11388
10. Naldini L, Blomer U, Gallay P et al (1996) In vivo gene delivery and stable transduction of nondividing cells by a lentiviral vector. Science 272:263–267

Chapter 9

Methods to Study the Proliferation and Differentiation of Cardiac Side Population (CSP) Cells

Konstantina-Ioanna Sereti, Angelos Oikonomopoulos, Kazumasa Unno, and Ronglih Liao

Abstract

Investigation of cardiac progenitor cell proliferation and differentiation is essential for both the basic understanding of progenitor cell biology as well as the development of cellular therapeutics for tissue regeneration. Herein, we describe techniques used for the analysis of CSP cell proliferation, cell cycle status, and cardiomyogenic differentiation.

Key words Stem/progenitor cells, Cell cycle, Proliferation, Ki67, Phospho-histone H3, BrdU, FUCCI, Cardiomyogenic differentiation

1 Introduction

Recent work has identified populations of progenitor cells, resident in terminally differentiated tissues, including the heart, that maintain regenerative potential [1–4]. This endogenous repair mechanism, however, is limited and is unable to regenerate cells lost following cardiac injury, such as myocardial infarction. While resident adult cardiac stem cells hold great potential for the development of cell-based therapies for cardiovascular disease, their utilization is limited by the small cell numbers obtained from single-patient biopsies [5]. Thorough investigation of the mechanisms regulating cardiac progenitor cell proliferation and differentiation may allow progenitor cell populations stimulation to enhance endogenous regeneration mechanisms and provide strategies for therapeutic regeneration.

In this chapter, we present detailed experimental techniques used for the analysis of cardiac side population (CSP) progenitor cell proliferation and cell cycle kinetics as well as methods to evaluate cardiomyogenic differentiation [6]. While the effects of a given intervention or condition on total CSP cell number can be

Race L. Kao (ed.), *Cellular Cardiomyoplasty: Methods and Protocols*, Methods in Molecular Biology, vol. 1036,
DOI 10.1007/978-1-62703-511-8_9,

determined by proliferation assays, changes in total cell number may result from altered cellular survival and/or altered cellular division. Therefore, proliferation assays should be accompanied by additional methods examining proliferation markers such as Ki67 [7, 8] or cell cycle status. Propidium iodide (PI) is the most commonly used DNA dye for cell cycle analysis and is often combined with staining for the phosphorylated form of histone-H3 (pH3) as well as BrdU incorporation as G2/M and S cell cycle phase markers, respectively [9]. More detailed monitoring of cell cycle kinetics can be obtained through the use of cell cycle reporter systems, including the FUCCI (Fluorescence Ubiquitination Cell Cycle Indicator) system developed by Sakaue-Sawano et al. [10], that allows for live monitoring of cellular division. These probes contain Cdt1-Kusabira-Orange or Geminin-Azami-Green fusion proteins that are temporally regulated by the ubiquitin E3 ligases APC^{Cdh1} and SCF^{Skp2}. Cdt1 expression peaks in G1 phase and is sustained through G1-S transition, while Geminin expression is activated during G1-S transition and remains elevated during S, G2, and M phases [10]. Several methods have been used to assess the cardiomyogenic differentiation of cardiac progenitor cells [11–14]. In CSP cells we have established a coculture system with neonatal rat ventricular cardiomyocytes that allows for monitoring of CSP differentiation into functionally mature cardiomyocytes [6].

2 Materials

2.1 Culture Media

All media must be stored at 4 °C and aliquots of media should be warmed to 37 °C, 15 min prior to use.

1. CSP expansion medium: α-MEM, 20 % heat-inactivated (HI) FBS, 2 mM L-glutamine, 1 % penicillin/streptomycin.
2. HEK-medium: DMEM, 10 % HI FBS, 1 % penicillin/streptomycin.
3. Synchronization medium: α-MEM, 0.1 % HI FBS, 2 mM L-GLUTAMINE, and 1 % penicillin/streptomycin.
4. Pre-culture medium: low glucose DMEM, 7 % HI FBS, 1 % penicillin/streptomycin, 100 μM BrdU, 1.5 mM vitamin B12.
5. Coculture medium: DMEM, 5 % HI FBS, 1 % penicillin/streptomycin, 10 μg/ml insulin, 10 μg/ml transferrin, 1.5 mM vitamin B12.

2.2 Kits

1. Cytofix/Cytoperm kit (BD Biosciences).
2. 5-Bromo-2′-deoxyuridine Labeling and Detection Kit I (Roche).

2.3 Staining Solutions

1. Paraformaldehyde solution: 4 % paraformaldehyde diluted in 1× PBS.
2. Blocking solution: 1 % BSA in 1× PBS.
3. Ethanol fixative: 30 ml glycine (50 mM), 70 ml 100 % ethanol.
4. Anti-BrdU working solution: anti-BrdU stock solution (provided) diluted 1:10 in incubation buffer (provided).
5. PI staining solution: 0.1 % Triton X-100, 2 μg/ml PI, 400 ng/ml RNase A in 1× PBS.

2.4 Solutions for Neonatal Rat Ventricular Myocyte (NRVM) Isolation

1. Trypsin solution: 15 mg of trypsin in 25 ml HBSS.
2. Collagenase B solution: 1 mg/ml collagenase B in HBSS.
3. Laminin solution: 0.0112 mg/ml laminin in 10 ml cold medium (DMEM, 1 % penicillin/streptomycin).

2.5 FUCCI Reporter System

FUCCI plasmids may be purchased from RIKEN BRC DNA Bank, Invitrogen, Clontech.

1. SIN plasmids: mKO2-hCdtl (30/120, Kusabira-Orange), mAG-hGeminin (1/110, Azami-Green).
2. Packaging plasmids: pCAG-HIVgp, pCMV-VSV-G-RSV-Rev.
3. 2× BBS solution: 50 mM BES, 280 mM NaCl, 1.5 mM Na_2HPO_4.
4. Transfection mix: 17 μg of each SIN plasmid, 10 μg of each packaging plasmid, 50 μl 2.5 M $CaCl_2$, 500 μl 2× BBS solution, low glucose DMEM to reach a total volume of 1 ml.

3 Methods

All experiments should be performed with CSP cells at passage 4–6 and incubated in 5 % CO_2 unless otherwise specified.

3.1 Proliferation Assay

1. Plate CSP cells in 60 mm dishes at a density of 4.76 cells/mm^2 and culture in expansion medium for 6 days (*see* **Note 1**). Change medium every 3 days.
2. At day 6, lift cells by trypsinization: rinse cells with serum free medium or sterile PBS, add trypsin (2 ml for a 6 mm dish) and incubate at 37 °C for 5 min. Inactivate the enzyme by the addition of 2 ml expansion medium and centrifuge at 530 g for 5 min at 4 °C (*see* **Note 2**).
3. Resuspend pellets in 1 ml expansion medium and isolate 10 μl of resuspended cells for cell counting with a hemocytometer (*see* **Note 3**).

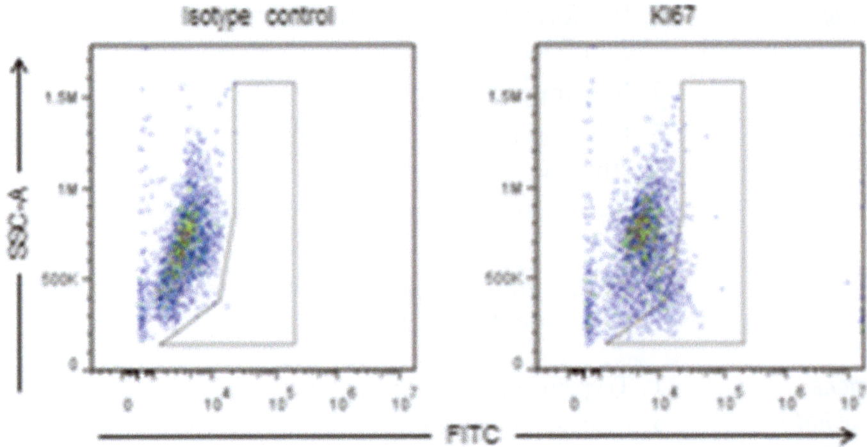

Fig. 1 Flow cytometric analysis of Ki67 staining. Isotype control is used for proper gating. Ki67$^+$ cells appear in the boxed area

3.2 Immunostaining for Proliferation Markers

3.2.1 Ki67 Staining for Flow Cytometric Analysis

1. Pellet cells from a proliferation assay by centrifugation (530 g, 5 min, 4 °C).
2. Thoroughly resuspend in 1 ml of 4 % paraformaldehyde solution. Incubate at 4 °C for 20–30 min and wash twice with 1× PBS (*see* **Notes 4** and **5**).
3. Permeabilize cells using the BD Cytofix/Cytoperm fixation/permeabilization solution kit.
4. Resuspend pellets in 1 ml 1× BD Perm/Wash buffer and incubate at 4 °C for 15 min.
5. Pellet cells by centrifugation (530 g, 5 min, 4 °C) and proceed to Ki67 staining.
6. Resuspend cells in 100 μl 1× BD Perm/Wash buffer containing a FITC-conjugated anti-Ki67 antibody (Santa Cruz) at a concentration of 4 ng/μl (1/50) and incubate at 4 °C for 30 min in the dark (*see* **Note 6**).
7. Wash cells twice with 1× PBS, resuspend in 100–200 μl of 1× PBS, and analyze by flow cytometry (Fig. 1).

3.2.2 Immunocytochemical Staining for Phospho-histone-H3 (pH3)

1. Resuspend CSP cells in expansion medium at a concentration of ~5,000 cells/ml.
2. Place a glass coverslip (20×40 mm) in a 60 mm dish and cover it with 1 ml of cell suspension (*see* **Note 7**).
3. Following 1 h incubation at 37 °C, add 2 ml of expansion medium in all dishes and culture for 5 days.
4. Aspirate medium, rinse cells with 3 ml 1× PBS, and cover cell layer with 3 ml of 4 % paraformaldehyde solution. Incubate for 20–30 min at room temperature (RT). Wash cells three times with 1× PBS.

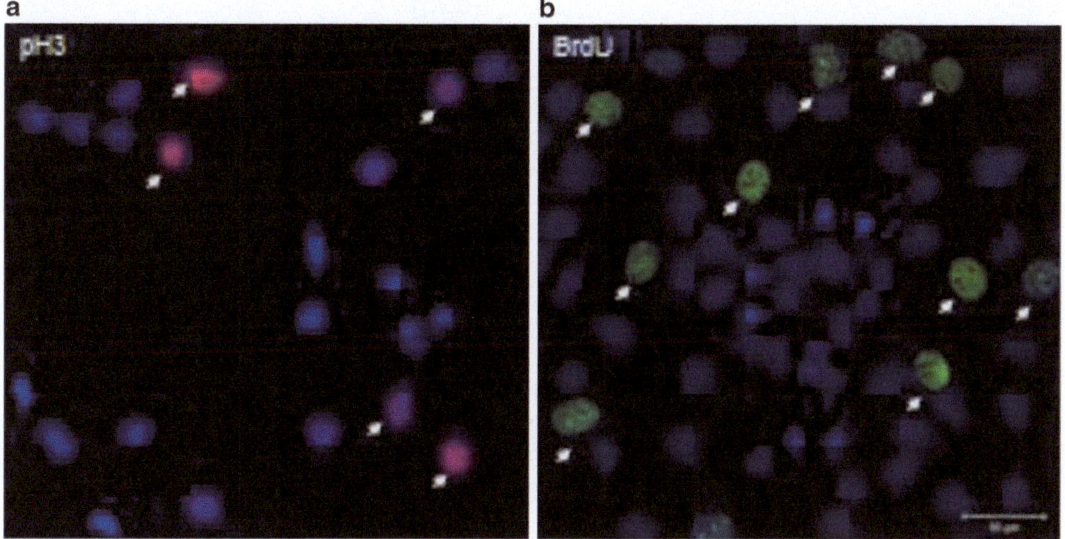

Fig. 2 Immunocytochemical staining for pH3 and BrdU. Representative fluorescent microscope images of (**a**) pH3⁺ and (**b**) BrdU⁺ CSP cells

5. Permeabilization: cover cell layer with 3 ml ice cold 100 % methanol and incubate for 25–30 min at −20 °C (*see* **Note 8**). Wash cells three times with 1× PBS.
6. Incubate cells with 3 ml blocking solution for 1 h at RT.
7. Staining: Remove blocking solution and cover cells with 200 μl primary antibody (rabbit anti-pH3 from Abcam, 1/200 dilution in blocking solution). Incubate for 2 h at RT. Wash cells three times with 1× PBS. Cover cells with 200 μl anti-rabbit fluorophore-conjugated secondary antibody solution (molecular probes, 1/200 dilution in blocking solution) and incubate for 2 h at RT. Wash cells three times with 1× PBS, thoroughly aspirate PBS, add one drop of DAPI-containing mounting medium (Vector Vectashield), and mount coverslips on slides (*see* **Note 9**).
8. Visualize cells with a fluorescent microscope (Fig. 2a).

3.2.3 Immunocytochemical Staining for 5-Bromo-2′-deoxyuridine (BrdU)

BrdU labeling and staining is performed using the 5-Bromo-2′-deoxyuridine Labeling and Detection Kit I from Roche.

1. Culture cells on coverslips as described in Subheading 3.2.2.
2. One hour prior to fixation, incubate cells with BrdU labeling solution added to the expansion medium (1:1,000 dilution) for 1 h at 37 °C. Wash cells three times with 1× PBS.
3. Cover cell layer with 3 ml ethanol fixative and incubate for 20 min at −20 °C. Wash three times with 1× PBS.

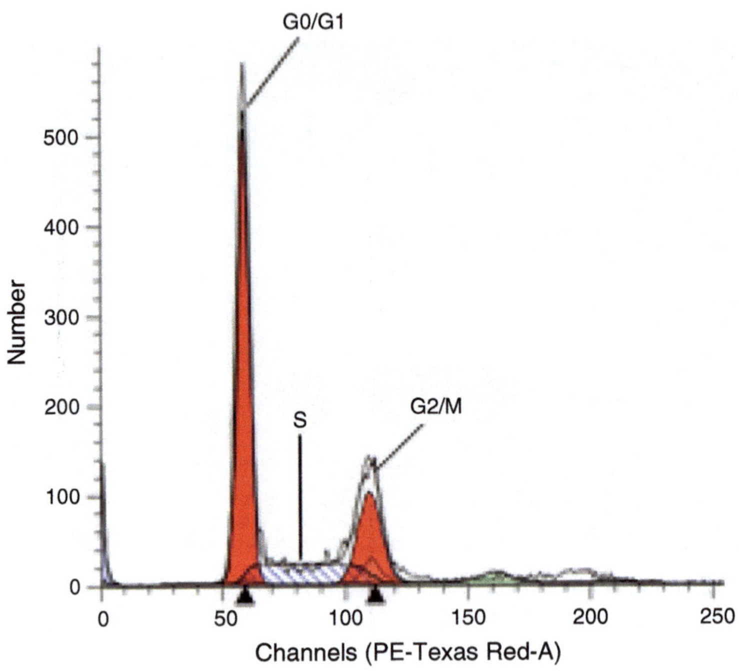

Fig. 3 Cell cycle analysis with PI staining. Representative flow cytometric analysis of CSP cells stained with PI. The first peak represents the G0/G1 fraction, the second peak corresponds to cells residing in the G2/M phases, and the area in between indicates cells in the S phase

4. Staining: Apply 200 μl of anti-BrdU working solution and incubate for 30 min at 37 °C. Wash three times with 1× PBS. Apply secondary antibody (1:10 dilution in 1× PBS) and incubate for 30 min at 37 °C (*see* **Note 10**). Wash three times with 1× PBS, add mounting medium, and mount coverslips on slides as described in Subheading 3.2.2 (*see* **Note 9**).
5. Visualize cells with a fluorescent microscope (Fig. 2b).

3.3 Cell Cycle Analysis

3.3.1 Propidium Iodide (PI) Staining for Flow Cytometric Analysis

1. Plate CSP cells in 60 mm dishes at a concentration of 4.76 cells/mm^2. Culture in expansion medium for 5 days.
2. Lift cells from culture dish by trypsinization as described in Subheading 3.1.
3. Resuspend cells in 300 μl ddH_2O, add dropwise in 700 μl 100 % ethanol, and incubate o/n at 4 °C. Wash twice with 1× PBS (*see* **Note 4**).
4. Resuspend cells in 1 ml PI staining solution and incubate for 1 h at 37 °C protected from light. Wash twice with 1× PBS (*see* **Note 4**) and analyze by flow cytometry (Fig. 3).
5. Data analysis may be performed with the ModFit Lt software by Verity House or other appropriate software.

3.3.2 Fluorescence Ubiquitination Cell Cycle Indicators (FUCCI)

1. Lentivirus production: Plate 5×10^6 HEK293-T cells in a 10 mm dish and culture in HEK-medium for 24 h at 37 °C in 10 % CO_2. At 24 h 75 % confluency must be reached.
2. Prepare the transfection mix and incubate for 15–20 min at RT.
3. Add transfection mix to the cells dropwise and incubate at 37 °C for 12–16 h in 3 % CO_2.
4. Replace HEK-medium with CSP expansion medium and incubate cells for additional 48 h at 37 °C in 10 % CO_2 (*see* **Note 11**).
5. Collect lentivirus-containing medium (*see* **Note 12**), filter through a 0.45 μm sterile filter, and aliquot in 1.5 ml cryotubes. Freeze in liquid nitrogen and store at –80 °C.
6. CSP cell lentiviral infection: Plate CSP cells in 100 mm culture dishes at a density of 54.5 cells/mm^2 (~3×10^5 cells) and culture in expansion medium until ~80 % confluency is reached (~24 h) (*see* **Note 13**).
7. Thaw 3 ml of each virus (mKO2 and mAG) for each 100 mm dish by placing the tubes directly from –80 °C into a 37 °C water bath for approximately 2 min.
8. Remove expansion medium from CSP cells, add 3 ml of virus supplemented with 6 μg/ml protamine sulfate (Sigma), and incubate for 3 h at 37 °C.
9. Add 7 ml of fresh expansion medium and incubate for 48 h (*see* **Note 14**).
10. Select and sort Azami-Green and Kusabira-Orange single- and double-positive CSP cells by FACS.
11. Plate cells at a density of 5–15 cells/mm^2 and culture in expansion medium until ~90 % confluency is reached.
12. Replace expansion medium with synchronization medium and incubate for 24 h at 37 °C.
13. Lift cells by trypsinization as described in Subheading 3.1 and proceed to flow cytometric analysis of the cell cycle [6] or live cell imaging [7].
14. Cell cycle monitoring by flow cytometry: Plate cells in 60 mm dishes at a density of 23.8 cells/mm^2 (50×10^3 cells) in expansion medium. Prepare triplicates for each time point to be analyzed.
15. At each desired time point, lift cells by trypsinization. Resuspend cells in 100 μl 1× PBS and analyze by flow cytometry for the expression of Cdtl (Kusabira-Orange, 548/559 nm) and/or Geminin (Azami-Green, 492/505 nm) (Fig. 4).

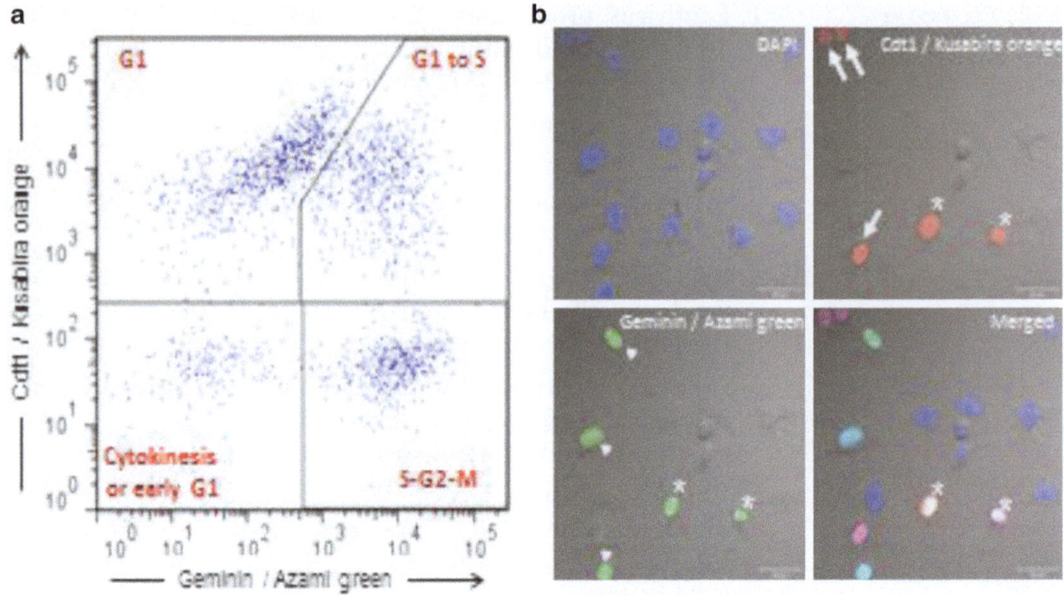

Fig. 4 Cell cycle analysis with the FUCCI indicators. (**a**) Representative flow cytometric analysis of CSP cells expressing the FUCCI probes. dt1 and Geminin single-positive fractions represent cells in G1 and S-G2-M phases, respectively. Double-positive cells correspond to cells residing in the G1 to S transition. The double-negative fraction indicates cells undergoing cytokinesis or in early G1. (**b**) A representative picture of FUCCI-expressing CSP cells. *Arrows* and *arrowheads* indicate cells in G1 and S-G2-M, respectively. Stars indicate cells in G1-S transition

16. Time lapse-live cell imaging: Plate cells in 2-well chamber slides at a density of 15 cells/mm^2 (*see* **Note 15**).
17. Perform live cell imaging at desired time point while maintaining cells at 37 °C in 5 °C, protected from light.

3.4 Cardiomyogenic Differentiation: Coculture Assay

All surfaces and equipment require sterilization prior use. All steps must be performed as quickly as possible to ensure cell quality and viability.

1. Neonatal rat ventricular cardiomyocytes isolation (NRVM): For NRVM isolation, use 1 litter of 1–2-day-old Wistar rats.
2. Sacrifice pups by decapitation. Open the sternum and remove the heart by pressing the scissors against the chest. Place heart in a 50 ml tube containing HBSS and store on ice. Proceed with the following pup.
3. Transfer hearts in a 60 mm dish containing ice cold HBSS, remove atria, and squeeze gently to wash out the blood. Transfer hearts to a clean 60 mm dish with fresh HBSS. Cut each heart in 6–8 pieces to facilitate digestion. Transfer all pieces to a clean 60 mm dish with fresh HBSS for a last wash (*see* **Note 16**).

4. Place hearts in 25 ml trypsin solution and incubate for 18 h at 4 °C (*see* **Note 17**).
5. Add 25 ml of pre-culture medium to inactivate trypsin solution and shake for 3 min at 38 °C (150 rpm).
6. Discard supernatant, add 10 ml collagenase B solution, and incubate for 3 min 45 sec under constant shaking at 38 °C.
7. Collect supernatant and store on ice. Incubate tissue with collagenase B solution for 4 min 45 sec under constant shaking. Repeat this step three additional times. During the last cycle, extend incubation time to 5 min. At each time, collect supernatant in the same tube and store on ice. The total collected volume should be approximately 50 ml, and by the last digestion step, almost all tissue should be gone (*see* **Note 18**).
8. Pellet cells by centrifugation at 200 × *g* for 5 min. Gently resuspend cells in 20 ml pre-culture medium to remove any remaining collagenase B solution. Pellet cells by centrifugation at 50–100 × *g* for 5 min.
9. Gently resuspend cells in 10 ml pre-culture medium and transfer them into a T75 flask. Incubate cells for 1.5 h at 37 °C. Transfer medium to a new T75 flask and incubate for an additional 1.5 h at 37 °C (*see* **Note 19**).
10. Collect medium and count cells.
11. Coculture of NRVM with GFP^+ CSP cells: At least 30 min prior to the completion of the second NRVM incubation in a T75 flask, prepare laminin-coated coverslips (20 × 20 mm). Place coverslip in a 35 mm dish and cover with 200 μl laminin solution. Leave inside a sterile culture hood until use.
12. Aspirate laminin solution from coverslips and plate NRVM at a density of 375 cells/mm^2 in no more than 200 μl of pre-culture medium. Leave at RT for 15 min, add 2 ml of pre-culture medium, and incubate for 48 h at 37 °C. Renew medium daily.
13. Aspirate pre-culture medium. Plate 100 μl coculture medium containing GFP^+ CSP cells on coverslip at a density of 37.5 cells/mm^2. Incubate for 1 h at 37 °C. Add 2 ml of coculture medium and incubate for 72 h at 37 °C. Renew medium daily.
14. Immunocytochemical staining for α-sarcomeric actinin: Fix and permeabilize cells as described in Subheading 3.2.2.
15. Incubate cells with blocking solution for 1 h at RT.
16. Staining: Cover cells with 200 μl of primary antibody solution containing mouse anti-α-sarcomeric actinin (Sigma, 1:800 dilution in blocking solution) and rabbit anti-GFP (Invitrogen, 1:150 dilution in blocking solution) and incubate for 2 h at RT. Wash three times with 1× PBS. Cover cells with 200 μl of fluorophore-conjugated anti-mouse and anti-rabbit secondary antibody solution (molecular probes, 1:200 dilution in blocking

solution) and incubate for 2 h at RT. Wash cells three times with 1× PBS, thoroughly aspirate PBS, add one drop of DAPI-containing mounting medium (Vector Vectashield), and mount coverslips on slides (*see* **Note 9**).

17. Visualize cells with a fluorescent microscope and score α-sarcomeric actinin⁺ GFP⁺ CSP cells.

4 Notes

1. This density corresponds to approximately 10,000 cells in a 60 mm culture dish. Larger or smaller dishes may be used as long as the density is kept constant. The duration of the proliferation assay may also be adjusted. It is important to keep in mind that the doubling time of CSP cells is approximately 28 h.
2. CSP cells grow under adherent conditions. CSP cells adhere to the plastic dish 4–6 h following plating. All media and buffers used for live cell processing such as trypsin, expansion medium, and PBS must be warmed to 37 °C, 15–20 min prior use.
3. Cells may be counted by other means including a Coulter counter or a flow-cytometry analyzer such as the Accuri C6 analyzer (BD Biosciences).
4. Perform all washes with 5–10 volumes of indicated washing solution. In the case of low cell number, limit washes to one.
5. Following fixation, cells can be stored for later use in 1× PBS at 4 °C for 72 h or in a solution consisting of FCS and DMSO at a 9:1 ratio at −80 °C for a longer period.
6. It is important to always use an isotype control for flow cytometric analysis.
7. For assays involving cells plated on coverslips, a higher cell concentration is used since a fraction of cells will not attach to the coverslips. Different sizes of coverslips and dishes may be used as long as the same cell density is maintained.
8. Incubation with methanol must not exceed 30 min. Cells tend to detach from coverslips when longer incubation periods are used.
9. Make sure to aspirate all solution (blocking or PBS) from dish and coverslip before addition of the antibody solution especially around the coverslip edges to avoid leaking. A hydrophobic barrier pen may be used to trace the coverslip's borders. In the case of different coverslip size, antibody solution volumes must be adjusted. Cells may be incubated with antibody solutions for 1 h at 37 °C. When mounting coverslips on slides, remove all air bubbles with the use of a clean plastic tip.

10. The secondary antibody is provided with the kit. Other anti-mouse antibodies may be used and correct concentration must be determined.
11. HEK-medium is replaced to allow virus collection in CSP expansion medium for later use in CSP infection.
12. New expansion medium may be added to the remaining HEK cells for collection of day 2 virus the following day.
13. After lentiviral infection cells will be passaged twice before they are ready to be used for cell cycle analysis. In order to avoid using cells beyond passage 6, it is preferable to start infection with CSP cells from earlier passages (3–4).
14. Medium can be replaced with fresh at 24 h.
15. For live cell imaging, use α-mem without phenol red pH indicator.
16. To transfer the hearts, cut the tip of a 5 ml or 10 ml plastic pipette and aspirate the contents of the dish. Let the tissue fall to the opening of the pipette by gravity and release it in the new dish/container.
17. Use a 100 ml specimen container for incubation with trypsin solution.
18. Avoid mixing the tissue. Collect supernatant with a 10 ml pipette without aspirating any tissue.
19. Transfer the medium to a new T75 flask carefully without disturbing attached cells. Cardiomyocytes do not attach on plastic very rapidly and therefore this double incubation allows the attachment of non-myocytes (fibroblasts) to the plastic flask and thus the purification of the cell preparation from contaminating cells.

Acknowledgements

This work was supported in part by NIH grants (HL086967 and HL093148) to R.L. K.-I.S. was supported by the Manasaki fellowship from the University of Crete-Greece.

References

1. Bergmann O, Bhardwaj RD, Bernard S et al (2009) Evidence for cardiomyocyte renewal in humans. Science 324:98–102
2. Beltrami A, Urbanek K, Kajstura J et al (2001) Evidence that human cardiac myocytes divide after myocardial infarction. N Engl J Med 344: 1750–1757
3. Linke A, MΓOller P, Nurzynska D et al (2005) Stem cells in the dog heart are self-renewing, clonogenic, and multipotent and regenerate infarcted myocardium, improving cardiac function. Proc Natl Acad Sci USA 102: 8966–9037
4. Hsieh P, Segers V, Davis M et al (2007) Evidence from a genetic fate-mapping study that stem cells refresh adult mammalian cardiomyocytes after injury. Nat Med 13: 970–974

5. Bolli R, Chugh A, D'Amario D et al (2011) Cardiac stem cells in patients with ischaemic cardiomyopathy (scipio): initial results of a randomised phase 1 trial. Lancet 378: 1847–1904
6. Pfister O, Fdr M, Jain M et al (2005) Cd31- but not cd31+ cardiac side population cells exhibit functional cardiomyogenic differentiation. Circ Res 97:52–113
7. Pfister O, Liao R (2008) Pump to survive: novel cytoprotective strategies for cardiac progenitor cells. Circ Res 102:998–1001
8. Sirish P, Lopez JE, Li N et al (2012) Microrna profiling predicts a variance in the proliferative potential of cardiac progenitor cells derived from neonatal and adult murine hearts. J Mol Cell Cardiol 52:264–272
9. Oikonomopoulos A, Sereti KI, Conyers F et al (2011) Wnt signaling exerts an antiproliferative effect on adult cardiac progenitor cells through igfbp3. Circ Res 109:1363–1374
10. Sakaue-Sawano A, Kurokawa H, Morimura T et al (2008) Visualizing spatiotemporal dynamics of multicellular cell-cycle progression. Cell 132:487–498
11. Beltrami A, Barlucchi L, Torella D et al (2003) Adult cardiac stem cells are multipotent and support myocardial regeneration. Cell 114:763–839
12. Oh H, Bradfute S, Gallardo T et al (2003) Cardiac progenitor cells from adult myocardium: homing, differentiation, and fusion after infarction. Proc Natl Acad Sci USA 100: 12313–12321
13. Matsuura K, Nagai T, Nishigaki N et al (2004) Adult cardiac sca-1-positive cells differentiate into beating cardiomyocytes. J Biol Chem 279:11384–11475
14. Martin C, Meeson A, Robertson S et al (2004) Persistent expression of the atp-binding cassette transporter, abcg2, identifies cardiac sp cells in the developing and adult heart. Dev Biol 265:262–337

Chapter 10

Immune Responses After Mesenchymal Stem Cell Implantation

Rony Atoui and Ray C.J. Chiu

Abstract

Stem cell transplantation is a promising approach for improving cardiac function after severe myocardial damage for which use of autologous cells have been preferred to avoid immune rejection. Recently, however, rodent as well as human mesenchymal stromal cells (MSCs) have been reported to be uniquely immune tolerant, both in in vitro as well as in vivo transplant models. In this chapter, we summarize the current understanding of the underlying immunologic mechanisms, which can facilitate the use of such cells as "universal donor cells."

Key words Marrow stem cell (MSC), Mesenchymal stem cell, Cellular cardiomyoplasty, Immunomodulatory properties, Cell transplantation, Universal donor cells, Xenograft, Allograft, Myocardial regeneration

1 Introduction

Myocardial infarction remains a widespread and important cause of morbidity and mortality among adults, accounting for more than 15 million new cases worldwide every year [1]. The loss of cardiomyocytes that results, combined with the limited endogenous repair mechanism, sets into play the remodeling process that ultimately leads to progressive heart failure. End-stage heart failure still has a grave prognosis with an estimated 5-year mortality of 70% [2].

Although current medical and surgical treatments have significantly altered the survival of these patients, none of these modalities contributes new contractile tissue to replace the myocardial scar. A promising approach, currently still under intensive investigation, is cellular transplantation which is directly aimed to overcome the problem of myocardial cell loss and improve the function of the injured myocardium through several mechanisms, including myogenesis [3], angiogenesis [4], and paracrine effects [5, 6], which may attenuate left ventricular function. Since the

Race L. Kao (ed.), *Cellular Cardiomyoplasty: Methods and Protocols*, Methods in Molecular Biology, vol. 1036,
DOI 10.1007/978-1-62703-511-8_10, © Springer Science+Business Media New York 2013

introduction of the concept of cellular transplantation in 1992 [7], several experimental models and preclinical studies have shown that the transplantation of a wide range of stem cells could contribute to the improvement in the cardiac function. Notable among such donor cells, are the satellite cells derived from skeletal muscle [8], embryonic stem cells [9], adult mesenchymal stem cells (MSCs) [10], adipose stem cells [11], umbilical cord stem cells [12], and hematopoietic stem cells CD34+. The observed beneficial effects of cell transplantation have led to numerous human clinical trials in the past several years [13].

The current preferred approach of using autologous stem cells aims to avoid immune rejection of donor cells, which can be expected after allogeneic or xenogeneic transplantation. Despite the promising early results, harvesting autologous cells from individual patients still poses significant logistic, economic, and timing constrains. Furthermore, most of the patients who could benefit from such therapy are elderly patients with multiple medical comorbidities. Unfortunately a number of recent studies have documented that MSCs obtained from elderly donors, and those with diabetes, renal failure, or severe ischemic heart disease, demonstrate significantly reduced capacity for proliferation, differentiation, and neovascularization, with increased levels of apoptosis in vitro and in vivo [14]. Such impaired autologous donor cells from sick elderly patients could therefore limit their therapeutic potential. Thus, there would be obvious clinical advantages if "universal donor cells" from healthy young donors could be used for stem cell allotransplantation without the need for immunosuppressive therapies.

In the last several years, increasing experimental findings have pointed towards a unique immunomodulatory property of the MSCs both in the in vitro and in vivo settings [15]. One intriguing property of MSCs is their ability to escape immune recognition and even actively inhibit immune responses. In this chapter, we will first review the general properties of MSCs, briefly comparing them to other cellular alternatives. We will then discuss in depth the evidence behind the role of MSCs in immunomodulation, both in vivo and in vitro, and to describe our current understanding of the possible underlying mechanisms by which it occurs and by which MSCs could be viewed as "universal donor cells."

2 Mesenchymal Stem Cells (MSCs) as Adult Stem Cells

Mesenchymal stem cells, also known as bone marrow stem cells, stromal stem cells, marrow progenitor cells, or marrow-derived adult stem cells, essentially represent a heterogeneous population of fibroblast-like cells, which can be found in the bone marrow stroma.

These cells were previously believed to play only supportive roles for hematopoiesis by expressing various cytokines, growth factors, and adhesion molecules. Cohnheim in the nineteenth century first suggested the presence of these cells in the blood and their possible role in wound repair [16]. Friedenstein and his group were the first in the early 1970s to better describe these MSCs in a number of species, including mice, rats, rabbits, guinea pigs, hamsters, and humans, showing their differentiation potential into cells of mesenchymal lineage including chondrocytes, osteoblasts, myocytes, and adipocytes [17]. Isolation of MSCs was then undertaken by Caplan who described a technique still used today by harvesting the cells that adhered to the bottom of the plates when the bone marrow cells are cultured in vitro [18]. MSCs have also been successfully isolated from various mid-gestational fetal tissue, including amniotic fluid [19] and first- and second-trimester fetal tissues [20]. Several in vivo and in vitro studies have confirmed the pluripotent potential of these cells and have observed the presence of injected MSCs in host adipose tissue, lung, cartilage, central nervous system, liver, spleen, thymus, and skeletal muscle [21]. Although the extent of their plasticity is still under investigation, studies within the last few years have demonstrated the capacity of these MSCs to differentiate into cells of lineages other than mesenchymal, such as hepatocytes, renal cells, and even early astrocytes [22, 23]. Because these cells do not have the ethical or tumorigenicity problems of ESCs, their plasticity have generated much excitement, giving hope to their therapeutic use in a wide range of diseases.

Besides the bone marrow, several sources of adult stem cells are known. Zuk and colleagues have demonstrated that adipose tissue contains both HSCs and MSCs [11]. Peripheral blood is also a source of HSCs and endothelial progenitor cells that have been used for cellular transplantation [13]. Skeletal myoblasts or satellite cells have been isolated from adult muscle, expanded in culture and even used in clinical trials [24].

3 MSCs Characteristics and Subpopulations

Although MSCs pluripotent potential has been demonstrated in many studies, controversy still exists as to what proportion of these cells is truly pluripotent. Thus, although they are collectively called marrow stromal cells, not all stromal cells are pluripotent [25]. In fact, it was reported that up to one-third of the initial adherent stromal colonies are truly polypotent [21]. Plating studies confirm the rarity of MSCs in the adult bone marrow, representing approximately 0.01–0.05% of the nucleated cells, being much less abundant than their hematopoietic counterpart [26].

Human MSCs can be cloned and expanded to greater than one million fold and still retain their ability to differentiate into several mesenchymal lineages [27]. Unlike hematopoietic cells, MSCs are CD34− and CD45−. Although still not fully indentified, other surface markers include CD29, CD44, CD71, CD90, CD106, SH2, SH3, and SH4-69 [25].

It is however important to note that some variation has been seen from laboratory to another. In fact, there is still considerable confusion regarding the exact composition of these cells. For this reason, no unique phenotype has been identified that allows the reproducible isolation of MSCs with predictable lineage differentiation. The reasons behind such uncertainty lie primarily in the experimental conditions used such as the heterogeneity of culture conditions, cell separation techniques, and different molecular cell markers used by various investigators. Thus, while the principle of clonal homogeneity is used by some experts to define these cells [21], others use a combination of molecular cell markers such as c-kit+/Lin− cells [26], sac1+Lin−/ckit+ cells [27], ckit+/cd34− cells [28], etc. Because of such differences, it is often difficult to compare the findings among different studies [29]. Standardization of such classifications is of paramount importance as it will be very helpful in the further exploration of the mechanisms of MSCs differentiation or engraftment. One possible reason behind this confusion might be because only fully mature cells can be characterized by a defined set of markers. In fact, because of their undifferentiated state, a constantly changing set of markers may be continuously defining the "labile" phenotype of MSCs.

4 MSCs as "Universal Donor Cells"

Recently there has been an explosive advance in our knowledge on adult stem cells for their use as donor cells for regenerative therapies. Associated with such advances are some unexpected and controversial findings which defy current scientific dogmas. One of such dilemma is a series of observations indicating that some populations of multipotent MSCs are immune privileged, able to survive and differentiate in immunocompatibility-mismatched allogeneic or even xenogeneic transplant recipients [15]. In fact, a number of laboratories have recently reported that MSCs may have a unique immunological property capable of inducing tolerance in immunocompetent allotransplants or even xenotransplant recipients [30, 31]. The mechanisms of such immunotolerance have been the subject of intense studies, and three interrelated candidate mechanisms are emerging [32, 33]. MSCs appear to evade rejection by: (1) being hypoimmunogenic, (2) modulating T-cell phenotype, and (3) immunosuppressing the local environment.

5 Evidence from In Vitro Studies

A large body of in vitro experiments involving coculture-mixed lymphocyte reactions supports the view that MSCs avoid allogeneic response [15, 31, 33, 34] and that the use of mismatched MSCs does not induce a proliferative T-cell response in allogeneic and xenogeneic coculture studies [30, 32, 35, 36]. Largely responsible for being hypoimmunogenic is a unique expression pattern of cell surface antigens on the MSCs. Although there is a continuous controversy surrounding the exact composition of these cell surface markers, most studies describe MSCs as MHC class I positive and MHC class II negative [37]. The expression of class I MHC is important because it protects these cells from certain NK-cell-mediated deletion. As MHC class II proteins are potent alloantigens, their lack of expression on MSCs allows them to escape recognition by effector CD4+ T cells. In addition to this, MSCs do not appear to express Fas-ligand nor co-stimulatory molecules such as B7-1 (CD80), B7-2 (CD86), CD40 for effector T-cell induction [21]. The presence of these cell surface markers, along with the findings that MSCs are customary residents of the bone marrow stroma, suggest that MSCs are hypoimmunogenic cells that play an important role in the immunoregulation provided by the bone marrow microenvironment by evading the recognition of alloreactive cells [33, 37].

There is also good in vitro evidence that MSCs can directly modulate the function of T cells. Pittenger and coworker reported that human MSCs constitutively secrete PGE2, hence altering the cytokine secretion profile of dendritic cells, naïve and cytotoxic T lymphocytes, as well as NK cells, namely, by inhibiting TNF-α and interferon-γ (INF-γ) and by stimulating IL-10 secretion to modulate the immune cell response [38]. By doing so, they inhibit the maturation and migration of various antigen-presenting cells, suppress B-cell activation, induce suppressor T-cell formation, and alter the expression of several receptors necessary for antigen capture and processing [33, 38]. Furthermore, through the release of IL-4, they accelerate a shift from a majority of proinflammatory Thl cells towards an increase in the anti-inflammatory Th2 cells [37]. We suspect that this anti-inflammatory property of MSCs may play an important role in the so-called paracrine effects associated with MSCs, as postulated by several investigators [5, 6].

Although still controversial, there is some evidence that MSCs do also exhibit immunosuppressive properties. Some reports show that MSCs do express mRNA for cytokines such as IL-1,6,-7,-8,-11,-12,-14,-15,-27, leukemia inhibitory factor, macrophage colony-stimulating factor, and stem cell factor [34, 38]. Although their role is still not fully understood, some of these cytokines provide critical cell-cell interactions and promote HSCs differentiation. Furthermore, IL-10 seems to be constitutively expressed by MSCs. This interleukin has a well-documented role in T-cell regulation and in the promotion of the suppressor phenotype and can also antagonize the action of IL-12 during induction of the inflammatory immune responses [37].

In addition to the proposed role of indoleamine 2,3-dioxygenase (IDO)-mediated tryptophan degradation [34], MSCs can also secrete other peptides such as hepatocyte growth factor (HGF) which may contribute to the creation of a local immunosuppressive environment [32, 39]. Similarly, transforming growth factor β1 (TGF-β1) seems also involved in T-cell suppression by working with HGF in promoting the allo-escaping phenotype. In fact, Di Nicola and his group showed that neutralizing antibodies to HGF and TGF-β1 restored the proliferative response in mixed lymphocytes reactions [32].

Zhang and associates provided further evidence that MSCs interfere with dendritic cell (DC) maturation, differentiation, and function by downregulating the expression of CD1a, CD40, CD80, CD86, and HLA-DR [40]. These findings were confirmed by Beyth and his group who suggested that human MSCs convert the DC into a suppressor cell thus locking it into an immature state and thereby inducing peripheral tolerance [41]. All these results suggest that MSCs may be mediating allogeneic tolerance by directing antigen-presenting cells (APC) toward a suppressor phenotype that ultimately results in an attenuated T-cell response [33, 34].

One can perhaps speculate that MSCs may play a role in what Chiu R. called "immunological homeostasis," since the signaling molecules secreted by these cells are predominantly anti-inflammatory cytokines [42]. When there is tissue injury, such as in acute myocardial infarction, inflammatory immune cells and cytokines are mobilized and expressed at the site of injury. It has been shown that excessive inflammatory response could aggravate the ventricular remodeling process. Mobilization of the MSCs with anti-inflammatory properties may then restore a measure of this "immunological homeostasis" by attenuating the inflammatory damage to facilitate the regenerative process, which may be one of the evolutionary roles for these adult stem cells [42]. Of course, this hypothesis is highly speculative at present. However, a recent clinical report demonstrating a better prognosis for patients with ischemic heart disease when their anti-inflammatory/proinflammatory cytokine ratio was higher in their blood appears consistent with such hypothesis [43]. Furthermore, these immunosuppressive properties had been shown to be partially mediated through the generation of CD8+ regulatory cells (T-regs) [38, 44–46] and by the inhibition of the cytotoxic T lymphocytes formation in a dose-dependent fashion [47].

Most studies have also shown that these immunosuppressive properties are broad, increase with increased concentration of MSCs [34], and are effective whether the stimulation is specific or nonspecific [32, 35, 36, 45], across species [45, 46] and across different populations of lymphocytes [39, 41, 46]. Together, these results suggest that these immunosuppressive mechanisms may even cross species barriers. In addition, increasing evidence has emerged that MSCs can also interact directly with T cells to suppress alloreactivity and direct CD4+ T cells to a suppressive phenotype. Di Nicola and his group [32] as well as Tse and associates [36] showed that MSCs strongly suppressed $CD4^{+}$ T cells in mixed lymphocyte reactions and attenuated the proliferation of T-cell subsets.

Some studies have also shown that MSCs can influence control over cell division cycle pathways in cells of immunological relevance. Glennie and his group have shown that T cells stimulated in cocultures with MSCs exhibited an extensive inhibition of cyclin-D2 and an upregulation of the cyclin-dependent kinase inhibitor p27kip1 [48]. Furthermore, the role of MSCs on $CD8^{+}$ T cells and NK cells has also been addressed [49]. There is evidence that MSCs inhibit the formation of $CD8^{+}$ T cells and appear to evade NK-cell targeting mechanisms [48]. Rasmusson and associates showed that NK cells in cocultures did not recognize MSCs although their lytic properties were still present [47]. Moreover, it has been suggested that MSCs reduce IL-2 induced NK-cell proliferation and INF-γ production [38, 47, 50]. Finally, another level at which MSCs may modulate immune responses is through the inhibition of B cells proliferation as well as their chemotactic behavior and antibody production [15, 48].

6 Evidence from In Vivo Studies

Although considerable data of in vitro findings support the immunomodulatory properties of MSCs, relatively little evidence is available on the immunogenicity of MSCs in vivo. Despite this, there is growing evidence that the in vitro observations may translate to the in vivo setting. Bartholomew et al. [35] group first demonstrated that the in vivo administration of allogeneic MSCs prolonged third party skin graft survival in immunocompetent baboons. This study, as well as many others, paved the way for the use of these cells in immune-mediated disorders [15, 31]. For example, Koc and coworkers showed no evidence of alloreactive T cells and no incidence of graft versus host disease (GVHD) when allogeneic MSCs were infused into patients with Hurler's syndrome or metachromatic leukodystrophy [51]. Horwitz and colleagues reported that donor MSCs contributed to bone remodeling after allogeneic stem cell transplantation in three children with osteogenesis imperfecta

[52]. Other groups have reported that it can also prevent the rejection of allogeneic B16 mouse melanoma cells in immunocompetent mice [46], successfully engraft in brains of albino rats [53], lead to significant improvement in symptoms in mice with autoimmune encephalomyelitis through the induction of peripheral tolerance [54], and attenuate GVHD in humans with grade IV acute GVHD [55]. It is important to note that several mechanisms involving specific factors have been proposed, mostly based on in vitro findings, but a clear consensus, based on in vivo experiments specifically targeting these particles, is still lacking [33].

Allogeneic MSCs transplanted into the myocardium between unrelated porcine donors and recipients was reported by Caparelli et al. [56] and by Makkar et al. [57]. The recipients underwent coronary ligation before allogeneic MSC implantation and received no immunosuppression. The implanted cells remained viable and differentiated without being rejected. Furthermore, the cardiac functions of transplanted hearts were significantly improved. In a swine and a rat model, Amado and his group [58] and Dai and associates [5] respectively reported the survival of allogeneic MSCs in infarcted myocardium without immunosuppression. Moreover, these cells were shown to differentiate and contribute to the functional improvement of the host myocardium [59].

In November 2000, a fascinating study by Liechty and coworkers was published in *Nature Medicine* [60]. Well-characterized human MSCs were implanted into fetal sheep early in gestation. In this xenogeneic system, the human MSCs engrafted and persisted in multiple tissues for as long as 13 months after transplantation, even after maturation of the fetal immune system. Furthermore, these cells underwent site-specific differentiation into multiple cell lineages including cardiomyocytes. Nevertheless, these experiments were carried out in fetal recipients.

In a series of studies at our laboratory, Saito and associates injected intravenously labeled mice MSCs into fully immunocompetent adult rats, successfully producing stable cardiac chimeras for at least 12 weeks without any immunosuppression and with no evidence of rejection [61]. It was confirmed that within days these mouse cells had homed into the bone marrow of the rats and upon coronary artery ligation, were recruited to the peri-infarcted myocardium. In the following 4–6 weeks, the labeled cells were seen to differentiate into various phenotypes. In subsequent studies, MacDonald and colleagues showed that not only stable chimeras were formed but also the overall ventricular function was significantly improved [62]. These findings were once again replicated by Luo and coworkers who confirmed the survival of pig MSCs implanted into fully immunocompetent rat myocardium for up to 6 months after xenotransplantation [63]. More recently, Atoui and associates were able to confirm the engraftment of human MSCs within the rat myocardium for at least 8 weeks after myocardial infarction and without the use of any immunosuppression [64]. Such xenotransplant significantly contributed to the improvement in the overall cardiac function and in attenuating left ventricular remodeling.

However, tolerance of MSCs across the MHC barrier might not be absolute. Grinnemo et al. [65] demonstrated that although the MSCs successfully engraft across allogeneic barriers, rejection occurs when a xenotransplant model is used. In their follow-up study, the same group demonstrated that the survival of human MSCs into ischemic rat myocardium is possible only when immunosuppression is used [66]. These findings were in direct contrast to those obtained in our laboratory. Despite the similarities between our two studies, there seems to be nonetheless subtle differences in the experimental designs. For instance, in their study, MSCs were harvested from the sternum of patients undergoing cardiac surgery. These cells were previously shown to have lower capacity for differentiation, survival, and even proliferation [14, 67]. It is of interest to note that in the in vitro studies, human MSCs were harvested from young healthy donors. Still, further studies are needed to better clarify these contradictory findings.

Other opposing findings were also reported showing that despite retaining their immunosuppressive properties in vitro, allogeneic murine MSCs can be immunogenic in immunocompetent animals [68, 69]. The discrepancy observed could be observed by differences in the experimental conditions such as the level of INF-γ [70], different stages of differentiation or species diversity [33]. For instance, a number of studies have shown that the amount of fetal calf serum present in the culture media can induce a significant immune response against cultured cells [71]. Finally, it should also be mentioned that murine and human MSCs differ in their immunosuppressive property. In fact, it was shown that the immunosuppressive effect of human MSCs, at least in vitro, is much stronger than that of murine MSCs [32, 39].

Such contradictory findings are perplexing, but not unique in this rapidly developing field of stem cell biology and regenerative medicine. Despite the substantive body of evidence from the in vitro literature confirming the immunomodulatory properties of MSCs, their importance in the in vivo setting remains controversial. Nevertheless, MSCs have already been introduced to clinical practice, especially in the autoimmune and hematological fields.

Furthermore, although the immunomodulatory effects of MSCs are now well documented, it provides no explanation as to why such tolerance persists even after the implanted stem cells differentiated into their targeted tissue phenotypes. In an attempt to explain this phenomenon, Chiu proposed the "stealth immune tolerance" hypothesis [32], which is in fact an application of the "danger model" theory described earlier by Matzinger [47], who suggested that the immune rejection of a transplanted organ is not due to the mismatch of MHC antigens alone but also due to the presence of a "danger signal" serving as a co-stimulant factor. Thus, although it is still hypothetical, the "stealth immune tolerance" hypothesis is based on the fact that the expression of new foreign recognition antigens (i.e., MHC antigens) on the gradually differentiating cells is dissociated in timing from the "danger signals" derived from the injury inflicted by the invasive implantation procedure. In other words, it takes weeks for the implanted cells to mature and fully express their MHC antigens. Thus, by the time these implanted cells differentiate, the effects to tissue injury would have subsided, so that the immune synapsis receives only the first "recognition" signal without the second "activation" signal [47]. According to the two-signal theory for immune synapsis, recognition without activation could then lead to T-cell anergy, such that the implanted cells, now fully differentiated, are tolerated and allowed to survive. It is important to note that presently this view remains hypothetical and needs to be further confirmed.

7 Clinical Trials Involving Allogeneic Stem Cells Transplantation

Interestingly, and based on the clinical and experimental data discussed previously, there have been two clinical trials so far that looked at the allogeneic use of MSCs in patients post myocardial infarction. The FDA recently approved an Osiris Inc. sponsored Phase I multicenter clinical trial in which allogeneic human MSCs were given intravenously, without immunosuppression, to patients following an acute myocardial infarction. The preliminary results after 6 months were recently presented and are highly encouraging [72] with evidence of significant improvement in the ventricular function. Similarly, the Revascor trial is another randomized, placebo-controlled multicenter trial that assesses the safety and feasibility of three different doses of allogeneic MSCs delivered into the myocardium of patients with chronic heart failure. After 3 months, their preliminary results were also reported online (http://www.angioblast.com) and described a significant improvement in the overall ventricular function [73].

8 Conclusion

The potential importance of these findings for the treatment of ischemic heart disease is apparent. In addition to their powerful replicative capacity, MSCs can easily be harvested from bone marrows, expanded ex vivo, and differentiated into many cell type lineages, if desired. Due to their immunotolerance property, the establishment of MSCs as effective "universal donor cells" [33] could then dramatically expand the therapeutic potential for cellular cardiomyoplasty. From a clinical perspective, these cells could be isolated and expanded from donors irrespective of their MHC haplotype, tested for their functional capabilities well in advance, and stored as an "off-the-shelf" cell population for immediate use when needed on any patient after an acute myocardial infarction. Such logistic advantages are not available with the use of autologous MSCs which is currently the cell source of choice. Perhaps more importantly, since such allogeneic MSCs can be obtained from young healthy donors, they could be of great value in patients with genetic cardiomyopathies and in elderly patients with multiple medical comorbidities whose own MSCs could be dysfunctional.

Despite the exciting preliminary results, further investigations are required to address many of the remaining controversial findings, as well as the important question of chronic rejection after cell transplantation. Although the preliminary results of allogeneic MSC transplantation described above seem quite promising, the trials enrolled only a limited number of patients who were evaluated relatively shortly after the treatment [74, 75]. Furthermore, further mechanistic studies and more quantitative assessment of MSCs engraftment are still needed before the therapeutic promise of these cells can be fully achieved [15, 33].

References

1. Orlic D, Hill J, Arai A (2002) Stem cells for myocardial regeneration. Circ Res 91:1092–1102
2. Nir S, David R, Zaruba M et al (2003) Human embryonic stem cells for cardiovascular repair. Cardiovasc Res 58:313–323
3. Orlic D, Kajstura T, Chimenti S et al (2001) Bone marrow cells regenerate infracted myocardium. Nature 401:701–705
4. Davani S, Marandin A, Mersin N et al (2003) Mesenchymal progenitor cells differentiate into an endothelial phenotype, enhance vascular density, and improve heart function in a rat cellular cardiomyoplasty model. Circulation 108II:253–258
5. Dai W, Hale S, Martin B et al (2005) Allogeneic mesenchymal stem cell transplantation in postinfarcted rat myocardium: short and long-term effects. Circulation 112:214–223
6. Tang Y, Zhao Q, Qin X et al (2005) Paracrine action enhances the effects of autologous mesenchymal stem cell transplantation on vascular regeneration in rat model of myocardial infarction. Ann Thorac Surg 80:229–237
7. Marelli D, Desrosiers C, El-Alfy M et al (1992) Cell transplantation for myocardial repair: an experimental approach. Cell Transplant 1:383–390
8. Chiu RCJ, Zibaitis A, Kao RL (1995) Cellular cardiomyoplasty: myocardial regeneration with satellite cell implantation. Ann Thorac Surg 60:12–18
9. Hodgson DM, Behfar A, Zingman LV et al (2004) Stable benefit of embryonic stem cell therapy in myocardial infarction. Am J Physiol 287:H471–H479
10. Wang JS, Shum-Tim D, Galipeau J et al (2000) Marrow stromal cells for cellular cardiomyoplasty: feasibility and clinical advantages. J Thorac Cardiovasc Surg 120:999–1006
11. Zuk P, Zhu M, Ashjian P et al (2002) Human adipose tissue is a source of multipotent stem cells. Mol Biol Cell 13:4279–4296
12. Lee OK, Kuo TK, Chen WM et al (2004) Isolation of multipotent mesenchymal stem cells from umbilical cord blood. Blood 103:1669–1675
13. Schachinger V, Erbs S, Elsasser A et al (2006) Intra-coronary bone marrow derived progenitor cells in acute myocardial infarction. N Engl J Med 355:1210–1221
14. Heeschen C, Lehman R, Honold J et al (2004) Profoundly reduced neovascularization capacity of bone marrow mononuclear cells derived

from patients with chronic ischemic heart disease. Circulation 109:1615–1622
15. Nauta AJ, Fibbe WE (2007) Immunomodulatory properties of mesenchymal stromal cells. Blood 110(10):3499–3506
16. Cohnheim J (1867) Ueber entzuendung und eiterung. Arch Path Anat Physiol Klin Med 40:1
17. Friedenstein AJ, Petrakova KV, Kurolesova AI et al (1968) Heterotopic of bone marrow. Analysis of precursor cells for osteogenic and hematopoietic tissues. Transplantation 6:230–247
18. Caplan AI (1991) Mesenchymal stem cells. J Orthop Res 9:641–650
19. De Coppi P, Bartasch G, Siddiqui MM et al (2007) Isolation of amniotic stem cell lines with potential for therapy. Nat Biotechnol 25(1):100–106
20. In't Anker PS, Noort WA, Scherjon SA et al (2003) Mesenchymal stem cells in human second-trimester bone marrow, liver, lung and spleen exhibit a similar immunophenotype but a heterogeneous multilineage differentiation potential. Haematologica 88(8):845–852
21. Pittenger MF, MacKay AM, Beck SC et al (1999) Multilineage potential of adult human mesenchymal stem cells. Science 284:143–147
22. Dezawa M, Ishikawa H, Itokazu Y et al (2005) Bone marrow stromal cells generate muscle cells and repair muscle degeneration. Science 309(5732):314–317
23. Brazelton TR, Rossi FM, Keshet GI et al (2000) From marrow to brain: expression of neuronal phenotypes in adult mice. Science 290:1775–1779
24. Menasche P, Hagege AA, Vilquin JT et al (2003) Autolougous skeletal myoblast transplantation for severe postinfarction left ventricular dysfunction. J Am Coll Cardiol 41:1078–1083
25. Pittenger MF, Mosca JD, McIntosh KR (2000) Human mesenchymal stem cells: progenitor cells for cartilage, bone, fat and stroma. Curr Top Microbiol Immunol 251:3–11
26. Pittenger M, Martin B (2004) Mesenchymal stem cells and their potential as cardiac therapeutics. Circ Res 95:9–20
27. Ringes-Lichtenberg SM, Jaeger MD, Fuchs M et al (2002) Sustained improvement of left ventricular function after myocardial infarction by intravenous application of Sca1+ Lin/ckit+ bone marrow derived stem cells. Circulation 106(Suppl):II-14
28. Mangi AA, Kong D, He H (2002) Genetically modified mesenchymal stem cells perform in vivo repair of damaged myocardium. Circulation 106(Suppl):II-131
29. Deans R, Moseley A (2000) Mesenchymal stem cells: biology and potential clinical uses. Exp Hematol 28:875–884
30. Le Blanc K, Tammik C, Rosendahl K et al (2003) HLA expression and immunologic properties of differentiated and undifferentiated mesenchymal stem cells. Exp Hematol 31:890–896
31. Leblanc K, Ringden O (2007) Immunomodulation by mesenchymal stem cells and clinical experience. J Intern Med 262:509–525
32. Di Nicola M, Carlo-Stella C, Magni M et al (2002) Human bone marrow stromal cells suppress T lymphocyte proliferation induced by cellular or non-specific mitogenic stimuli. Blood 99:3838–3843
33. Atoui R, Shum-Tim D, Chiu RCJ (2008) Myocardial regenerative therapy: immunologic basis for the potential "universal donor cells". Ann Thorac Surg 86:327–334
34. Rasmusson I (2006) Immune modulation by mesenchymal stem cells. Exp Cell Res 312:2169–2179
35. Bartholomew A, Sturgeon C, Satskas M et al (2002) Mesenchymal stem cells suppress lymphocyte proliferation in vitro and prolong skin graft survival in vivo. Exp Hematol 30:42–48
36. Tse WT, Pendleton JD, Beyer WM et al (2003) Suppression of allogeneic T-cell proliferation by human marrow stromal cells: implication in transplantation. Transplantation 75:389–397
37. Ryan J, Barry F, Murphy J, Mahon B (2005) Mesenchymal stem cells avoid allogeneic rejection. J Inflamm 2(8):1–11
38. Aggarwal S, Pittenger M (2005) Human mesenchymal stem cells modulate allogeneic immune cell responses. Blood 105:1815–1822
39. LeBlanc K, Tammik L, Sundberg B et al (2003) Mesenchymal stem cells inhibit and stimulate mixed lymphocyte cultures and mitogenic responses independently of the major histocompatibility complex. Scand J Immunol 57:11–20
40. Zhang W, Ge W, Li C et al (2004) Effects of mesenchymal stem cells on differentiation, maturation, and function of human monocyte-derived dendritic cells. Stem Cell Dev 13:263–271
41. Beyth S, Borovsky Z, Mevorach D et al (2005) Human mesenchymal stem cells alter antigen-presenting cell maturation and induce T cell unresponsiveness. Blood 105:2214–2219
42. Yen BLJ, Yen ML, Liu KJ, Chiu RCJ (2008) In: Columbus F (ed) Immune tolerance research development, Nova science Publishers, Inc., Hauppauge, NY. Recent

Advances in Immune Tolerance in Stem Cells, pp 151–166
43. Anguera I, Miranda-Guardiola F, Bosch X et al (2002) Elevation of serum levels of anti-inflammatory cytokine interleukin-10 and decreased risks of coronary events in patients with unstable angina. Am Heart J 144:811–817
44. Prevosto C, Zancolli M, Canevali P et al (2007) Generation of CD4+ or CD8+ regulatory T cells upon mesenchymal stem cell–lymphocyte interaction. Haematologica 92(7):881–888
45. Maccario R, Podesta M, Moretta A et al (2005) Interaction of human mesenchymal stem cells with cells involved in alloantigen-specific immune response favors the differentiation of CD4+ T-cell subsets expressing a regulatory/suppressive phenotype. Haematologica 90:516–525
46. Djouad F, Plence P, Bony C et al (2003) Immunosuppressive effect of mesenchymal stem cells favors tumor growth in allogeneic animals. Blood 102:3837–3844
47. Rasmusson I, Ringden O, Sundberg B et al (2003) Mesenchymal stem cells inhibit the formation of cytotoxic T lymphocytes, but not activated cytotoxic T lymphocytes or natural killer cells. Transplantation 76:1208–1213
48. Glennie S, Soeiro I, Dyson PJ et al (2005) Bone marrow mesenchymal stem cells induce division arrest anergy of activated T cells. Blood 105(7):2821–2827
49. Kassis I, Vaknin-Dembinsky A, Karussis D (2011) Bone marrow mesenchymal stem cells: agents of immunomodulation and neuroprotection. Curr Stem Cell Res Ther 6(1):63–68
50. Spaggiari GM, Capobianco A, Becchetti S et al (2006) Mesenchymal stem cell–natural killer cell interactions: evidence that activated NK cells are capable of killing MSCs, whereas MSCs can inhibit IL-2 induced NK-cell proliferation. Blood 107(4):1484–1490
51. Koc ON, Day J, Nieder M et al (2002) Allogeneic mesenchymal stem cell infusion for treatment of metachromatic leukodystrophy and Hurler syndrome. Bone Marrow Transplant 30:215–222
52. Horwitz EM, Gordon PL, Koo WK et al (2002) Isolated allogeneic bone marrow-derived mesenchymal cells engraft and stimulate growth in children with osteogenesis imperfecta: implications for cell therapy of bone. Proc Natl Acad Sci 99:8932–8937
53. Azizi SA, Stokes D, Augelli BJ et al (1998) Engraftment and migration of human bone marrow stromal cells implanted in the brains of albino rats: similarities to astrocyte grafts. Proc Natl Acad Sci 95:3908–3913
54. Zappia E, Casazza S, Pedemonte E et al (2005) Mesenchymal stem cells ameliorate experimental autoimmune encephalomyelitis inducing T-cell anergy. Blood 106:1755–1761
55. LeBlanc K, Rasmusson J, Sundberg B et al (2004) Treatment of severe acute graft-versus-host disease with third party haploidentical mesenchymal stem cells. Lancet 363:1439–1441
56. Caparelli DJ, Cattaneo SM, Shake JG et al (2001) Cellular cardiomyoplasty with allogeneic mesenchymal stem cells results in improved cardiac performance in a swine model of myocardial infarction. Circulation 104:II-59
57. Makkar RR, Price M, Lill M et al (2005) Intramyocardial injection of allogeneic bone marrow-derived mesenchymal stem cells without immunosuppression preserves cardiac function in a porcine model of myocardial infarction. J Cardiovasc Pharmacol Ther 10(4):225–233
58. Amado LC, Saliaris AP, Schuleri KH et al (2005) Cardiac repair with intramyocardial injection of allogeneic mesenchymal stem cells after myocardial infarction. Proc Natl Acad Sci 102:11474–11479
59. Chiu R (2005) "Stealth immune tolerance" in stem cell transplantation: potential for "universal donors" in myocardial regenerative therapy. J Heart lung transpl 24(5):511–516
60. Liechty KW, Mackenzie TC, Shaaban AF et al (2000) Human mesenchymal stem cells engraft and demonstrate site-specific differentiation after *in utero* transplantation in sheep. Nat Med 11:1282–1286
61. Saito T, Kuang JQ, Bittira B et al (2002) Xenotransplant cardiac chimera: immune tolerance of adult stem cells. Ann Thorac Surg 74:19–24
62. MacDonald D, Saito T, Shum-Tim D et al (2005) Persistence of marrow stromal cells implanted into acutely infarcted myocardium: observations in a xenotransplant model. J Thorac Cardiovasc Surg 130:1114–1121
63. Luo J, Shum-Tim D, Chiu RCJ (2009) Marrow stromal cells as universal donor cells for cardiac regenerative therapy: fact or fancy. In: Dimarakis I (ed) Stem cell therapy in ischemic heart disease. Imperial College Press, London, pp 117–137
64. Atoui R, Asenjo JF, Duong M et al (2008) Marrow stomal cells as "universal donor cells" for myocardial regenerative therapy: their unique immune tolerance. Ann Thorac Surg 85:571–580
65. Grinnemo K, Mansson A, Dellgren D et al (2004) Xenoreactivity and engraftment of human mesenchymal stem cells transplanted

into infracted rat myocardium. J Thorac Cardiovasc Surg 127:1293–1300

66. Grinnemo KH, Mansson-Broberg A, Leblanc K et al (2006) Human mesenchymal stem cells do not differentiate into cardiomyocytes in a cardiac ischemic xenomodel. Ann Med 38:144–153
67. Stolzing A, Scutt A (2006) Age-related impairment of mesenchymal progenitor cell function. Aging Cell 1:1–12
68. Eliopoulos N, Stagg J, Lejeune L et al (2005) Allogeneic marrow stromal cells are immune rejected by MHC class I- and class II-mismatched recipient mice. Blood 106:4057–4065
69. Nauta AJ, Westerhuis G, Kruisselbrink AB et al (2006) Donor-derived mesenchymal stem cells are immunogenic in an allogeneic host and stimulate donor graft rejection in a nonmyeloablative setting. Blood 108:2114–2120
70. Stagg J, Pommey S, Eliopoulos N et al (2006) Interferon-γ-stimulated marrow stromal cells; a new type of nonhematopoietic antigen-presenting cell. Blood 107:2570–2577
71. Javazon EH, Beggs KJ, Flake AW (2004) Mesenchymal stem cells: paradoxes of passaging. Exp Hematol 32:414–425
72. Zambrano J, Traverse J, Henry T et al (2007) The impact of intravenous human mesenchymal stem cells (Provacel™) on ejection fraction in patients with myocardial infarction. Circulation 116(Suppl 16):II-202
73. Kinkaid HY, Huang XP, Li RK et al (2010) What's new in cardiac cell therapy? Allogeneic bone marrow stromal cells as "universal donor cells". J Card Surg 25:359–366
74. Wei HM, Wong P, Hsu LF et al (2009) Human bone marrow-derived adult stem cells for post myocardial infarction cardiac repair: current status and future directions. Singapore Med J 50(10):935–942
75. Chen SL, Fang WW, Ye F et al (2004) Effect on left ventricular function of intracoronary transplantation of autologous bone marrow mesenchymal stem cells in patients with acute myocardial infarction. Am J Cardiol 94:92–95

Chapter 11

Route of Delivery, Cell Retention, and Efficiency of Polymeric Microcapsules in Cellular Cardiomyoplasty

Alice Le Huu, Arghya Paul, Satya Prakash, and Dominique Shum-Tim

Abstract

Stem cell transplantation has been considered as a major breakthrough for treating ischemic heart disease. However, survival and retention of transplanted cells at the site of infarction remains tenuous. This chapter details a method of creating polymeric microcapsules for cell delivery, resulting in increased retention of transplanted cells at the target site, while achieving minimal mechanical trauma and cell loss. Simultaneously biocompatible and biodegradable, polymeric microcapsules have important implications in regenerative cell therapy.

Key words Microcapsules, Stem cells, Regenerative medicine, Cell therapy, Myocardial infarction

1 Introduction

1.1 Scope of the Disease

In 2008, 7.3 million deaths were attributed to coronary artery disease; by the year 2030, it is estimated that 23.6 people will perish from cardiovascular disease [1]. The statistics are daunting, but the development of percutaneous, surgical, and pharmacological interventions has improved the management of an acute myocardial infarction (MI) [2–4]. In hospital mortality following an MI has dropped considerably but remains disquieting at 10.8 % [5]. Mortality rates remain elevated due to the devastating pathophysiology of an MI: an acute rupture of an atherosclerotic plaque results in sudden thrombosis and occlusion of artery [6]. Impaired blood flow leads to oxygen deprivation and cardiomyocyte death within 20 minutes, which precludes the patient's arrival at a medical facility [7]. Cellular necrosis then activates an intense inflammatory response, mediated by cytokines, attracting leucocytes to the ischemic area [8]. The reaction is essential for the debridement of dead tissue and the formation of a collagen scar; however, it may also harm viable heart tissue, leading to expansion of the MI. The rapid and sustained inflammatory response can be tempered by rapid medical

Race L. Kao (ed.), *Cellular Cardiomyoplasty: Methods and Protocols*, Methods in Molecular Biology, vol. 1036,
DOI 10.1007/978-1-62703-511-8_11, © Springer Science+Business Media New York 2013

intervention. This creates an interesting paradox: the mortality rates following an MI are lower, but the number of patients surviving with damaged, weakened myocardium has increased. Presently, the therapeutic modalities for congestive heart failure are aimed at palliation of symptoms.

1.2 Cellular Cardiomyoplasty: Clinical and Cellular Limitations

The use of stem cell therapy to regenerate infracted myocardium has been in development since 1992 [9]. The scientific model for cellular cardiomyoplasty is simple: following an acute MI, stem cells are harvested from patients and expanded in vitro, before being implanted via intramyocardial or intracoronary route to the damaged tissue [10, 11]. Results from clinical trials show modest improvement in heart function, collectively averaging between 3.3 and 5.9 % amelioration in left ventricular ejection fraction [11–14]. Although intriguing, the benefits of cellular cardiomyoplasty are severely hampered by marginal retention of stem cells: less than 10 % remain 24 hours after implantation. Cell loss has been hypothesized to be the result of cell death or through mechanical factors inherent to a beating heart. Implementation of stem cells into recently infracted tissue is problematic due to inadequate tissue perfusion, coupled with extensive free radical formation and apoptosis caused by necrotic cells. Mechanical factors such as forceful, continuous contractions of the heart may expel cells from the myocardium and may contribute to cell loss. Additionally, intramyocardial injection of cells can lead to leakage through the injection tract created by the needle puncture, while intracoronary infusion results in rapid washout through the coronary venous system [15–18].

Widespread clinical application of cellular cardiomyoplasty is further hindered by the necessity of performing an autologous harvest of the bone marrow cells to prevent a profound immunological reaction. Stem cells obtained from elderly patients with multiple comorbidities are often frail, demonstrating slow proliferation and early apoptosis [19]. Consequently, these cells may be unsuitable for cellular cardiomyoplasty.

1.3 Microcapsules as a Method of Delivery

To alleviate these limitations, current research is focused on developing efficacious methods of delivery. A particularly promising concept consists of microencapsulation, which consists of a thin, semipermeable polymer membrane, surrounding the stem cells. The size of the micropores allows stem cells to secrete cytokines to the exterior of the membrane, while simultaneously preventing the influx of immunoglobulins into the capsule [20]. Microencapsulation would prevent an immune reaction from occurring, concurrently protecting cells from the harsh environment prevalent after an MI. The semipermeable membrane enables the diffusion of oxygen and nutrients into the cell environment while permitting cellular waste products to exit. Microencapsulation will prevent stem cell loss by enhancing the retention of the

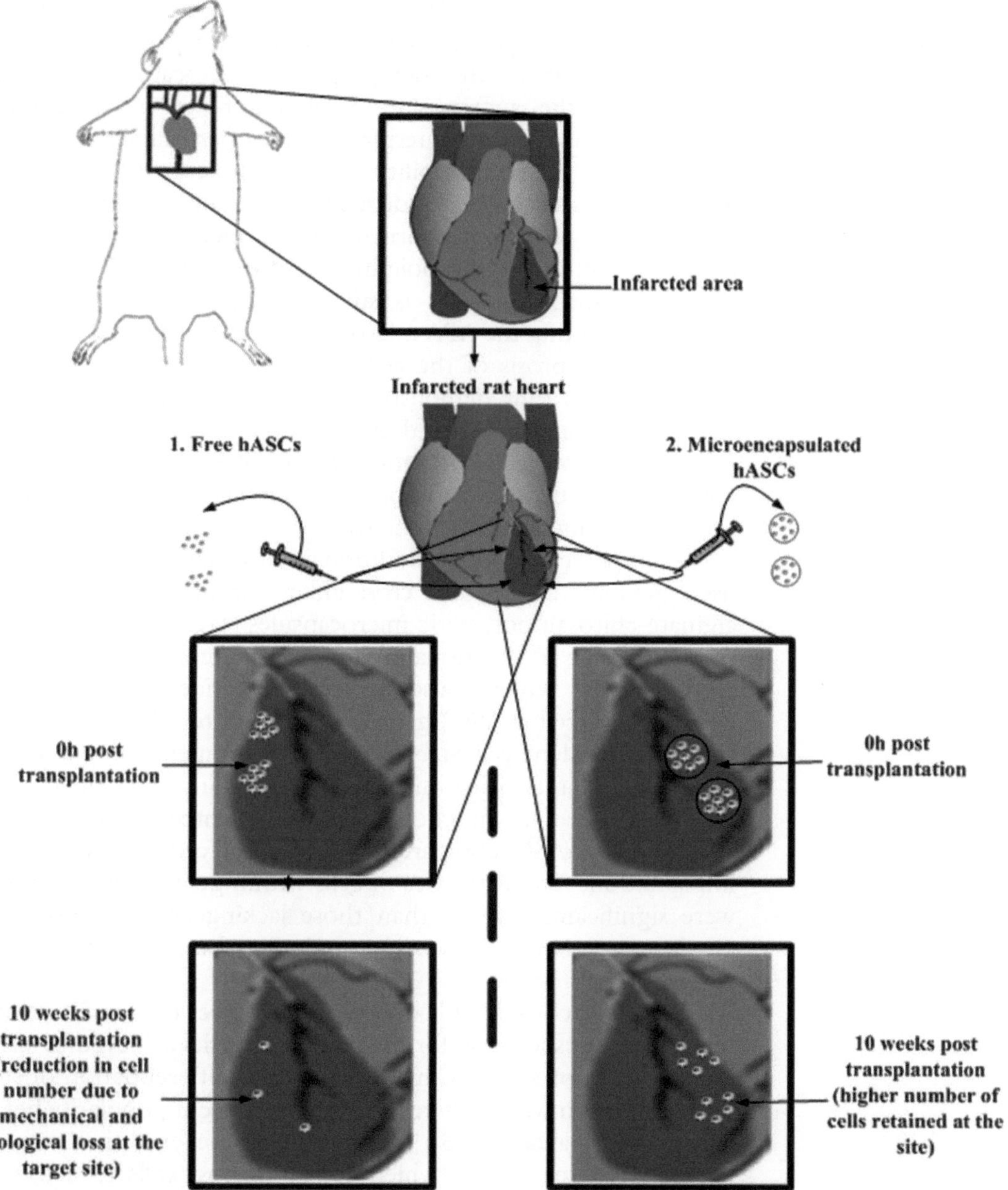

Fig. 1 Schematic representation of direct intramyocardial delivery of microencapsulated adipose stem cells (hASCs) at the peri-infarct sites in comparison to free hASCs. We hypothesized that compared to nonencapsulated free hASCs (Method 1), the microencapsulated hASCs (Method 2) can better retain the transplanted cells at the infarct site, reduce massive mechanical cell washouts into microcirculation and inhibit biological cell losses induced by the beating heart. The higher retention of transplanted viable cells at the infarct site (in this study, 10 weeks post transplantation) can eventually facilitate superior functional improvement of the infracted heart [34]

transplanted at the site (Fig. 1). Blood vessels in the heart are less than 200 μm in diameter. Accordingly, intramyocardial injection of microspheres with diameters above this threshold are more likely to be retained within the myocardium [21, 22].

1.4 Types of Microcapsules

Two different types of microcapsules have been utilized in cellular cardiomyoplasty, alginate-poly-L-lysine-alginate (APA) and genipin cross-linked alginate-chitosan polymeric microcapsules (GCAC). Selection of the appropriate membrane for a microcapsule is governed by an intricate interplay between permeability, structural stability, and biocompatibility [23]. APA capsules are widely investigated as a method for disseminating continuous therapeutics and are used to deliver pharmacological agents, as well as islets, mesenchymal, and erythropoietin secreting cells [24–27]. Presently, complete biocompatibility is still pending; as an inflammatory reaction, targeting the APA microcapsule has been noted leading to premature apoptosis of the cells within the membrane [28, 29]. These capsules thus demonstrate poor long-term viability as the structure is deformable and demonstrate cell leakage [30, 31]. Some studies suggest that implantation of APA microcapsules in conjunction with dexamethasone may temper the immune response, prolonging functionality of the structure [27, 32].

As an alternative to a traditional APA membrane, Paul et al. used genipin, a nontoxic cross-linker for proteins, to develop alginate-chitosan polymeric microcapsules (GCAC). GCACs were more resistant to rotational and osmotic pressures compared to APA capsules. GCAC also achieved superior human adipose-derived stem cell (hASC) growth compared to APAs while maintaining equivalent cell viability [33]. Subsequent in vivo studies suggest that rats with infracted myocardium benefited from improved cardiac function when implanted with genipin-encapsulated hASC, compared to unenclosed cells. Ten weeks after implantation, retention rates of cells within genipin microcapsules were significantly higher than those lacking an enclosure [34]. Genipin is a relatively new compound; therefore, its biocompatibility remains untested.

Presently, considerable debate remains over the precise cellular mechanisms responsible for the clinical benefits achieved by cellular cardiomyoplasty. Two hypotheses, transdifferentiation of stem cells and fusion with host cells, enjoyed transient popularity before falling out of favor [35, 36]. Currently, it is believed that stem cell release paracrine factors which act upon host cells to activate a regenerative process [37, 38]. The use of microcapsules transcends this controversy. Microcapsules are a viable delivery method in the event that transdifferentiation or fusion is the primary mechanism for cellular cardiomyoplasty. Conversely, biocompatible polymeric microcapsules may provide sustained release of cytokines from encapsulated cells to promote myocardial angiogenesis, as demonstrated in our recent study [34]. Moreover, microcapsules have important implications in the delivery of pharmacological drugs, conferring universal appeal, beyond the scope of regenerative medicine.

2 Materials

2.1 APA Microcapsules

1. 2-Ethoxyethyl acetate 98 %.
2. Phosphate-buffered saline (PBS, Invitrogen).
3. 1 % alginate acid: Mix 0.9 % saline with alginic acid (200 cps, Sigma Laboratories).
4. 0.1 M calcium chloride.
5. 0.1 % poly-L-lysine (Mw 27.4 kDa).
6. 1.5 % sodium alginate solution (low viscosity).
7. Saturated sodium citrate.
8. Saturated ethylenediaminetetraacetic acid (Fisher, ACS grade).
9. 2-Ethoxyethyl acetate.
10. Molecular Probes (Invitrogen, Calsbad, CA, USA).
11. Encapsulator (Innotech Biotechnologies Ltd, Basel Switzerland).
    - 100 μm nozzle.
12. Filter (0.22 μm pore size).
13. Spectrophotometer.

2.2 GCAC Microcapsules

1. 1.5 % sodium alginate solution with deionized water.
2. Alginic acid sodium (Sigma Chemicals, St. Louis, MO).
3. Poly-L-lysine hydrobromide (Sigma Chemicals, St. Louis, MO).
4. Chitosan (Wako BioProducts, USA).
5. Encapsulator (Innotech Corp).
    - 200 μm nozzle.
6. Filter (0.22 μm).
7. 0.1 M $CaCl_2$.
8. Acetic acid.
9. Genipin (Wako Chemicals USA Inc).

2.3 Transduction of Cells with Lac Z Gene

1. Polybrene 4 μg/ml (Sigma).
2. E86 retroviral vector carrying Lac Z gene.
3. Filter (0.80 μm).
4. Fresh culture medium (DMEM supplemented with 10 % serum).
5. Chromogenic X-gal staining substrate solution (Invivogen, San Diego, CA).

2.4 GCAC Microcapsules Encapsulating Stem Cells

1. 1.5 % sodium alginate solution with stem cells (0.5×10^6 cells/ml) within 0.1 M $CaCl_2$.
2. hASC (Invitrogen).
3. Encapsulator (Innotech Corp).
   - 200 μm Nozzle.
4. 0.89 % saline physiological solution.
5. Sodium alginate (low viscosity).
6. Chitosan (Sigma, low viscosity: $Mv = 7.2 \times 10^4$ by viscometry).
7. Genipin (Wako Chemicals USA Inc).

2.5 APA Microcapsules Encapsulating Stems Cells

1. hASCs (Invitrogen).
2. Encapsulator.
   - 200 μm Nozzle size.
3. Physiological solution.
4. Sodium alginate.
5. Fresh culture medium (DMEM supplemented with 10 % serum).

2.6 Monitoring Cell Growth Within GCAC and APA Microcapsules

1. PBS (Invitrogen).
2. 27 mM NaCl solution with 100 mM sodium citrate with 10 mM MOPS (Sigma-Aldrich).
3. EthD-III Cell Viability Assay (Biotium, Inc., Hayward, USA).
4. Calcein AM Cell Viability Assay (Biotium, Inc., Hayward, USA).

2.7 Intramyocardial Injections of Microspheres into Rat Myocardium

1. PBS (Invitrogen).
2. Saturated sodium nitrate.
3. Ethylenediaminetetraacetic acid (EDTA).
4. Anesthetic for rats.
5. 27 or 25 gauge needles.
6. Restraining Tube.
7. Clean Gauze.

2.8 Quantitative Analysis of Microspheres

1. 4 M Ethanolic KOH (Commercial Alcohol Inc., Ontario, Canada) and KOH Sigma, ACS grade.
2. TWEEN 80.
3. Saturated sodium citrate.
4. EDTA.
5. Deionized water.
6. 2-Ethixyethyl acetate.

2.9 Histological Analysis of Heart (Lac Z Staining)

1. X-gal chromogenic solution.
2. Incubator set at 37 °C.
3. PBS.
4. 2 % paraformaldehyde.
5. Paraffin.
6. Microtome.
7. Eosin dye.

2.10 PCR Analysis of Heart When Employing Gender-Mismatched Stem Cells

1. DNeasy (Qiagen, Valencia, CA).
2. Microsatellite sequence within the human Y chromosome (DYS390).
3. Taq DNA polymerase (Invitrogen).
4. The following primers [39, 40]:
   - Forwardprimer: 5′TATATTTTACACATTTTTGGGCC3′.
   - Reverseprimer: 5′TGACAGTAAAATGAACACATTGC3′.
5. Agarose gel.

3 Methods

3.1 APA Microcapsule Preparation to Encapsulate Microspheres

1. Create a standard regression line to determine the number of microspheres/fluorescence unit (diameter 10 μm, similar to cell size in suspension). Microspheres with a diameter of 10 μm will be used as an example for the calculation. Each vial of Molecular Probes (Invitrogen) contained 36 million microspheres/fluorescence unit.
2. Pipette seven samples of 50 μl of microspheres (180,000 U) and dissolve each sample in 3 ml of 2-ethoxyethl acetate 98 %.
3. Allow the samples to stand for 24 h.
4. Perform the following dilutions: 1:50, 1:100, 1:200, and 1:400 diluted in physiological saline solution. Take 200 μl from each sample.
5. Have the microtiter spectrophotometer read each sample twice.
6. Use the averaged values to construct a standard regression curve of fluorescence versus microspheres.
7. Depending on number of microspheres required, centrifuge the suspension at 2,000 × *g* for 15 min.
8. Mix pelleted microspheres with 0.89 % saline and alginic acid (200 cps, Sigma Laboratories), so that the final concentration of alginate obtained is 1 % (*see* **Notes 1** and **2**).

9. Run the solution through the encapsulator (Innotech Biotechnologies Ltd, Basel Switzerland), employing the 100 μm nozzle (*see* **Notes 3** and **4**). Use the following parameters:
   - Frequency at 2,000 Hz.
   - Voltage at 0.917 V.
   - Speed at 4.0 min^{-1}.
10. Collect the microcapsules (diameter of 200–250 μm), and solidify for 10 min within a stirred solution of 0.1 M of calcium chloride (*see* **Note 5**).
11. Filter the solidified beads by immersing the beads in 0.1 % poly-L-lysine and then in 0.1 % alginate for 10 min.
12. The formed microcapsules are then suspended within a saline solution.
13. Depolymerize the APA microcapsule to release the microspheres contained within. This will enable the determination of microsphere content per milliliter of encapsulated solution.
14. Pipette samples consisting of 50 μl of microcapsules.
15. Dissolve each sample in 10 ml of saturated sodium citrate for 1 h.
16. Centrifuge the solution.
17. Dissolve the pellet in saturated ethylenediaminetetraacetic acid (Fisher, ACS grade).
18. Centrifuge the solution again.
19. Wash with deionized water.
20. Dissolve pellets in 3 ml of 2-ethoxyethyl acetate.
21. Run samples through spectrophotometer twice to determine the number of microspheres per milliliter of encapsulated solution using the standard regression curve.
22. Alternatively, 400 μm microcapsules can be produced with prepared by changing the following parameters for the encapsulator, at **step 5**.
   - Use the 200 μm nozzle.
   - Frequency at 2,066 Hz.
   - Voltage at 1,332 V.
   - Speed at 14.2 m/min.

The remaining steps for filtration and washing remain unchanged.

3.2 GCAC Microcapsule Preparation

1. Prepare 1.5 % sodium alginate solution in deionized water, then sterile filter the solution through a 0.22-μm filter.
2. Extrude the solution through an encapsulator (Innotech Corp), employing a 200 μm nozzle.

3. Gelate the solution in 0.1 M $CaCl_2$ solution for 20 min.
4. Dissolve chitosan solution (2 %) in saline solution with pH adjusted to 5.2 using dilute acetic acid.
5. Immerse the core alginate beads in the chitosan solution for 30 min.
6. Wash the beads with normal physiological solution twice.
7. Immerse the beads in genipin solution (5 mg/ml) solution for 24 h at 37 °C, promoting cross-linking with the chitosan layer.

3.3 Transduction of Cells with Lac Z Gene Before Encapsulation

1. Transductions may be performed on the cells using the E86 retroviral vector containing the Lac Z gene or similar Lac Z gene delivery vehicle to transfect the cells before in vivo transplantation.
2. Filter the viral supernatants through 0.80 μm filters, and then infect the desired cells.
3. Add 10 ml of viral supernatant and 4 μg/ml polybrene (Sigma) to the cells, and allow 24 h to elapse. After the appropriate time delay, remove the medium containing the viral supernatant, and replace with fresh medium.
4. Repeat the previous step.
5. To confirm the efficiency of transduction, replate an aliquot of transduced cells in a 6-well plate, and stain with the chromogenic substrate X-gal to detect for β-galactosidase activity. Transduction rates should range from 70 to 80 %.

3.4 Preparation of GCAC Containing Transduced Stem Cells

1. Use an encapsulator (Innotech Corp) with a 200 μm nozzle, to dispense droplets of 1.5 % sodium alginate solution containing cells (0.5×10^6 cells/ml) into a solution of 0.1 M $CaCl_2$, under constant stirring.
2. After 20 min of stirring, take the newly formed beads and immerse the beads in a chitosan solution for 30 min (*see* **Note 6**).
3. Wash the microcapsules with normal physiological solution twice.
4. Immerse the microcapsules in genipin solution (5 mg/ml) solution for 24 h at 37 °C, promoting cross-linking with the chitosan layer.

3.5 Preparation of APA Microcapsules Containing Stem Cells

1. Resuspend stem cells (0.5×10^6 cells/ml) in alginate solution, and extrude through the nozzle (200 μm) on the stirring 0.1 M of calcium chloride.
2. Wash the APA capsules with physiological solution twice.
3. Immerse the formed beads in 0.1 % poly-L-lysine for 5 min and then in 0.1 % alginate for another 5 min.

4. Wash the resulting APA microcapsules in saline solution, and replenish them with fresh media in a culture flask (*see* **Note 7**).
5. Place the flask containing microencapsulated cells in an incubator at 37 °C, containing 5 % CO_2 for further culture of the encapsulated cells (*see* **Note 8**).

3.6 Monitoring Cell Growth Within GCAC and APA Microcapsules

1. Take 1,000 GCAC and 1,000 APA stem cell containing microcapsules and wash with PBS.
2. Treat the microcapsules with 27 mM NaCl solution containing: 100 mM sodium citrate, and 10 mM MOPS (Sigma-Aldrich) for 1 h at room temperature. This will break the microcapsules, allowing for retrieval of the cells contained within.
3. Centrifuge the broken and dissolved microcapsules at 800 rpm for 7 min to recover the free cells from the pellet. Discard the sodium citrate and capsular fragments in the supernatant.
4. Wash the cells three times with PBS to get rid of the excess sodium citrate solution and polymeric debris.
5. Stain the cells with viability assay kits, EthD-III and calcein AM according to the manufacturer's protocol (available from Biotium, Inc., Hayward, USA). EthD-III enters cells with damaged membranes, binds to nucleic acids, and produces bright red fluorescence in deceased cells. Calcein AM dye is a nonfluorescent, cell-permanent, poly-anionic substance converted by intracellular esterase to fluorescent green. The suggested concentrations are 2 μM calcein AM in PBS and 4 μM EthD-III in PBS.
6. Quantify the number of viable cells with hemocytometer and fluorescence microscope (*see* **Note 9**).

3.7 Intramyocardial Injection of Microencapsulated Stem Cells into Rat Myocardium

1. Take 1.5×10^6 Lac Z gene-transduced hASCs (male donor) encapsulated in microcapsules suspended within 150 μl media, and divide into three injections. Use a 27 or 25 gauge needle for implantation (*see* **Notes 10–13**).
2. Perform three intramyocardial injections into the left ventricle of female rats (*see* **Note 14**).
3. Sacrifice the rats after 10 weeks and section a part of the ventricular region for histological analysis and Lac Z staining to trace the transplanted cells (Fig. 2a).
4. Store another part of the heart tissue sample for PCR analysis to trace the Y chromosome of transplanted male donor cells in gender-mismatched female rats (Fig. 2b).

3.8 Histological Analysis of Heart (Lac Z Staining)

1. Add the X-gal chromogenic solution to the harvested rat hearts.
2. Incubate the specimens for 8 h at 37 °C.

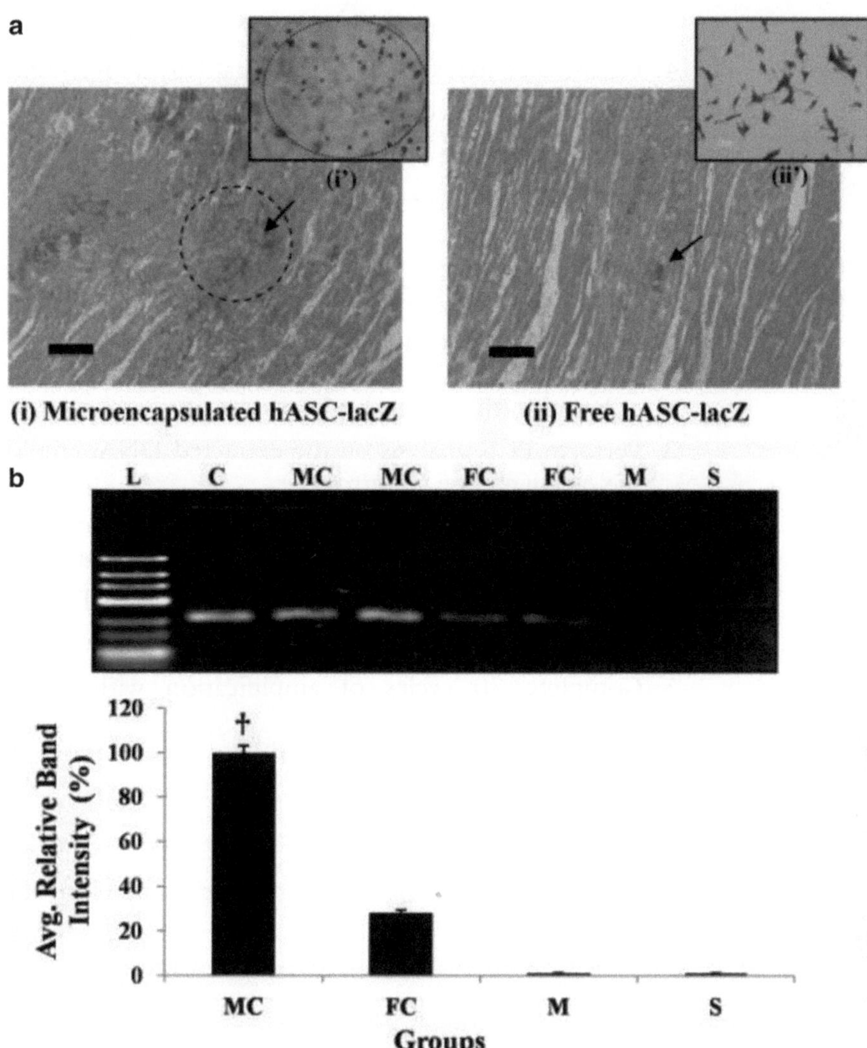

Fig. 2 Higher retention of adipose stem cells (hASCs) in the *left* ventricular myocardium using microcapsules 10 weeks post transplantation. Histological sections of the *left* ventricular heart stained with X-gal in (**ai**) encapsulated hASCs group and (**aii**) free hASCs group. The transplanted hASCs are indicated by the *arrows*. **ai**′ represents the X-gal stained microencapsulated hASCs, with stable Lac Z expression, which were used for transplantation in microencapsulated hASC group. This positive X-gal staining illustrates that the encapsulated cells were viable and express the Lac Z transgene from within the microcapsules. **aii**′ represents the X-gal-stained monolayer hASC culture, stably transduced with Lac Z gene, which were used for transplantation in free hASC group. The scale bars indicate 100 μm. (**b**) PCR products (250 bp) specific for the human Y chromosome (DYS390 sequence) as detected in 2 % agarose gel. There were clear and distinct bands in all the female rat hearts with microencapsulated male hASCs at 10 weeks (MC). These band intensities were much lower in free hASC groups (FC). Two PCR products from each group are shown here. The Image J analysis of the band intensities show the FC group with average 28 % band intensity taking the band intensity of MC group as 100 %. *C* represents the positive control for the in vitro cultured male hASCs, whereas *M* represents the negative control for the group M treated with empty microcapsules and *S* represents the myocardium for the sham group S. *Statistically significant between microencapsulated hASCs and free hASCs [34]

3. Remove the specimens from the incubator and wash with PBS.
4. Fix the specimens in 2 % paraformaldehyde overnight.
5. Once fixation is complete, embed the myocardium in paraffin.
6. Use a microtome to cut ribbon sections of the tissue.
7. Stain the specimens with eosin dye.

3.9 PCR Analysis of Heart When Employing Gender-Mismatched Stem Cells

1. Following the manufacturer's instructions, use DNeasy (Qiagen, Valencia, CA) to purify the genomic DNA.
2. Use the microsatellite sequence within the human Y chromosome (DYS390) to confirm the presence of viable human male cells within the female rat hearts.
3. Perform PCR analysis on the extracted DNA, employing Taq DNA polymerase (Invitrogen).
4. The following primers, with an amplicon size of 250 bp, were used to detect the specific gene product [39, 40]:
   - Forward primer: 5′TATATTTTACACATTTTTGGGCC3′.
   - Reverse primer: 5′TGACAGTAAAATGAACACATTGC3′.
5. Complete 30 cycles of amplification with the following parameters:
   - Denaturation: 94 °C for 15 s.
   - Annealing 54 °C for 20 s.
   - Extension 72 °C for 20 s.
6. Run the PCR products in agarose gel using electrophoresis to trace the DNA bands.

4 Notes

1. It has been seen that filtered alginate, rather than autoclaved alginate, produces superior, uniform shaped microcapsules.
2. If the capsules have a tendency to break during preparation, increasing the concentration of alginate may be beneficial.
3. Choose a nozzle diameter smaller than the desired microcapsule size.
4. If the microencapsulator nozzle gets blocked, wash it with 0.1 (M) NaOH solution.
5. Decreasing the number of cell loading may alleviate microcapsule fracture during preparation.
6. If the outer morphology of the capsules is irregular and there is debris in the suspending media, preparing fresh coating reagents will be helpful. In case of APA microcapsules, this may be because of old PLL stock solution which needs to be stored

properly at 4 °C. Reducing the chitosan and genipin coating time in GCAC preparation may also be beneficial.

7. If the media turns yellow within a day in culture, then there must be some contamination while preparing the microcapsules. Use antibiotics and antimycotic agents in media. Also make sure to sterilize all the components of the microencapsulator. You may also refilter the alginate solution prior to next use.
8. While maintaining the microencapsulated cells in cell culture flasks, make sure that you add enough media to submerge the microcapsules.
9. If the cells start losing their viability too early, then there can be some problem with coating procedure or inefficient nutrient/oxygen supply leading to a hypoxic condition and apoptosis. You may reduce the concentration of coating reagents to allow more media and oxygen to pass through the microcapsule membrane.
10. For in vivo studies, try using freshly prepared microencapsulated cells. If you get suboptimal results, you may want to increase the number of cells for the study.
11. For intravenous administration, you have to use smaller microcapsules (less than 100 μm) as bigger capsules can lead to artery blockage or embolism.
12. While administering the microcapsules, make sure to use syringes with proper needle size. Else this mechanical stress may damage the capsular surface leading to unwanted release and loss of viable cells.
13. Depending on the design of the experiment, suspending the microencapsulated cells in media of PBS before injecting the into experimental animals may be necessary.
14. For repeated administration of microencapsulated cells, it is preferable to maintain a gap of at least 6 weeks between injections, to allow for the capsules to be degraded.

Acknowledgments

This work is supported in part by research grant (to D Shum-Tim and S Prakash) from Natural Sciences and Engineering Research Council, Canada. A Paul acknowledges postdoctoral award from Fonds Québécois de la Recherche sur la Nature et les Technologies (FRSQ, Canada).

References

1. WHO Media Center (2012) Cardiovascular disease. http://www.who.int/mediacentre/factsheets/fs317/en/index.html
2. Roth GJ, Calverley DC (1994) Aspirin, platelets, and thrombosis: theory and practice. Blood 83:885–898
3. Shepherd J, Cobbe SM, Ford I, Isles CG, Lorimer AR, Macfarlane PW, McKillop JH, Packard CJ (1995) Prevention of coronary heart disease with pravastatin in men with hypercholesterolemia. N Eng J Med 333:1301–1308
4. DeWood MA, Spores J, Notske RN, Lang HT, Shields JP, Simpson CS, Rudy LW, Grunwald R (1979) Medical and surgical management of myocardial infarction. Am J Cardiol 44:1356–1364
5. Kuch B, Bolte HD, Hoermann A, Meisinger C, Loewel H (2002) What is the real hospital mortality from acute myocardial infarction? Epidemiological vs clinical view. Eur Heart J 23:714–720
6. Lilly L (2003) Pathophysiology of heart disease. Lippincott Williams & Wilkins, Baltimore, MD
7. Taki J, Higuchi T, Kawashima A, Tait JF, Kinuya S, Muramori A, Matsunari I, Nakajima K, Tonami N, Strauss HW (2004) Detection of cardiomyocyte death in a rat model of ischemia and reperfusion using 99mTc-labeled annexin V. J Nucl Med 45:1536–1541
8. Ono K, Matsumori A, Shioi T, Furukawa Y, Sasayama S (1998) Cytokine gene expression after myocardial infarction in rat hearts: possible implication in left ventricular remodeling. Circulation 98:149–156
9. Marelli D, Desrosiers C, el-Alfy M, Kao RL, Chiu RC (1992) Cell transplantation for myocardial repair: an experimental approach. Cell Transplant 1:383–390
10. Traverse JH, Henry TD, Ellis SG, Pepine CJ, Willerson JT, Zhao DX, Forder JR, Byrne BJ, Hatzopoulos AK, Penn MS, Perin EC, Baran KW, Chambers J, Lambert C, Raveendran G, Simon DI, Vaughan DE, Simpson LM, Gee AP, Taylor DA, Cogle CR, Thomas JD, Silva GV, Jorgenson BC, Olson RE, Bowman S, Francescon J, Geither C, Handberg E, Smith DX, Baraniuk S, Piller LB, Loghin C, Aguilar D, Richman S, Zierold C, Bettencourt J, Sayre SL, Vojvodic RW, Skarlatos SI, Gordon DJ, Ebert RF, Kwak M, Moyé LA, Simari RD (2011) Effect of intracoronary delivery of autologous bone marrow mononuclear cells 2 to 3 weeks following acute myocardial infarction on left ventricular function the LateTIME randomized trial. JAMA J Am Med Assoc 306(19):2110-211 9. Epub 2011 Nov 14
11. Abdel-Latif A, Bolli R, Tleyjeh IM, Montori VM, Perin EC, Hornung CA, Zuba-Surma EK, Al-Mallah M, Dawn B (2007) Adult bone marrow-derived cells for cardiac repair: a systematic review and meta-analysis. Arch Intern Med 167:989–997
12. Schächinger V, Erbs S, Elsässer A, Haberbosch W, Hambrecht R, Hölschermann H, Yu J, Corti R, Mathey DG, Hamm CW, Süselbeck T, Assmus B, Tonn T, Dimmeler S, Zeiher AM (2006) Intracoronary bone marrow-derived progenitor cells in acute myocardial infarction. N Eng J Med 355:1210–1221
13. Wollert K, Meyer G, Lotz J, Ringes-Lichtenberg S, Lippolt P, Breidenbach C, Fichtner S, Korte T, Hornig B, Messinger D, Arseniev L, Hertenstein B, Ganser A, Drexler H (2004) Intracoronary autologous bone-marrow cell transfer after myocardial infarction: the BOOST randomised controlled clinical trial. Lancet 364:141–148
14. Meyer GP, Wollert KC, Lotz J, Steffens J, Lippolt P, Fichtner S, Hecker H, Schaefer A, Arseniev L, Hertenstein B, Ganser A, Drexler H (2006) Intracoronary bone marrow cell transfer after myocardial infarction. Circulation 113:1287–1294
15. Müller-Ehmsen J, Whittaker P, Kloner RA, Dow JS, Sakoda T, Long TI, Laird PW, Kedes L (2002) Survival and development of neonatal rat cardiomyocytes transplanted into adult myocardium. J Mol Cell Cardiol 34:107–116
16. Retuerto MA, Schalch P, Patejunas G, Carbray J, Liu N, Esser K, Crystal RG, Rosengart TK (2004) Angiogenic pretreatment improves the efficacy of cellular cardiomyoplasty performed with fetal cardiomyocyte implantation. J Thorac Cardiovasc Surg 127:1041–1050
17. Zhang M, Methot D, Poppa V, Fujio Y, Walsh K, Murry CE (2001) Cardiomyocyte grafting for cardiac repair: graft cell death and anti-death strategies. J Mol Cell Cardiol 33:907–921
18. Teng CJ, Luo J, Chiu RCJ, Shum-Tim D (2006) Massive mechanical loss of microspheres with direct intramyocardial injection in the beating heart: implications for cellular cardiomyoplasty. J Thorac Cardiovasc Surg 132:628–632
19. Stolzing A, Scutt A (2006) Age-related impairment of mesenchymal progenitor cell function. Aging Cell 5:213–224
20. Christensen L, Dionne K, Lysaght M (1993) Biomedical application of immobilized cells. CRC Press, Boca Raton, FL
21. Al-Kindi A, Chen G, Asenjo J (2007) Microencapsulation to reduce mechanical loss of microspheres: implication in myocardial cell

therapy. Canadian Cardiovascular Congress, Quebec City, QC

22. Al Kindi AH, Asenjo JF, Ge Y, Chen GY, Bhathena J, Chiu RCJ, Prakash S, Shum-Tim D (2011) Microencapsulation to reduce mechanical loss of microspheres: implications in myocardial cell therapy. Eur J Cardiothorac Surg 39:241–247
23. Prakash S, Jones ML (2005) Artificial cell therapy: new strategies for the therapeutic delivery of live bacteria. J Biomed Biotechnol 1:44–56
24. Elliott RB, Escobar L, Calafiore R, Basta G, Garkavenko O, Vasconcellos A, Bambra C (2005) Transplantation of micro- and macroencapsulated piglet islets into mice and monkeys. Transplant Proc 37:466–469
25. Baruch L, Benny O, Gilert A, Ukobnik M, Ben Itzhak O, MacHluf M (2009) Alginate-PLL cell encapsulation system Co-entrapping PLGA-microspheres for the continuous release of anti-inflammatory drugs. Biomed Microdevices 11:1103–1113
26. Ding HF, Liu R, Li BG, Lou JR, Dai KR, Tang TT (2007) Biologic effect and immunoisolating behavior of BMP-2 gene-transfected bone marrow-derived mesenchymal stem cells in APA microcapsules. Biochem Biophys Res Commun 362:923–927
27. Murua A, de Castro M, Orive G, Hernández RM, Pedraz JL (2007) In vitro characterization and in vivo functionality of erythropoietin-secreting cells immobilized in alginate-poly-L-lysine-alginate microcapsules. Biomacromolecules 8:3302–3307
28. De Groot M, Schuurs TA, Van Schilfgaarde R (2004) Causes of limited survival of microencapsulated pancreatic islet grafts. J Surg Res 121:141–150
29. de Vos P, Bučko M, Gemeiner P, Navrátil M, Švitel J, Faas M, Strand BL, Skjak-Braek G, Morch YA, Vikartovská A, Lacík I, Kolláriková G, Orive G, Poncelet D, Pedraz JL, Ansorge-Schumacher MB (2009) Multiscale requirements for bioencapsulation in medicine and biotechnology. Biomaterials 30:2559–2570
30. Chen H, Ouyang W, Jones M, Metz T, Martoni C, Haque T, Cohen R, Lawuyi B, Prakash S (2007) Preparation and characterization of novel polymeric microcapsules for live cell encapsulation and therapy. Cell Biochem Biophys 47:159–167
31. Orive G, Maria Hernández R, Rodriguez Gascón A, Calafiore R, Swi Chang TM, Vos P, Hortelano G, Hunkeler D, Lacík I, Luis Pedraz J (2004) History, challenges and perspectives of cell microencapsulation. Trends Biotechnol 22:87–92
32. Říhová B (2000) Immunocompatibility and biocompatibility of cell delivery systems. Adv Drug Deliv Rev 42:65–80
33. Paul A, Cantor A, Shum-Tim D, Prakash S (2011) Superior cell delivery features of genipin crosslinked polymeric microcapsules: preparation, in vitro characterization and pro-angiogenic applications using human adipose stem cells. Mol Biotechnol 48:116–127
34. Paul A, Chen G, Khan A, Rao VT, Shum-Tim D, Prakash S (2012) Genipin-crosslinked microencapsulated human adipose stem cells augment transplant retention resulting in attenuation of chronically infracted rat heart fibrosis and cardiac dysfunction. Cell Transplant 21(12):2735–2751. Epub 2012 Apr 10
35. Nygren J, Jovinge S, Breitbach M, Säwén P, Röll W, Hescheler J, Taneera J, Fleischmann B, Jacobsen S (2004) Bone marrow-derived hematopoietic cells generate cardiomyocytes at a low frequency through cell fusion, but not transdifferentiation. Nat Med 10:494–501
36. Noiseux N, Gnecchi M, Lopez-Ilasaca M, Zhang L, Solomon SD, Deb A, Dzau VJ, Pratt RE (2006) Mesenchymal stem cells overexpressing Akt dramatically repair infarcted myocardium and improve cardiac function despite infrequent cellular fusion or differentiation. Mol Ther 14:840–850
37. Gnecchi M, He H, Liang OD, Melo LG, Morello F, Mu H, Noiseux N, Zhang L, Pratt RE, Ingwall JS, Dzau VJ (2005) Paracrine action accounts for marked protection of ischemic heart by Akt-modified mesenchymal stem cells. Nat Med 11:367–368
38. Gnecchi M, Zhang Z, Ni A, Dzau VJ (2008) Paracrine mechanisms in adult stem cell signaling and therapy. Circ Res 103:1204–1219
39. Atoui R, Asenjo J-F, Duong M, Chen G, Chiu RCJ, Shum-Tim D (2008) Marrow stromal cells as universal donor cells for myocardial regenerative therapy: their unique immune tolerance. Ann Thorac Surg 85:571–579
40. Kayser M, Caglià A, Corach D, Fretwell N, Gehrig C, Graziosi G, Heidorn F, Herrmann S, Herzog B, Hidding M, Honda K, Jobling M, Krawczak M, Leim K, Meuser S, Meyer E, Oesterreich W, Pandya A, Parson W, Penacino G, Perez-Lezaun A, Piccinini A, Prinz M, Schmitt C, Schneider PM, Szibor R, Teifel-Greding J, Weichhold G, de Knijff P, Roewer L (1997) Evaluation of Y-chromosomal STRs: a multicenter study. Int J Legal Med 110:125–133

Chapter 12

Angiogenic Nanodelivery Systems for Myocardial Therapy

Arghya Paul, Dominique Shum-Tim, and Satya Prakash

Abstract

Despite outstanding progress in the area of cardiovascular diseases, significant challenges remain in designing efficient delivery systems for myocardial therapy. Nanotechnology provides the tools to explore such frontiers of biomedical science at cellular level and thus offers unique features for potential application in the field of cardiac therapy. This chapter focuses on the methodology, based on the work done in our lab, to prepare and investigate two kinds of biocompatible nanoparticles (NPs) that can be useful for sustained delivery of single or multiple angiogenic growth factors to damaged sites, such as in myocardially infarcted heart to promote myocardial angiogenesis and reduce scar area.

Key words Nanoparticles, Myocardial therapy, Angiogenesis, Biotherapeutics, Nanomedicine

1 Introduction

1.1 Myocardial Infarction and Therapeutics

Congestive heart disease is one of the leading causes of death worldwide [1]. It mainly includes acute myocardial infarction which leads to left ventricular remodeling, including expansion or aneurysm formation due to cardiomyocyte death in infarcted regions and left ventricular dilation associated with hypertrophy and fibrosis of non-infarcted regions [2, 3]. A promising therapeutic approach to treat congestive heart diseases is administration of therapeutic growth factors, either as recombinant protein or by gene transfer [4–9]. The treatment process includes several corroborated mechanisms, such as induction of neovascularization and myocyte formation for improved cardiac function and limited ventricular remodeling. But these methods are limited by inefficient drug delivery strategies and suboptimal therapeutic effect due to loss of bioactivity of the proteins at the target site. A major problem for treatment of myocardial infarction is the limited access to the ischemic myocardium by protein or drug molecules in an active form. Delivering therapeutics, such as growth factors, bone marrow-derived hematopoietic stem cells, and stem cell-derived growth factors, remains a challenging process as most of these

Race L. Kao (ed.), *Cellular Cardiomyoplasty: Methods and Protocols*, Methods in Molecular Biology, vol. 1036, DOI 10.1007/978-1-62703-511-8_12, © Springer Science+Business Media New York 2013

substances do not remain at the site of interest which is the infarcted tissue zone. Potential causes include differences between animal models, the delivery approaches, and biological and mechanical loss of biotherapeutics due to beating nature of the heart. Additionally, it has been suggested that the failure to deliver sufficient growth factors into damaged hearts or lack of a consistently high number of growth materials in the site of injury could be the main reason for the inability to detect differentiated cardiac structures in damaged myocardium [10]. On the other hand, active pharmaceutical agents used for myocardial infarction therapy have severe side effects when used at cardioprotective doses which hinders their translation into clinical practice [11].

1.2 Nanoparticles: Their Unique Features and Potential in Delivery of Biotherapeutics

To address these problems, research towards the application of nanomaterials as vehicles for the delivery of therapeutic growth factors and agents in congestive heart and cardiovascular diseases is increasingly gaining importance [11–16]. Designing new biotherapeutic nanosystems, which are able to deliver therapeutics to the right place in a controlled manner, at appropriate times, and at the right dosage with minimal drug degradation, is an exciting area of current research. NP and microparticles composed of biodegradable polyester have been the most suitable and preferred system for such purpose [17–19]. This includes the use of polyisohexylcyanoacrylate and polyisobutylcyanoacrylate NP for the delivery of granulocyte colony-stimulating factor [17] and oligonucleotides [18] and the use of *N*-trimethyl chitosan NP as a vehicle for the nasal administration of ovalbumin [19]. Stromal cell-derived factor-1 is a well-characterized chemokine for attracting stem cells and thus a strong candidate for promoting regeneration. However, SDF-1 is cleaved by exopeptidases and matrix metalloproteinase-2 when injected directly in the host body. Self-assembling peptides which form nanofibers were generated for this purpose to make them resistant protease. Intramyocardial delivery of this nanoformulation after myocardial infarction recruited stem cells, increased capillary density, and improved cardiac function [20]. Currently, similar approaches are under intense research to explore its other unique characteristics such as targeting a specific tissue/or organ, antibody-mediated active targeting [21, 22], and cell-penetrating peptides [23, 24] for myocardial therapy.

Several factors need to be considered when designing delivery systems for biotherapeutics molecule such as proteins. It includes the methods of delivery (whether invasive or noninvasive), the stability of the protein (in vitro as well as in vivo), retention of biological function of the protein in the formulation (on the shelf as well as post delivery), and the dosage of the protein required for therapeutic efficiency. In addition, the nanomaterial needs to be nontoxic, biodegradable, non-immunogenic, and stable in presence of serum, has long half-life, can carry and release large amount of cargo to the target site, and should have features for controlled drug delivery. These factors determine the parameters of the controlled release formulation to be used. Moreover, the size, surface characteristics, and shape of an NP have a key role in its in vivo biodistribution. NPs smaller than 500 nm, such as dendrimers and short carbon nanotubes, are typically internalized via receptor-mediated endocytosis and particles less than 200 nm via clathrin mediated and others mostly via caveolae mediated [25]. On the other hand, microparticles (diameter 1–10 μm) are often processed via macropinocytic/phagocytic pathways. Intermediate-sized carriers (0.5–1 μm) are internalized via a mix of both modalities [26]. Other relevant criteria include choosing right material to enhance the shelf life. This includes materials such as synthetic biodegradable polymers, natural biopolymers, lipids, and polysaccharides which are safe as well as nontoxic upon degradation in the host system.

1.3 Albumin-Based Nanoparticles: Introduction and Overview of Protocol

Albumin, a versatile protein carrier for delivery of therapeutics, is a nontoxic, non-immunogenic, biocompatible, and biodegradable material [27]. Albumin NPs have gained considerable attention due to their high drug binding capacity and absence of any serious side effects. Among albumins from different origin, human serum albumin (HSA) is the most abundant plasma protein (~50 g/L of human serum) with an average half-life of 19 days. HSA is a very soluble globular monomeric protein consisting of 585 amino acid residues with a molecular weight of 66.5 kDa. Upon degradation, the amino acids from HSA provide nutrition to peripheral tissues. These properties as well as its preferential uptake in inflamed tissue, ready availability, bioresorbability, and lack of toxicity make it an ideal candidate for delivery of therapeutics [28]. The protocols to prepare albumin NP can be classified into three principal techniques; desolvation [5, 29], emulsification [30], nano spray drying, and clinically relevant nab Technology are currently used [27, 31–33].

Here we describe, in details, a widely used desolvation procedure [5] to prepare NP for efficient delivery of angiogenic growth factor proteins. Angiogenic growth factors, human vascular endothelial growth factor (VEGF), and human angiopoietin-1 (Ang1) are known to prevent vascular endothelial cell apoptosis and stimulate human vascular endothelial cell (HUVEC) proliferation for eventual myocardial angiogenesis in infarcted region of damaged heart. Here we documented a protocol to develop HSA NP, co-encapsulating VEGF and Ang1, and study the combined effect of these bioactive proteins for endothelial proliferation and evaluate the potential application of this delivery system towards therapeutic angiogenesis.

1.4 Alginate-Based Nanoparticles: Introduction and Overview of Protocol

Alginates are random, linear, and anionic polysaccharides consisting of linear copolymers of α-L-guluronate and β-D-mannuronate residues. This natural biopolymer has been widely used in numerous biomedical applications, including cell and drug delivery, as they are biodegradable, biocompatible, and mucoadhesive polymers [34]. Alginate polymers are also hemocompatible and have not been found to accumulate in any major organs and show evidence of in vivo degradation [35]. Research using alginate polymer as biotherapeutic drug delivery system has illustrated that the latter can maintain the structure and activity of biomolecules, are non-immunogenic, release the therapeutic agent in a sustained manner over time, and degrade to nontoxic metabolites that are either absorbed or excreted.

The interaction between amine groups of biodegradable cationic polymer, such as chitosan and polylysine, and carboxyl groups of anionic alginate biopolymers forms polyionic hydrogels, which have favorable characteristics for drug entrapment and delivery. Chitosan and polylysine, being cationic polymers, have been successfully used for the generation of microspheres and NP by ionotropic gelation with negatively charged alginate for delivery of drugs, proteins, DNA, and other therapeutic molecules [3, 36–38]. In addition, due to its nontoxic nature, repeated administration of therapeutic agents is possible. Here we report a detailed procedure to encapsulate pro-angiogenic growth factor, placental growth factor (PIGF), and a 50 kDa homodimeric glycoprotein sharing 53 % sequence homology at the amino acid level with VEGF, for efficient delivery of active protein molecules to the target infarct site in order to promote myocardial angiogenesis [16].

2 Materials

Prepare all solutions using ultrapure deionized water (using efficient purifying system such as Barnstead Reverse Osmosis system) and analytical grade reagents. Prepare and store all reagents at room temperature (unless indicated otherwise) and try to use them as fresh as possible for the experiments. In order to sterilize the prepared reagent stocks or working solutions, either filter them through 0.22 μm filter papers or autoclave them based on the nature of the reagents. Follow material safety data sheet and waste disposal regulation guidelines while working and disposing the reagents.

2.1 Albumin Nanoparticles

1. Human serum albumin (HSA; fraction V, purity 96–99 %) (Sigma Chemical Company, St. Louis, MO, USA). Store at 4 °C.
2. 10 mM NaCl solution.
3. 0.1 N NaOH for pH adjustment.

4. Recombinant proteins: human Ang 1 and VEGF 165 (R&D Systems, Minneapolis, MN).
5. Anhydrous ethyl alcohol. Store at RT.
6. 5 wt% glutaraldehyde solution (Sigma Chemical Company, St. Louis, MO, USA) Page 6.
7. Ultracentrifuge machine and centrifuge tubes (Beckman Coulter Inc, Ontario, Canada).
8. 5 mL scintillation glass vials.
9. Magnetic stirrer with magnetic bar (Fisher Scientific, Ontario, Canada).
10. Human VEGF and human Angl enzyme-linked immunosorbent assay (ELISA) kits (R&D systems Minneapolis, MN). Store at −4 °C.
11. CellTiter 96 Aqueous Non-Radioactive Cell Proliferation MTS Assay kit (Promega, Madison, USA). Store at −4 °C.
12. Multilabel Counter (Victor3TM, Perkin Elmer, Woodbridge, Canada).
13. 1× Phosphate buffered saline, pH 7.2 (Invitrogen, Burlington, Canada). Store at RT.
14. 96-well assay plates – tissue culture treated (Corning Incorporated, NY, USA).

2.2 Alginate Nanoparticles

1. Low viscosity alginic acid sodium salt (viscosity: ~250 cP, 2 % in water at 25 °C) from Sigma Chemicals (St. Louis, MO).
2. Chitosan (low viscosity, Mv = 7.2 × 104 by viscometry, degree of deacetylation at 73.5 % by titration) from Wako BioProducts (Richmond, VA).
3. Calcium chloride was bought from Sigma-Aldrich Canada Ltd (Oakville, Canada).
4. Magnetic stirrer with magnetic bar (Fisher Scientific, Ontario, Canada).
5. Ultracentrifuge machine and centrifuge tubes (Beckman Coulter Inc, Ontario, Canada).
6. Recombinant human PlGF and ELISA kit (R&D Systems Inc, Minneapolis, MN). Store at −4 °C.
7. Ultrasonic water bath sonicator (Branson 2510; Cleveland, OH).

3 Methods

3.1 Preparation of Albumin NP Co-encapsulating Vegf and Ang1 Angiogenic Proteins

Carry out all procedures at room temperature unless otherwise specified.

1. Add 100 mg of human serum albumin protein to 2 mL of 10 mM NaCl solution in a glass vessel.

2. Mix the solution at room temperature.
3. Adjust the pH of the solution to 8 by the adding 0.1 N NaOH (*see* **Note 1**).
4. Dissolve 14 μL of 0.5 mg/mL of Ang-1, 1 μL of 0.5 mg/mL human VEGF, and 1 μL of 0.5 mg/mL of bovine serum albumin in endothelial cell medium.
5. Add the growth factor cocktail into the human serum albumin solution.
6. Slowly add 4 mL of 100 % ethanol dropwise to the aqueous phase at a constant rate of 1 mL/min to form the NP by desolvation method (*see* **Notes 2–4**).
7. The clear protein solution slowly turns turbid by addition of alcohol, which confirms the generation of albumin NP (*see* **Notes 5–8**).
8. Stabilize the generated NP by adding 40 μL of 5 % glutaraldehyde and leave it for 4 h under stirring condition (*see* **Note 9**).
9. Ultracentrifuge the turbid solution at 20,000 × *g* for 30 min.
10. Disperse the formed NP pellets in double-distilled water using ultrasonicator for 15 min.
11. Repeat **steps 8** and **9** twice to completely wash the NP and make them completely dispersed in the solution. Figure 1 represents an anticipatory NP characterization study example, following the above-mentioned albumin NP preparation procedure (*see* **Notes 10** and **11**).
12. Lyophilize/free-dry the generated NP.
13. Store the dehydrated NP powder at −80 °C for term preservation.

3.2 Procedure to Analyze In Vitro Protein Release Kinetics of NP

1. Suspend the VEGF and Ang1 loaded NP in 5 mL of cell medium with 1 % penicillin/streptomycin and placed in a thermostatic environment at 37 °C with constant horizontal shaking (100 rpm) (*see* **Note 12**).
2. At appropriate time intervals, remove 0.4 mL of the buffer solution and replace with the same quantity of media in order to maintain same volume.
3. Centrifuge the collected buffer solution at 20,000 × *g* for 10 min to get rid of any particle debris or aggregates and store the NP supernatant, containing the released proteins, at −80 °C.
4. Thaw the frozen samples and measure the concentrations of VEGF and Ang1 released at different times using VEGF and Ang1 enzyme-linked immunosorbent assay (ELISA) (R&D Systems Inc) according to the manufacturer's instructions.

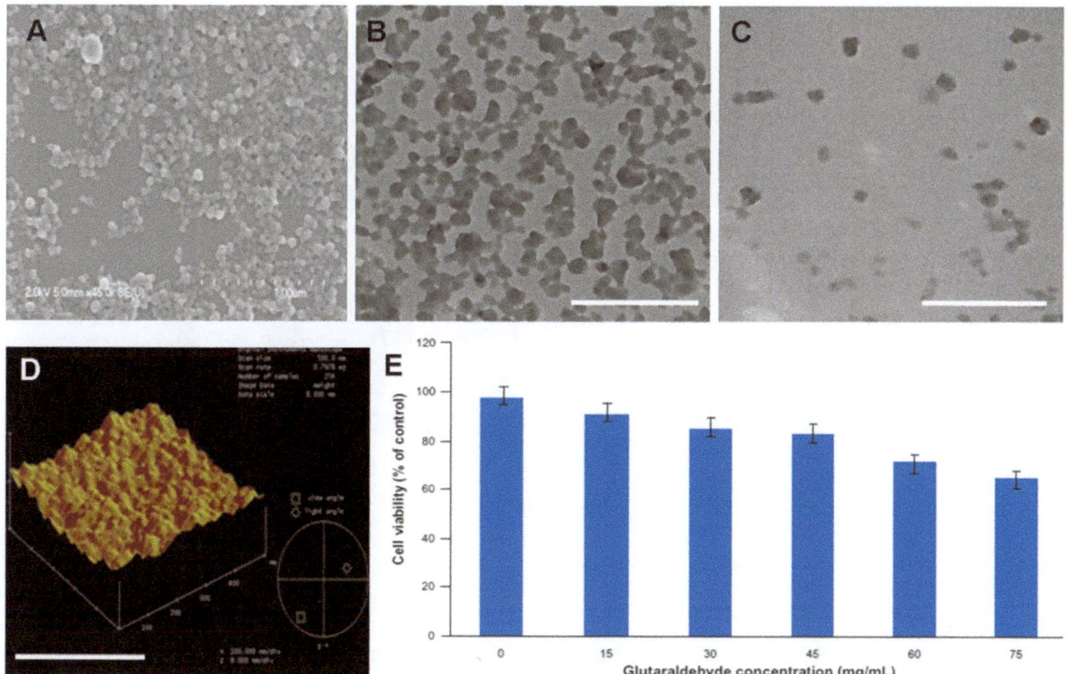

Fig. 1 (**a**) Scanning electron microscope (SEM) image of albumin NP prepared according to the procedure outlined. Transmission electron microscope (TEM) images of the albumin NP before (**b**) and after (**c**) final sonication step, showing evenly dispersed NP without any aggregate. (**d**) Three-dimensional atomic force microscopic image of prepared NP. Scale bar: 1,000 nm. (**e**) Albumin NPs exhibit no significant toxicity in vitro. The cytotoxicity of the blank NPs cross-linked with a series of glutaraldehyde concentrations was studied by incubating HUVECs for 96 h with the NPs. Percent cell viability over initial number of HUVECs treated with NPs for up to 96 h is shown. MTS cell proliferation assay was used to determine the cell viability after exposure to the NPs. NPs without glutaraldehyde coating showed a cell viability of above 90 % after 96 h. Increasing the amount of glutaraldehyde in the particle preparation increased the cytotoxicity of the NPs to the seeded HUVECs [5]

5. Make sure to perform the experiments in triplicate.
6. Repeat the above-described procedure to detect the release kinetics of only VEGF and only Ang1 encapsulating NP. Take bovine serum albumin loaded NP as the negative control.

Figure 2a, b represents anticipated VEGF and Ang1 release profiles (example) of the co-encapsulated NPs following the above-described procedure.

3.3 Endothelial Cell Proliferation Assay to Confirm Bioactivity of the Angiogenic NP

1. Seed 2×104 HUVEC cells/well in a 96-well plate with fresh medium.
2. After 24 h, remove the endothelial cell medium and wash the cells twice with PBS.
3. Quickly add 100 mL of NP supernatants from different groups, collected on different days from release kinetics study, to each well containing the washed seeded HUVEC.

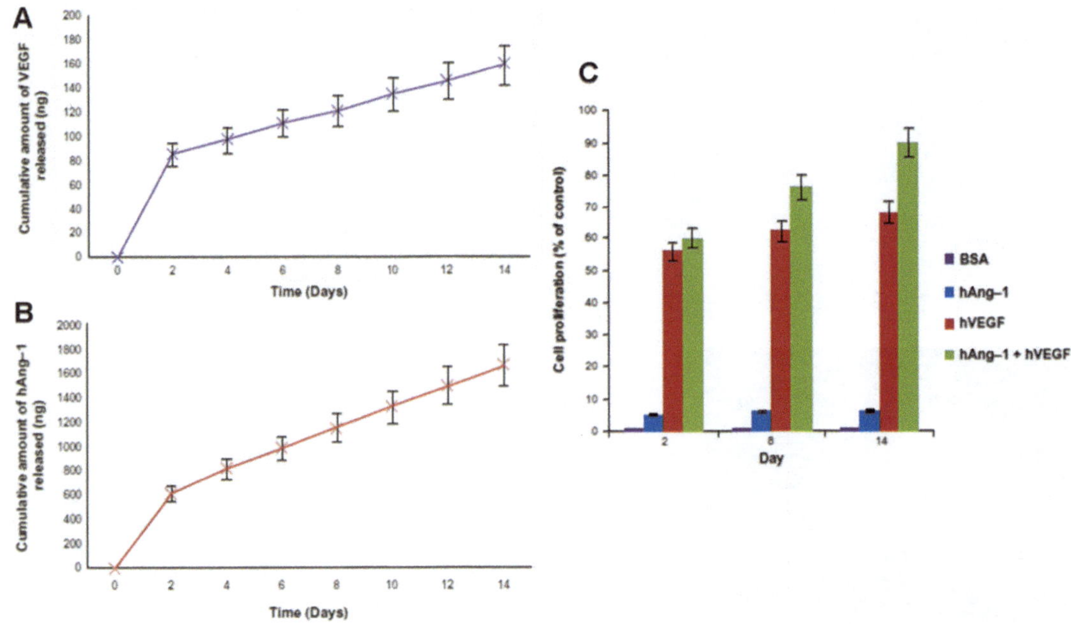

Fig. 2 Albumin NPs sustain in vitro protein release. (**a**, **b**) Cumulative amount of hAng-1 and hVEGF released from the NPs over a time period of 2 weeks. At the end of the 2-week incubation period, it was observed that ~49 % of hAng-1 and ~59 % of hVEGF had been released from the NPs. (**c**) Bioactivity of hAng-1 and hVEGF loaded in albumin NPs. The proliferation of HUVECs in response to the NP supernatant was observed. HUVECs were seeded in a 96-well plate and the media were replaced with NP supernatants from different groups containing VEGF, Ang1, Ang1 + VEGF, or control bovine serum albumin (BSA)-loaded NPs. After 96 h of culture, the results were illustrated as the percent increase in cell proliferation relative to the unstimulated control. Least cell proliferation is observed with hAng-1 and maximum proliferation is observed in supernatant with a combination of both hAng-1 and hVEGF. The supernatant with negative control BSA showed negligible effect as expected. An increasing cell proliferation is observed over the 2-week incubation period [5]

4. Incubate the cells for 96 h in cell culture incubator.
5. Wash the HUVECs twice with PBS.
6. Add 100 mL fresh endothelial cell medium to each well.
7. Add 20 mL of MTS solution to each well.
8. Incubate the cells for 4 h at 37 °C.
9. Measure the absorbance of each well using Multilabel Counter at 490 nm.
10. Analyze the data and plot the cell proliferation with respect to unstimulated control group. Figure 2c represents an anticipatory result (example) on assessing the bioactivity of the pro-angiogenic proteins after getting released from the NPs, following the above-mentioned procedure (*see* **Note 13**).

3.4 Preparation of Alginate NP Encapsulating PIGF Angiogenic Proteins

1. Add 10 mg of PIGF to 10 mL of 0.6 mg/mL aqueous sodium alginate solution (*see* **Notes 14** and **15**).
2. Dropwise add the 2 mL calcium chloride (0.67 mg/mL) to 10 mL of aqueous sodium alginate (0.6 mg/mL) while sonicating with an ultrasonic water bath sonicator (Branson 2510; Cleveland, OH) at 40 kHz for 60 min.
3. Transfer the resultant calcium alginate pre-gel to a 100 mL beaker and stir for 30 min with a magnetic bar.
4. Add 2 mL of 0.3 mg/mL solution of chitosan, dissolved in 3 % v/v acetic acid, into the beaker and stir for an additional 30 min to allow NP to have complete and uniform chitosan coating.
5. Collect the generated NP by ultracentrifugation at 20,000 × *g* for 60 min at 4 °C.
6. Disperse the resultant pellet NP in distilled water by sonicating in water bath sonicator for 2 min.
7. Wash the NP twice in water by ultracentrifugation by repeating **steps 5** and **6**. Figure 3 shows the scheme, mode of action, and implication of these NPs for efficient myocardial therapy by promoting rapid vasculogenesis.
8. Lyophilize/free-dry the generated NP and keep at −80 °C for term storage (*see* **Note 16**).
9. Follow the same procedure to prepare control empty NP without PIGF.

4 Notes

1. While preparing the albumin solution, it is important to adjust the pH as suggested. Improper pH adjustment may lead to formation albumin aggregates.
2. It is important to add the alcohol slowly and dropwise while preparing the albumin NPs. A fast addition of alcohol leads to incomplete NP formation which results in white albumin aggregates at the side of vial.
3. Stop adding the alcohol if the solution turns turbid, and wait until it becomes transparent again. If not, then do not add any more alcohol.
4. The magnetic stirrer speed can be optimized to achieve varied NP diameters to fit different applications.
5. If there still remain clumps of NP after ultracentrifugation, please reduce the centrifuge time and increase the sonication time to obtain evenly dispersed NP suspension.
6. The albumin concentration to prepare the NP will vary based on the molecular weight, charge, and other physical and biochemical properties of the protein molecules to be loaded.

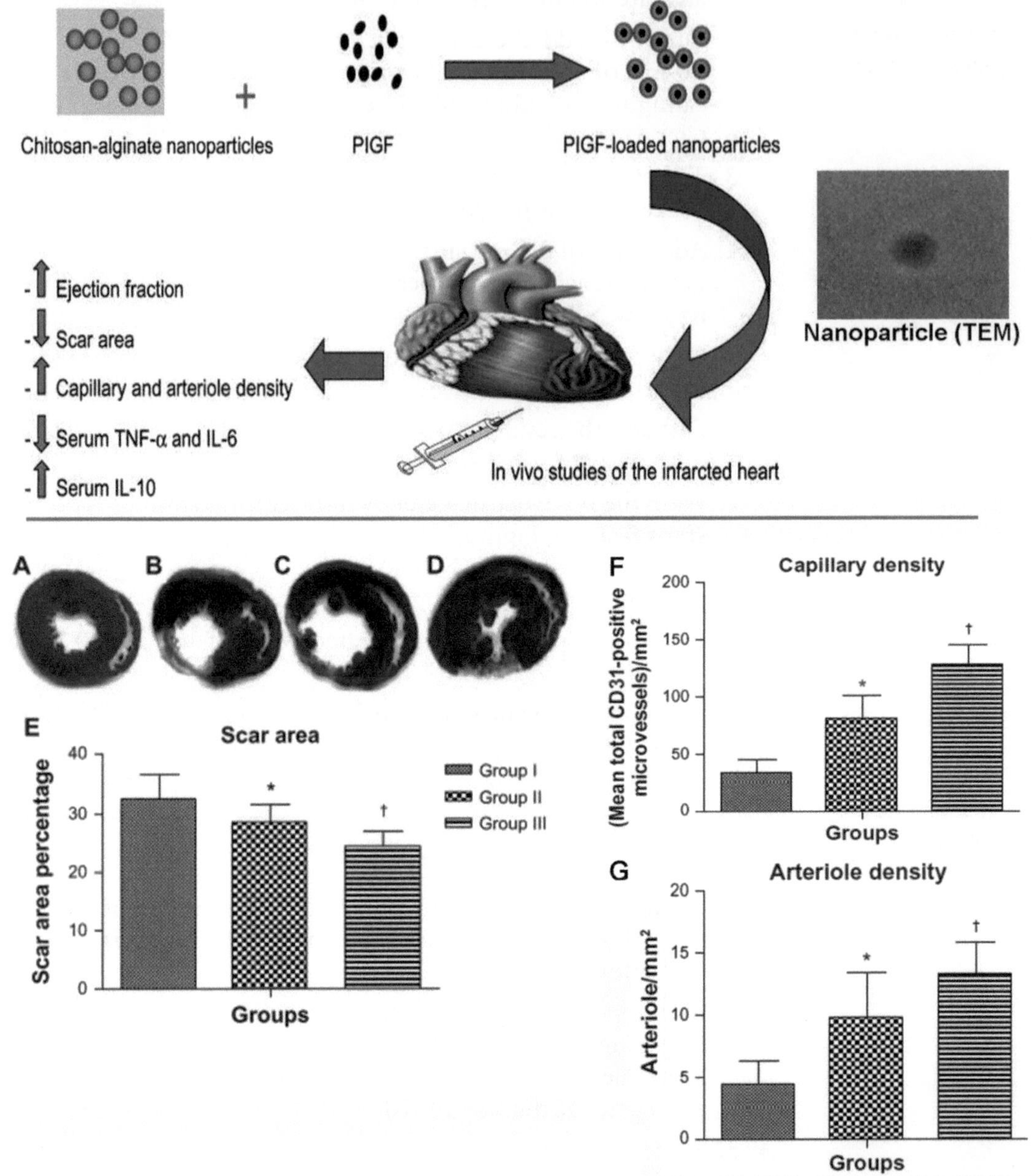

Fig. 3 Schematic representation of placental growth factor (PlGF) encapsulation with chitosan-alginate NPs and subsequent intramyocardial delivery to the infarcted rat heart. Its therapeutic effects include decrease in ventricle scar area formation (**a–e**: Masson's trichrome staining), increase in angiogenesis (**f**) and arteriogenesis (**g**), increase in cardiac function, and favorable effect in serum cytokine profile [group I (empty NPs), group II (free PlGF), and group III (NP + PlGF)]. Data represents mean ± standard deviation. *$P < 0.01$ versus group I; †$P < 0.01$ versus group II [16], p 12

7. The albumin and glutaraldehyde concentration can be varied to modulate the release kinetics of the encapsulated therapeutics based on the application type.
8. While choosing multiple protein molecules, it is ideal to have proteins of similar sizes or molecular weights to obtain evenly release of both the proteins from NPs.
9. As an alternate, the generated albumin NP can be stabilized with glutaraldehyde by leaving it for 12 h under stirring condition at 4 °C.
10. To determine the encapsulation efficiency of NPs, they need to be centrifuged at 20,000 × g for 15 min just after preparation to separate the NPs from the supernatant. Percentage encapsulation efficiency can be calculated as [(amount of initial growth factor loaded − amount of growth factor in supernatant)/amount of initial growth factor loaded] × 100.
11. It is beneficial to mix BSA with the therapeutic protein while preparing the NPs. This gives stability, helps retain bioactivity of the entrapped therapeutic proteins, as well as reduces the mechanical stress caused by the NP preparation process using sonicator, stirrer, ultracentrifugation, etc.
12. While co-encapsulating two or more proteins in NPs, the ratio of concentration of different proteins added during the NP preparation process is very important. In this preparation, the optimized amount of protein ratio used was optimized based on the fact that a ratio of 10:1 of Ang1 to VEGF gave best angiogenic and antiapoptotic results in vitro [5].
13. The MTS assay, used here for detecting HUVEC cell proliferation, can be used for analyzing the toxicity of different NP preparations as described in Fig. 1e and reported in earlier studies [5].
14. The alginate concentration to prepare the NP will vary based on the size, molecular weight, and other physical and chemical properties of the protein molecules to be entrapped.
15. NP containing bovine serum albumin as standard protein molecule works as a good negative control for such studies.
16. Similar procedures, as mentioned with albumin NPs, can be followed to study the protein release kinetics and confirm the bioactivity of the angiogenic alginate NP.
17. The NP described here is ideal for passive targeting and direct intramyocardial delivery. For other routes of administration and active targeting to the infarcted myocardium, the NPs can be surface functionalized with different targeting moieties that binds site-specifically to the cells in the infarcted region, such as antibodies or peptides against highly expressed cell surface receptors at the infarct site.

18. These nanodelivery systems can be readily modified to produce features such as fluorescence and radiography for imaging diagnostics, surface bio-functionalized for targeted delivery, and as adjuvants or alternatives to existing drug delivery methods.

Acknowledgments

This work is supported in part by research grant from Canadian Institutes of Health Research and Natural Sciences and Engineering Research Council, Canada. A. Paul acknowledges postdoctoral award from Fonds Québécois de la Recherche sur la Nature et les Technologies (FRSQ, Canada).

References

1. Lloyd-Jones D, Adams RJ, Brown TM et al (2010) Heart disease and stroke statistics-2010 update a report from the American Heart Association. Circulation 121:E46–E215
2. Reynolds HR, Srichai MB, Iqbal SN et al (2011) Mechanisms of myocardial infarction in women without angiographically obstructive coronary artery disease. Circulation 124:1414–1425
3. Paul A, Ge Y, Prakash S et al (2009) Microencapsulated stem cells for tissue repairing: implications in cell-based myocardial therapy. Regen Med 4:733–745
4. Yoon YS, Johnson IA, Park JS et al (2004) Therapeutic myocardial angiogenesis with vascular endothelial growth factors. Mol Cell Biochem 264:63–74
5. Khan AA, Paul A, Abbasi S et al (2011) Mitotic and antiapoptotic effects of nanoparticles coencapsulating human VEGF and human angiopoietin-1 on vascular endothelial cells. Int J Nanomedicine 6:1069–1081
6. Ko YT, Hartner WC, Kale A et al (2009) Gene delivery into ischemic myocardium by double-targeted lipoplexes with anti-myosin antibody and TAT peptide. Gene Ther 16:52–59
7. Paul A, Binsalamah ZM, Khan AA et al (2011) A nanobiohybrid complex of recombinant baculovirus and Tat/DNA nanoparticles for delivery of Ang-1 transgene in myocardial infarction therapy. Biomaterials 32:8304–8318
8. Shim WSN, Li W, Zhang L et al (2006) Angiopoietin-1 promotes functional neovascularization that relieves ischemia by improving regional reperfusion in a swine chronic myocardial ischemia model. J Biomed Sci 13:579–591
9. Takahashi K, Ito Y, Morikawa M et al (2003) Adenoviral-delivered angiopoietin-1 reduces the infarction and attenuates the progression of cardiac dysfunction in the rat model of acute myocardial infarction. Mol Ther 8:584–592
10. Kajstura J, Rota M, Whang B et al (2005) Bone marrow cells differentiate in cardiac cell lineages after infarction independently of cell fusion. Circ Res 96:127–137
11. Galagudza M, Korolev D, Postnov V et al (2012) Passive targeting of ischemic-reperfused myocardium with adenosine-loaded silica nanoparticles. Int J Nanomedicine 7:1671–1678
12. Riehemann K, Schneider SW, Luger TA et al (2009) Nanomedicine-challenge and perspectives. Angew Chem Int Ed 48:872–897
13. Paulis LE, Geelen T, Kuhlmann MT et al (2012) Distribution of lipid-based nanoparticles to infarcted myocardium with potential application for MRI-monitored drug delivery. J Control Release 162:276–285
14. Binsalamah ZM, Paul A, Prakash S et al (2012) Nanomedicine in cardiovascular therapy: recent advancements. Expert Rev Cardiovasc Ther 10:805–815
15. Paul A, Shao W, Shum-Tim D et al (2012) The attenuation of restenosis following arterial gene transfer using carbon nanotube coated stent incorporating TAT/DNA(Ang1+Vegf) nanoparticles. Biomaterials 33:7655–7664
16. Binsalamah ZM, Paul A, Khan AA et al (2011) Intramyocardial sustained delivery of placental growth factor using nanoparticles as a vehicle for delivery in the rat infarct model. Int J Nanomedicine 6:2667–2678
17. Gibaud S, Rousseau C, Weingarten C et al (1998) Polyalkylcyanoacrylate nanoparticles as carriers for granulocyte-colony stimulating factor (G-CSF). J Control Release 52:131–139

18. Fattal E, Vauthier C, Aynie I et al (1998) Biodegradable polyalkylcyanoacrylate nanoparticles for the delivery of oligonucleotides. J Control Release 53:137–143
19. Amidi M, Romeijn SG, Borchard G et al (2006) Preparation and characterization of protein-loaded N-trimethyl chitosan nanoparticles as nasal delivery system. J Control Release 111:107–116
20. Segers VFM, Tokunou T, Higgins LJ et al (2007) Local delivery of protease-resistant stromal cell derived factor-1 for stem cell recruitment after myocardial infarction. Circulation 116:1683–1692
21. Jaracz S, Chen J, Kuznetsova LV et al (2005) Recent advances in tumor-targeting anticancer drug conjugates. Bioorg Med Chem 13:5043–5054
22. Torchilin VP (2004) Targeted polymeric micelles for delivery of poorly soluble drugs. Cell Mol Life Sci 61:2549–2559
23. Gupta B, Levchenko TS, Torchilin VP (2005) Intracellular delivery of large molecules and small particles by cell-penetrating proteins and peptides. Adv Drug Deliv Rev 57:637–651
24. Lochmann D, Jauk E, Zimmer A (2004) Drug delivery of oligonucleotides by peptides. Eur J Pharm Biopharm 58:237–251
25. Rejman J, Oberle V, Zuhorn IS et al (2004) Size-dependent internalization of particles via the pathways of clathrin-and caveolae-mediated endocytosis. Biochem J 377:159–169, p 14
26. Decuzzi P, Godin B, Tanaka T et al (2010) Size and shape effects in the biodistribution of intravascularly injected particles. J Control Release 141:320–327
27. Elzoghby AO, Samy WM, Elgindy NA (2012) Albumin-based nanoparticles as potential controlled release drug delivery systems. J Control Release 157:168–182
28. Kratz F (2008) Albumin as a drug carrier: design of prodrugs, drug conjugates and nanoparticles. J Control Release 132:171–183
29. Abbasi S, Paul A, Shao W et al (2012) Cationic albumin nanoparticles for enhanced drug delivery to treat breast cancer: preparation and in vitro assessment. J Drug Deliv 2012:686108
30. Yang L, Cui F, Cun DM et al (2007) Preparation, characterization and biodistribution of the lactone form of 10-hydroxycamptothecin (HCPT)-loaded bovine serum albumin (BSA) nanoparticles. Int J Pharm 340:163–172
31. Conlin AK, Seidman AD, Bach A et al (2010) Phase II trial of weekly nanoparticle albumin-bound paclitaxel with carboplatin and trastuzumab as first-line therapy for women with HER2-overexpressing metastatic breast cancer. Clin Breast Cancer 10:281–287
32. Cortes J, Saura C (2010) Nanoparticle albumin-bound (nab (TM))-paclitaxel: improving efficacy and tolerability by targeted drug delivery in metastatic breast cancer. EJC Suppl 8:1–10
33. Lee SH, Heng D, Ng WK et al (2011) Nano spray drying: a novel method for preparing protein nanoparticles for protein therapy. Int J Pharm 403:192–200
34. Motwani SK, Chopra S, Talegaonkar S et al (2008) Chitosan-sodium alginate nanoparticles as submicroscopic reservoirs for ocular delivery: formulation, optimisation and in vitro characterisation. Eur J Pharm Biopharm 68:513–525
35. Rajaonarivony M, Vauthier C, Couarraze G et al (1993) Development of a new drug carrier made from alginate. J Pharm Sci 82:912–917
36. Paul A, Shum-Tim D, Prakash S (2010) Investigation on PEG integrated alginate-chitosan microcapsules for myocardial therapy using marrow stem cells genetically modified by recombinant baculovirus. Cardiovasc Eng Technol 1:154–164
37. Paul A, Shao W, Abbasi S et al (2012) PAMAM dendrimer–baculovirus nanocomplex for microencapsulated adipose stem cell-gene therapy: in vitro and in vivo functional assessment. Mol Pharm 9:2479–2488, p 15
38. Paul A, Nayan M, Khan AA et al (2012) Angiopoietin-1-expressing adipose stem cells genetically modified with baculovirus nanocomplex: investigation in rat heart with acute infarction. Int J Nanomedicine 7:663–682

Chapter 13

Bio-hybrid Tissue Engineering for Cellular Cardiomyoplasty: Future Directions

Juan Carlos Chachques

Abstract

Cardiomyopathy induces geometric alteration of the ventricular cavity, which changes from a natural elliptical (conical) to a spherical shape. Ventricular chamber dilatation and spherical deformation are important causes of morbidity and mortality among patients with congestive heart failure. In addition, diastolic dysfunction is an important clinical problem in these cases because there is no medical or surgical specific treatment. Myocardial tissue engineering associating stem cells represent a new road and fresh hope for this heart failure population.

Key words Heart failure, Ischemic heart disease, Cardiomyoplasty, Stem cell transplantation, Myocardial tissue engineering, Bioartificial myocardium, Chagas heart disease, Ventricular support bioprostheses

1 Background

Since intrinsic myocardial regeneration takes places but is reduced during a normal life span, it needs to be assisted by extrinsic bioactive procedures, like stem cell transplantation and tissue-engineered implants [1–3]. Extracellular matrix remodeling in myocardial diseases is related to excessive matrix degradation and myocardial fibrosis, contributing to left ventricular (LV) dilatation and progressive cardiac dysfunction [4].

Cell transplantation to the diseased heart has emerged as a promising strategy for refractory heart failure that cannot successfully be treated by conventional therapies. There is a growing body of evidence that when transplanting mesenchymal stem cells as a part of cardiac therapies, observed beneficial effects are mainly due to angiogenic and myogenic effects as well as paracrine factors secreted by the stem cells that are antiapoptotic and promote revascularization, cardiomyocyte survival, and reduction of fibrosis at the level of the infarcted tissue [5, 6].

Race L. Kao (ed.), *Cellular Cardiomyoplasty: Methods and Protocols*, Methods in Molecular Biology, vol. 1036,
DOI 10.1007/978-1-62703-511-8_13, © Springer Science+Business Media New York 2013

Among paracrine factors that could be responsible for the beneficial effect of the stem cell therapy, the most significant are believed to be vascular endothelial growth factor (VEGF), insulin-like growth factor 1 (IGF-1), and basic fibroblast growth factor that interestingly are upregulated by hypoxia. In fact, it has been demonstrated that hypoxic preconditioning of stem cells prior to implantation promotes their therapeutic potential as determined by their proangiogenic properties. Also, the stem cells have important anti-inflammatory properties, which may play a significant role in protection against ischemia reperfusion injuries [7, 8].

Current limitations of cell-based myocardial regenerative treatments can be summarized as follows:

- Cell bio-retention and engraftment within scar tissue is low.
- Mortality of implanted cells in ischemic myocardium is high.
- In ischemic heart disease the extracellular matrix (ECM) is pathologically modified.

Periodically repeated cell injections in poor responsive patients seem to be a solution for these problems [9] as well as tissue engineering for ECM replacement [10].

2 Myocardial Tissue Engineering

The stem cell niche, a specialized environment surrounding native and grafted stem cells, provides crucial support needed for stem cell maintenance. Compromised niche function may lead to the selection of stem cells that no longer depend on self-renewal factors produced by its environment. Stem cells seeded into a natural or synthetic structure capable of supporting 3D tissue formation can be injected into the myocardium or grafted onto the ventricular wall surface [2, 10].

Experimental and clinical studies in ischemic heart disease have showed that combining cell transplantation with matrix scaffolds offer further benefits with respect to cell therapy alone [11, 12]. Unfortunately patches of collagen, gelatin, and hydrogels are compromised by the short-term biodegradation of the grafted material. Thus, nanomaterials are emerging as the main candidates to ensure the achievement of a proper instructive cellular niche. The main purpose of these materials is to display structural and functional properties similar to extracellular matrices, containing truly 3D nanonetworks.

Reduced oxygen tension used to expand cells in the cultures points to an important potential in the treatment of ischemic myocardium, since like this the cells are preconditioned to survive in ischemic environment.

3 MAGNUM Clinical Trial (Myocardial Assistance by Grafting a New Bioartificial Upgraded Myocardium)

A new emerging therapeutic approach for ischemic heart disease consists in associating stem cell transplantation with tissue engineering for myocardial repair procedure using efficient scaffolds to reestablish a beneficial milieu for cell survival, multiplication, differentiation, and function.

Progenitor cells may provide the biological substrate for myocardial repair. Cell transplantation for myocardial regeneration is limited by poor graft viability and low cell retention. The stem cell niche is a specialized environment surrounding stem cells and supplies crucial support needed for stem cell maintenance. If the stem cell niche has aged or has been modified by a disease, it might not be capable of supporting stem cells grafted for local myocardial treatments.

3.1 Preclinical Study

Experimental studies performed in myocardial ischemic rodent models showed that the association between the cell-loaded collagen type 1 matrix and the intrainfarct cell implants was the most efficient approach to limiting postischemic ventricular dilation and remodeling. Ejection fraction improved in cell-treated groups; the collagen matrix alone did not improve LV function and remodeling. Histology showed fragments of the collagen matrix thickening and protecting the infarct scars. Segments of the matrix were consistently aligned along the LV wall, and cells were assembled within the collagen fibers in large populations [11].

In summary, the use of a cell-seeded scaffold combined with cell injections prevents ventricular wall thinning and limits postischemic remodeling. This tissue engineering approach seems to improve the efficiency of cellular cardiomyoplasty and could emerge as a new therapeutic tool for the prevention of adverse remodeling and progressive heart failure.

3.2 MAGNUM Trial

The goal of this clinical study was to evaluate intrainfarct cell therapy associated with a 3D cell-seeded collagen scaffold grafted onto infarcted ventricles (Fig. 1). In 20 patients (aged 55.2 ± 3.9 years) presenting LV postischemic myocardial scars and with indication for a single OP-CABG, autologous mononuclear bone marrow cells (BMC) were implanted during surgery in the scar. A 3D type I collagen matrix (5 cm × 7 cm × 0.6 cm) seeded with BMC was added on top of the scarred area (Fig. 2).

There was no mortality and any related adverse events (follow-up 25 ± 3.8 months). NYHA FC improved from 2.3 ± 0.5 to 1.3 ± 0.3 ($p = 0.005$). LV end-diastolic volume evolved from 142 ± 24 to 115 ± 3 mL ($p = 0.03$); LV filling deceleration time (Doppler mitral valve flow) improved from 162 ± 7 ms to 198 ± 7 ms

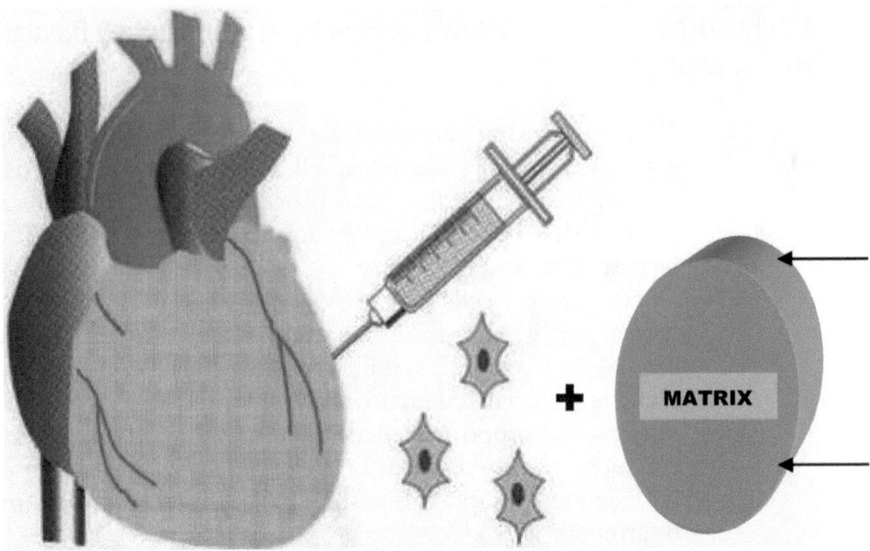

Fig. 1 MAGNUM Clinical Trial: Tissue engineering approach designed for myocardial support and regeneration. In the same procedure the myocardial infarction scar is treated both by the injection of stem cells and a cell-seeded collagen matrix

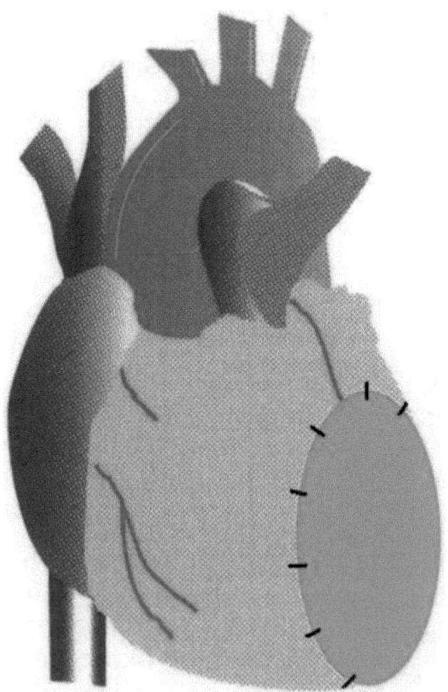

Fig. 2 MAGNUM Trial: The LV infarcted area is covered by a tridimensional biodegradable collagen scaffold (size: 7 cm × 5 cm × 0.6 cm) fixed to the epicardium by single sutures

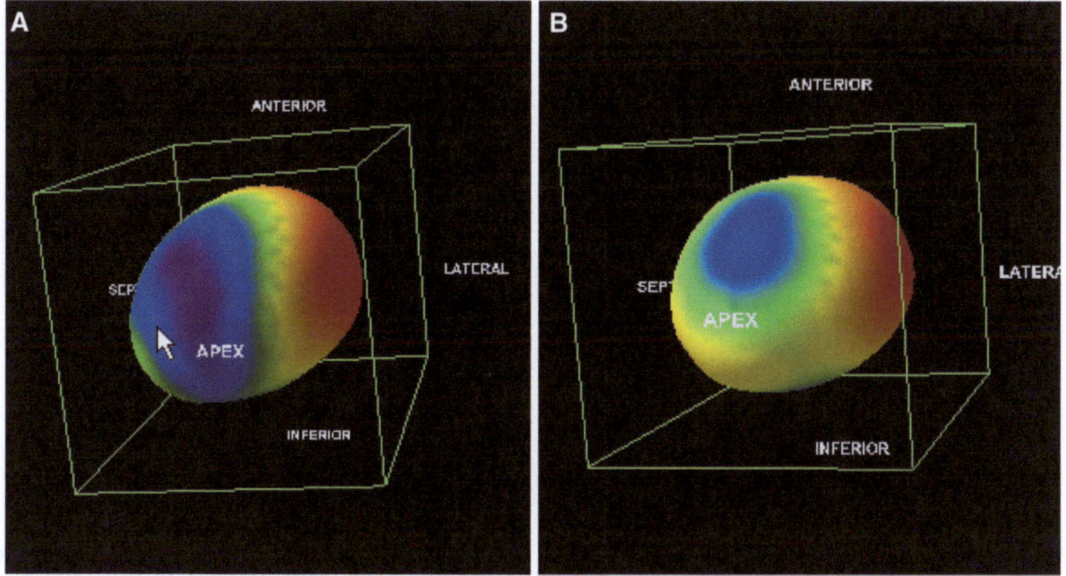

Fig. 3 (**a**) MAGNUM Trial: 3D representation of the preoperative radioisotopic SPECT Tc^{99m} sestamibi imaging, showing the chronic infarction area (*blue stain*). (**b**) Same patient, follow-up at 2 years showing the improvement of myocardial viability and function (62 % of reduction of the infarcted area, in *blue*)

($p=0.01$). Scar area thickness progress from 6 ± 1.4 to 9 ± 1.8 mm ($p=0.005$). EF improved from 25 ± 7 to 34 ± 5.2 % ($p=0.04$) (Fig. 3a, b).

In conclusion, simultaneous injection of BMC and fixation of a cell-seeded matrix onto the epicardium is feasible and safe. The matrix seems to increase the thickness of the scar with viable tissues and help to normalize wall stress in injured regions (scaffold effect), thus limiting ventricular remodeling and improving diastolic function. Associating stem cell transplantation with tissue engineering for myocardial repair seems to be beneficial to reestablish an efficient milieu for cell survival, multiplication, differentiation, and function [12].

4 RECATABI European Project (REgeneration of CArdiac Tissue Assisted by Bioactive Implants)

"Bioactive implants" for myocardial regeneration and ventricular support are developed in the RECATABI European Study http://www.recatabi.com/. This approach includes an elastomeric microporous membrane (bio-hybrid patch) having one synthetic nondegradable polymer and one partially degradable polymer (biological or synthetic) all associated with a peptide nanofiber hydrogel and stem cells (Figs. 4 and 5). This "bioactive implant" should provide

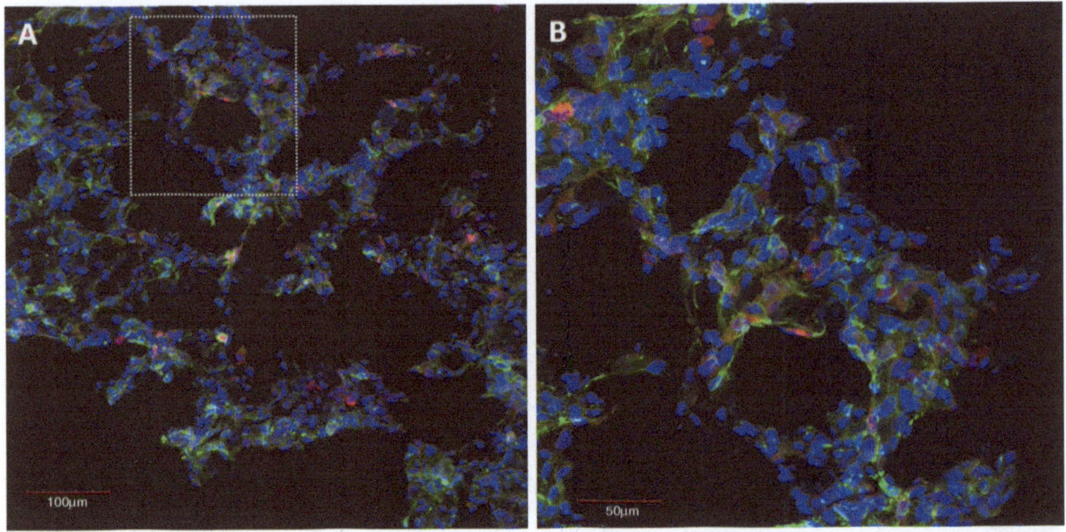

Fig. 4 Confocal microscopy of bio-hybrid scaffold (50-μm-thick slices) after 1 day of cell seeding, showing the transfected cells (nuclei in *red*), cytoplasm in *green* (phalloidin stain) and nonmarked cells (*blue* DAPI stain)

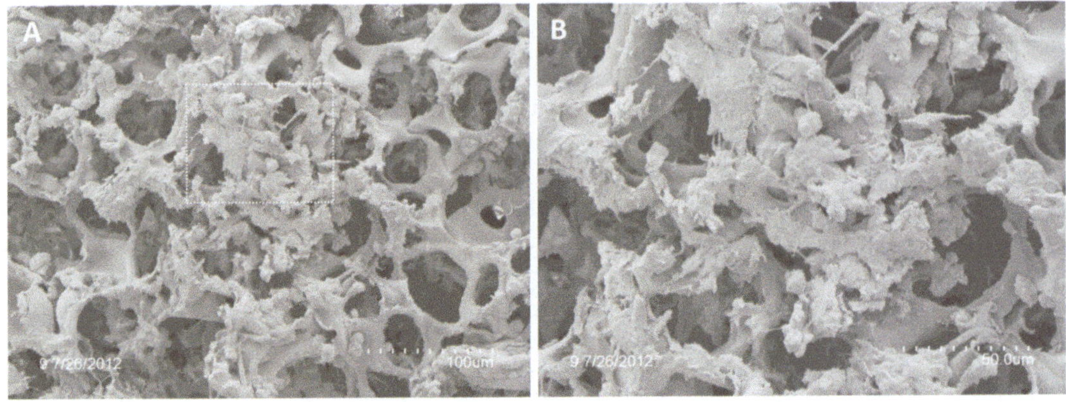

Fig. 5 Scanning electron microscopy (SEM) showing the 3D arrangement of scaffold's fibers. Stem cells are lodged into the niches after 1 day of implantation

a suitable environment for cell homing, growth, and differentiation (myocardial repair), as well as mechanical support to the heart [2, 13–15].

The combination of degradable and nondegradable polymers should be advantageous because cells implanted in niches will organize, connect, and contract more easily if they are surrounded by material that degrades with time. This partial degradation of the implant should reduce chronic fibrosis and the risk of diastolic function restriction. However, some nondegradable prosthetic fibers that remain seem necessary to avoid progressive heart dilatation (Fig. 6).

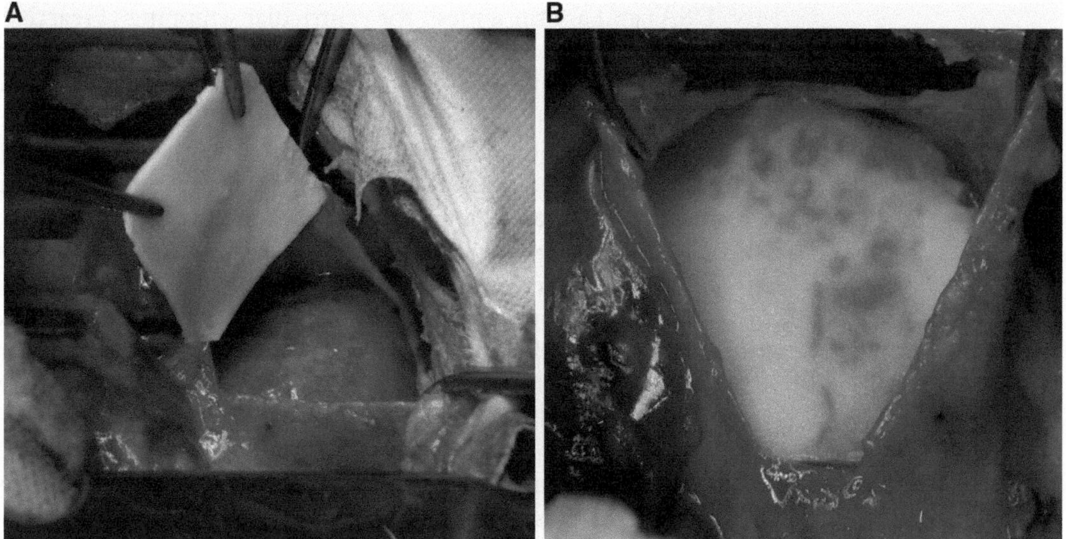

Fig. 6 Bioactive implant therapy: surgical implantation of bio-hybrid scaffold on the infarcted left ventricle

5 Ventricular Constraint Therapy

In the 1980s our group developed cardiomyoplasty, a procedure in which the heart was wrapped with a latissimus dorsi muscle flap and stimulated to contract with systole [16]. Although the procedure was effective at reducing myocardial oxygen consumption (mVO_2), wall stress, and adverse remodeling, these benefits persisted even if the muscle flap was not stimulated, that is, these effects remained with simply a passive muscle wrap. Passive prosthetic wraps were therefore developed, and ventricular restraint therapy was born.

Limitation of cardiac enlargement and reduction in mechanical ventricular wall stress was observed experimentally and clinically in cases treated with biological restraint-constraint therapy, i.e., latissimus dorsi dynamic cardiomyoplasty. This autologous source of circulatory assistance in which an electrically stimulated grafted skeletal muscle works in concert with myocardium requires a rather long and complex surgical procedure. For this reason less invasive alternative approaches have been proposed like ventricular restraint therapy using polyester or nitinol devices and more recently biological approaches for myocardial support and regeneration such as stem cell transplantation associated with tissue-engineered scaffolds.

Ventricular constraint therapy has been used to prevent and reverse the progression of heart failure in ischemic and nonischemic cardiomyopathies. Two devices have been used clinically: a polyester multifilament mesh (CorCap device, Acorn, St. Paul,

MN, USA) and a nitinol mesh for ventricular wrapping (HeartNet device, Paracor, Sunnyvale, CA, USA). But these devices failed to demonstrate clear positive effects on cardiopulmonary exercise testing and survival [17–19]. Adverse effects like restriction in diastolic function (mainly of the RV) seem to be the drawback of these devices. Diastolic dysfunction is actually a fairly common, dynamic process that, when it further deteriorates, increases the risk of dying by almost 80 %. Diastolic dysfunction, aside from being a marker of increased risk, seems also to be a direct contributor to the adverse progression of heart failure by limiting cardiac output reserve, accelerating neuroendocrine activation, increasing symptoms of breathlessness, and promoting physical inactivity, deconditioning, and frailty.

An adjustable and measurable restraint balloon device was recently evaluated in an ovine model of ischemic cardiomyopathy [20]. This device is a half-ellipsoidal balloon constructed from medical grade polyurethane sheets, filled with fluids. The device is placed around the heart and sutured to the atrioventricular groove such that both ventricles are covered. The balloon access line is connected to an implantable catheter (Port-A-Cath) which is placed in the chest wall. The port can be accessed for measuring the pressure within the balloon, restraint level is changed by adding or removing fluid from the balloon. The true risk of this ventricular restraint device placed in the pericardial sac concerns the restraint of the four chambers. Thus, clinical application of this device may result in cardiac tamponade [21].

6 Development of Bioartificial Myocardium

Cardiac tissue engineering emerges as a new therapeutic tool and provides even more amazing possibilities of cell therapies in cardiology, becoming a promising way for the creation of a "bioartificial myocardium."

By electrostimulation of 3D biocompatible scaffolds seeded with stem cells, we underwent a research program associating electrophysiology with stem cell therapy. Electrostimulation (ES) can be defined as a safe physical method to induce stem cell differentiation. We evaluated the effectiveness of ES on bone marrow mesenchymal stem cells (BMSCs) seeded in collagen scaffolds in terms of proliferation and differentiation into cardiomyocytes [22].

BMSCs were isolated from femur and tibia of 2-month-old Wistar rats and seeded into 3D collagen type 1 templates measuring 25 mm × 25 mm × 6 mm. In vitro bipolar electrostimulation of cell-seeded collagen scaffolds was performed during 21 days using two electrodes having curved needles for easy insertion, fixed into the opposites borders of the templates. Both electrodes were connected to bipolar pacemakers (transform model, Medtronic Inc, MN, USA). The cell-seeded collagen was stimulated using single pulses at a frequency of 120 impulses per minute (rate 2 Hz), pulse amplitude of 7 V, and pulse width of 5 ms.

Collagen matrixes were analyzed after 1 and 3 weeks of electrostimulation, electrical impedance and cell proliferation were measured, and expression of cardiac markers was assessed by immunocytochemistry. Viscoelasticity of collagen matrix was evaluated.

6.1 Results

These studies showed a good electrical conductivity of collagen matrix; values of resistance were low (234 ± 41 Ohms). Cell proliferation at 570 nm significantly increased in ES groups after 7 days (ES 0.129 ± 0.03 vs. non-stimulated control matrix 0.06 ± 0.01, $p = 0.002$) and after 21 days(ES 0.22 ± 0.04 vs. control 0.13 ± 0.01, $p = 0.01$). Immunocytochemistry of BMSCs after 21-day ES showed positive staining of cardiac markers, troponin I, connexin 43, sarcomeric alpha-actinin, slow myosin, fast myosin, and desmin [22].

In conclusion, electrostimulation of cell-seeded collagen matrix changed stem cell morphology and biochemical characteristics, increasing the expression of cardiac markers. Thus, stem cells grafted in biological scaffolds underwent differentiation by electrostimulation. This might result in a convenient tissue engineering source for myocardial diseases. The association of a multielectrode network for local pacing should improve the coupling of stem cells and scaffolds with host cardiomyocytes, becoming a dynamic tissue-engineered support [23].

7 Stem Cell Treatment for Chagas Heart Disease

Chagas disease is the infection with the protozoan parasite Trypanosoma cruzi, a form of trypanosomiasis endemic in Central and South America. It is named after the Brazilian physician Carlos Chagas discovered the parasite. Four main pathogenetic mechanisms explain the development of chronic Chagas heart disease: autonomic nervous system derangements, microvascular disturbances, parasite-dependent myocardial aggression, and immune-mediated myocardial injury. In the last decades, millions of people from South and Central America have migrated to the United States and Europe (mainly to Spain and Portugal) changing the scenario of acute Chagas disease associated with the risk of transmission of the disease during blood transfusions in the USA and Europe. France is affected by Chagas infections detected in the French Guiana territory; this population is part and frequently lives in the European Union.

At long term patients develop severe cardiac arrhythmias, dilated cardiomyopathy, and heart failure. In Chagasic patients who undergo heart transplantation and immunosuppression, the risk of late reactivation of Chagas disease by means of an isolated organ lesion is important. The performance of stem cell transplantation in patients presenting Chagasic cardiomyopathies is under evaluation in several medical centers [24–26].

8 Development of Bio-hybrid Ventricular Support Bioprostheses

The development of cardiac support bioprostheses for ventricular restoration and myocardial regeneration is in progress. The combination of myocardial tissue engineering together with stem cell-based myocardial regeneration seems to be a promising way for the treatment of heart failure patients [15, 27–30]. The application of bioactive molecules and the recent development of nanobiotechnologies should open the door for the creation of a new ventricular bioprosthesis, in a form of a semi-degradable device designed according with the concept of "helical ventricular myocardial band" [31]. It should be manufactured in different models for "adapted ventricular wrapping" of the left and/or right ventricle, capable of controlled stability or degradation in response to physiological conditions of the left or right heart (Fig. 7). Bio-hybrid implants should contribute to myocardial regeneration, improving systolic and diastolic functions and reducing adverse spherical cardiac dilatation in heart failure patients [32].

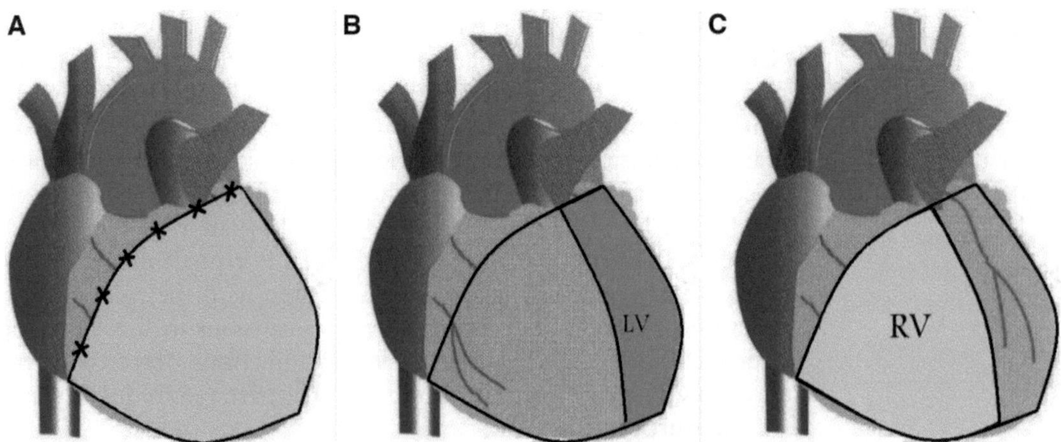

Fig. 7 Adaptative ventricular wrapping for left and/or right heart pathologies

References

1. Chachques JC (2009) Cellular cardiac regenerative therapy in which patients? Expert Rev Cardiovasc Ther 7:911–919
2. Soler-Botija C, Bago JR, Bayes-Genis A (2012) A bird's-eye view of cell therapy and tissue engineering for cardiac regeneration. Ann N Y Acad Sci 1254:57–65
3. Herreros J, Trainini JC, Chachques JC (2011) Alternatives to heart transplantation: integration of biology with surgery. Front Biosci 3:635–647
4. Dixon JA, Spinale FG (2011) Myocardial remodeling: cellular and extracellular events and targets. Annu Rev Physiol 73:47–68
5. Kao RL, Browder W, Li C (2009) Cellular cardiomyoplasty: what have we learned? Asian Cardiovasc Thorac Ann 17:89–101
6. Huang G, Pashmforoush M, Chung B et al (2011) The role of cardiac electrophysiology in myocardial regenerative stem cell therapy. J Cardiovasc Transl Res 4:61–65
7. Rasmussen JG, Frøbert O, Pilgaard L et al (2011) Prolonged hypoxic culture and trypsinization increase the pro-angiogenic potential of human adipose tissue-derived stem cells. Cytotherapy 13:318–326
8. Hu X, Yu SP, Fraser JL et al (2008) Transplantation of hypoxia-preconditioned mesenchymal stem cells improves infarcted heart function via enhanced survival of implanted cells and angiogenesis. J Thorac Cardiovasc Surg 135:799–808
9. Gavira JJ, Nasarre E, Abizanda G et al (2010) Repeated implantation of skeletal myoblast in a swine model of chronic myocardial infarction. Eur Heart J 31:1013–1021
10. Dai W, Hale SL, Kay GL et al (2009) Delivering stem cells to the heart in a collagen matrix reduces relocation of cells to other organs as assessed by nanoparticle technology. Regen Med 4:387–395
11. Cortes-Morichetti M, Carpentier AF, Chachques JC et al (2007) Association between a cell-seeded collagen matrix and cellular cardiomyoplasty for myocardial support and regeneration. Tissue Eng 13:2681–2687
12. Chachques JC, Trainini JC, Carpentier A et al (2008) Myocardial assistance by grafting a new bioartificial upgraded myocardium (MAGNUM trial): clinical feasibility study. Ann Thorac Surg 85:901–908
13. Mari-Buye N, Semino CE (2011) Differentiation of mouse embryonic stem cells in self-assembling peptide scaffolds. Methods Mol Biol 690:217–237
14. Arnal-Pastor M, Valles-Lluch A, Keicher M et al (2011) Coating typologies and constrained swelling of hyaluronic acid gels within scaffold pores. J Colloid Interface Sci 361:361–369
15. Chachques JC (2010) Development of bioartificial myocardium using stem cells and nanobiotechnology templates. Cardiol Res Pract 2010:806795
16. Chachques JC (2009) Cardiomyoplasty: is it still a viable option in patients with end-stage heart failure? Eur J Cardiothorac Surg 35:201–203
17. Lee LS, Ghanta RK, Mokashi SA et al (2010) Ventricular restraint therapy for heart failure: the right ventricle is different from the left ventricle. J Thorac Cardiovasc Surg 139:1012–1018
18. Olsson A, Bredin F, Franco-Cereceda A (2005) Echocardiographic findings using tissue velocity imaging following passive containment surgery with the Acorn CorCap cardiac support device. Eur J Cardiothorac Surg 28:448–453
19. Dixon JA, Goodman AM, Gaillard WF 2nd et al (2011) Hemodynamics and myocardial blood flow patterns after placement of a cardiac passive restraint device in a model of dilated cardiomyopathy. J Thorac Cardiovasc Surg 142:1038–1045
20. Lee LS, Ghanta RK, Mokashi SA et al (2013) Optimized ventricular restraint therapy: adjustable restraint is superior to standard restraint in an ovine model of ischemic cardiomyopathy. J Thorac Cardiovasc Surg 145:824–831
21. Kwon MH, Cevasco M, Schmitto JD et al (2012) Ventricular restraint therapy for heart failure: a review, summary of state of the art, and future directions. J Thorac Cardiovasc Surg 144:771–777
22. Haneef K, Lila N, Chachques JC et al (2012) Development of bioartificial myocardium by electrostimulation of 3D collagen scaffolds seeded with stem cells. Heart Int 7:e14
23. Shafy A, Lavergne T, Chachques JC et al (2009) Association of electrostimulation with cell transplantation in ischemic heart disease. J Thorac Cardiovasc Surg 138:994–1001
24. Vilas Boas LG, Bestetti RB, Otaviano AP et al (2012) Outcome of Chagas cardiomyopathy in comparison to ischemic cardiomyopathy. Int J Cardiol. Feb 22 [Epub ahead of print]
25. Andrade JP, Marin Neto JA, Paola AA et al (2011) I Latin American guidelines for the diagnosis and treatment of Chagas' heart

disease: executive summary. Arq Bras Cardiol 96:434–442

26. Vilas-Boas F, Feitosa GS, Soares MB et al (2011) Bone marrow cell transplantation in Chagas' disease heart failure: report of the first human experience. Arq Bras Cardiol 96:325–331
27. Al Kindi AH, Chiu RC, Shum-Tim D et al (2011) Microencapsulation to reduce mechanical loss of microspheres: implications in myocardial cell therapy. Eur J Cardiothorac Surg 39:241–247
28. Giraud MN, Guex AG, Tevaearai HT (2012) Cell therapies for heart function recovery: focus on myocardial tissue engineering and nanotechnologies. Cardiol Res Pract 2012: 971614
29. Sekine H, Shimizu T, Okano T (2012) Myocardial tissue engineering: toward a bioartificial pump. Cell Tissue Res 347:775–782
30. Habib M, Shapira-Schweitzer K, Caspi O et al (2011) A combined cell therapy and in-situ tissue-engineering approach for myocardial repair. Biomaterials 32:7514–7523
31. Torrent-Guasp F, Kocica MJ, Corno AF et al (2005) Towards new understanding of the heart structure and function. Eur J Cardiothorac Surg 27:191–201
32. Shafy A, Fink T, Chachques JC et al (2013) Development of cardiac support bioprostheses for ventricular restoration and myocardial regeneration. Eur J Cardiothorac Surg 43: 1211–1219

Chapter 14

Decellularized Whole Heart for Bioartificial Heart

Hug Aubin, Alexander Kranz, Jörn Hülsmann, Artur Lichtenberg, and Payam Akhyari

Abstract

Whole-organ decellularization has opened the gates to the creation of 3D extracellular matrix (ECM) templates that mimic nature's design to a degree that—as for today—is not reproducible with any synthetic materials. Here, we describe a whole-heart decellularization approach through software-controlled automated coronary perfusion with standard decellularization detergents, enabling us to create native ECM-derived 3D templates that preserve the basic anatomy, vascular network, and critical ECM characteristics of the native heart. Such a cardiac ECM platform directly derived from nature itself might help us to better understand and reproduce cardiac biology and may even lay the grounds for the construction of a bioartificial heart in the future.

Key words Bioartificial heart, Decellularized heart, Cardiovascular regenerative medicine, Engineered heart tissue, Cardiac 3D templates, Myocardial extracellular matrix, Myocardial tissue engineering, Whole-organ decellularization

1 Introduction

Whole-organ decellularization experiences an increasing level of attention and popularity in the fields of tissue engineering and regenerative medicine. Starting from bradytrophic tissues such as the cartilage in the early stages up to functionally more complex tissues such as muscle and nerve tissue, today we are able to decellularize almost every organ in toto [1]. Since macro- and microscopic architecture can be preserved in the decellularization process, such decellularized whole organs result in 3D extracellular matrix (ECM) templates that mimic nature's design to a degree that—as for today—is not reproducible with any synthetic material. Through whole-organ decellularization we are not only able to create organ-specific extracellular environments that, e.g., can serve for in vitro stem cell studies [2], but we might also have created a platform which may break new grounds in the fields of

Race L. Kao (ed.), *Cellular Cardiomyoplasty: Methods and Protocols*, Methods in Molecular Biology, vol. 1036,
DOI 10.1007/978-1-62703-511-8_14,

regenerative medicine leading the way to the creation of functional bioartificial organs [3].

Since Ott et al. introduced the whole-heart decellularization concept in 2008 [4], it has become possible to generate *native-derived*, acellular 3D ECM templates that preserve the basic anatomy, vascular network, and critical ECM characteristics of the native heart [5]. However, using a whole-heart template to create a one-to-one mimicry of a native heart still poses an insuperable challenge today because of its tremendous biological complexity. Nonetheless, a 3D platform directly derived from nature itself might help us to better understand and reproduce cardiac biology and may lay the grounds for the construction of a bioartificial heart in the future.

Four major steps are classically needed for the decellularization of native tissues:

1. Lysis of the cell membranes
2. Separation of the cellular components from the ECM
3. Solubilization of cytoplasmatic and nuclear components
4. Removal of cell debris

Ideally, all this has to be achieved without altering the 3D ultrastructure, the biochemical composition, and the mechanical properties of the ECM while warranting high biocompatibility of the decellularized scaffold. The decellularization methods commonly used vary from physical, over chemical, to enzymatic decellularization or the combination thereof [6]. While native tissues can be decellularized through sole dynamic incubation in decellularization agents, well-perfused organs are most commonly decellularized through organ perfusion taking advantage of the native vascular system that guarantees sufficient perfusion with the decellularization agents through the whole tissue, allowing for in toto decellularization [7]. Therefore, whole-heart decellularization is usually carried out through retrograde aortic perfusion allowing for coronary perfusion in an open or closed perfusion cycle with either pump- or gravity-driven perfusion flow. However, the decellularization protocols used to create acellular myocardial scaffolds vary widely throughout the published literature. Although cytocompatibility seems to remain high, so far no protocol has proved as entirely ideal for the generation of an optimal decellularized biological matrix, in the sense of template that is not only free of donor cell material but also highly preserves all the critical extracellular matrix components [5]. Depending on the protocol used, there are striking differences concerning the decellularization efficacy and its undesirable effects, ranging from differences in the remaining DNA quantities to differences in the macro- and microcomposition of the ECM on the histological and biochemical level. Hence, decellularization—using common cell removal agents—cannot be achieved without some degree of ECM alteration and ultrastructural disruption. However, a number of different protocols seem more or less suitable for myocardial decellularization depending on the template characteristics that are valued most. Nonetheless, a lot of important questions remain unanswered yet. For instance, there are no reliable in vivo data yet available to enable us to predict how much donor cell material left in a decellularized scaffold will provoke a critical adverse immunogenic reaction in a given host organism [8–10]. In addition, the efficacy of the protocols alters considerably depending on the tests applied for analysis. Standardized test for the confirmation of decellularization efficacy and for the evaluation of the extracellular matrix qualities needs to be implemented.

The experiences we have gained in the last years with the decellularization and processing of heart valves [11–17] have helped us translating the decellularization process to the myocardium as a whole [5]. Here we present a detailed protocol for whole-heart decellularization through automated software-controlled coronary perfusion in a closed perfusion cycle that, additionally to preserving basic anatomy of the myocardium and the vascular system—using our standard analysis tests—has proved to be reliable on high degree of donor cell removal, as well as on high extent of ECM conservation from basic collagen and glycosaminoglycan (GAG) matrix components up to critical base membrane proteins (e.g., laminin and collagen IV). Standard analysis performed in our laboratory includes hematoxylin and eosin (H&E) stain, DNA quantification assay and immunohistological staining for cytoplasmatic protein (sarcomeric α-actin) for confirmation of efficient cell removal, as well as standard assays to evaluate the GAG content and histological and immunohistological stainings revealing specific extracellular matrix proteins (including collagenous and elastic fibers as well as basement membrane proteins such as laminin and collagen IV) for the confirmation of optimal preservation of template components. Nonetheless, it should be noted that a simplified protocol that we successfully use for the decellularization of heart valves [11] might also be sufficient for the generation of standardized myocardial templates. However, the user has to determine for himself—using above-mentioned tests—which protocol and which possible modifications will meet the standards needed for his experimental setup. The selected decellularization protocol may also vary depending on template application, while, e.g., a potential in vivo use may demand complete removal of potentially immunogenic cellular remnants, in vitro cell studies may benefit from milder protocols with higher degree of ECM protein conservation.

Considering time and material basis, a rodent model seems to be the most convenient experimental frame for the mass production of myocardial templates for basic myocardial ECM-oriented scientific research. Thus, we describe an efficient method for decellularization of whole rat hearts, which though can theoretically be modified to fit other animal species, as well.

2 Materials

2.1 Heart Explantation

1. Ketanest.
2. Xylazine.
3. 27 gauge needle.
4. 1 ml syringe.
5. Unfractioned heparin.
6. 14 gauge cannula.
7. Surgical suture material.
8. Ringer's solution.

2.2 Whole-Heart Decellularization Through Coronary Perfusion: Automated Software-Controlled Organ Perfusion

1. 100 ml glass flask, GL45, modified with one inlet through the cap and two outlets at the bottom of the flask (*see* **Note 1**).
2. Silicon tubes.
3. Bubble trap (*see* **Note 2**).
4. Peristaltic pump (Stöcker).
5. Data acquisition device, ADAM-4018 Remote-I/O-Modul (Advantech).
6. Analog input/output model, ADAM-4024 Remote-I/O--Modul (Advantech).
7. Pressure transducer, LogiCal MX 960 (Medex).
8. Operational computer (Dell).
9. Control software (engine GmbH).

2.3 Whole-Heart Decellularization Through Coronary Perfusion: Decellularization Solutions

1. Phosphate buffered saline.
2. Penicillin–streptomycin. Storage at −20 °C.
3. Unfractioned heparin.
4. Adenosine.
5. Deionized water.
6. Glycerol anhydrous (AppliChem).
7. EDTA disodium salt dihydrate p. A. (AppliChem).
8. 0.9 % NaCl solution.
9. Magnesium chloride hexahydrate puriss. p.a. (Fluka).
10. DNase I (Roche). Storage at −20 °C.
11. Sodium azide (Carl Roth). Store at room temperature. Highly toxic and very dangerous for the environment. Harmful if swallowed. Irritating to eyes and skin. Do not inhale dust.

12. Desoxycholic acid sodium salt (DCA) ultrapure (Sigma). Store at room temperature. Harmful if swallowed. Irritating to eyes and skin. Do not inhale dust.
13. Sodium dodecyl sulfate (SDS) ultrapure (Carl Roth). Store at room temperature. Harmful if swallowed. Irritating to eyes and skin. Do not inhale dust.
14. Saponin (Sigma). Store at room temperature. Harmful if swallowed. Irritating to eyes and skin. Do not inhale dust.

2.4 H&E Staining

1. Acetone (J.T. Baker).
2. Hematoxylin (Merck).
3. Eosin (Merck).
4. Ethanol.
5. Xylol.
6. Eukitt (Sigma).

2.5 Movat's Pentachrome Staining

1. Alcian blue (Waldeck–Chroma).
2. Ammonia.
3. Ethanol.
4. Acetic acid.
5. Weigert's iron hematoxylin (Waldeck–Chroma).
6. Brilliant crocein (Waldeck–Chroma).
7. Acid fuchsin (Waldeck–Chroma).
8. Phosphotungstic acid (Merck).
9. Saffron du Gâtinais (Waldeck–Chroma).
10. Xylol.
11. Eukitt (Sigma).

2.6 Immunohistochemical Staining Using Fast Red/DAB

1. Sarcomeric α-actin: Actin, muscle specific Ab.4 (Clone HHF35), monoclonal mouse antibody (IgG1/kappa) (Thermo Scientific). Store at 2–8 °C.
2. Collagen IV: COL4A2 (T-15), polyclonal rabbit antibody (Santa Cruz). Store at 2–8 °C.
3. Laminin: Laminin Ab.1, polyclonal rabbit antibody (IgG) (Thermo Scientific). Store at 2–8 °C.
4. Protease XXV (LabVision).
5. Citrate buffer, pH 6.0 (Thermo Scientific).
6. Wash buffer: To make 1,000 ml buffer, dilute 876 mg NaCl (58.4 g/mol; Merck) in 588 mg Tris–HCl (157.6 g/mol; Merck) and in 100 ml distilled H_2O each, mix and add distilled H_2O up to 1,000 ml.

7. Antibody dilution buffer: 1 % bovine serum albumin (BSA) in wash buffer.
8. UltraVision LP Detection System—AP Polymer & Fast Red Chromogen (Thermo Scientific). Store at 2–8 °C. Each component is stable for up to 18 months.
   - Ultra V Block.
   - Primary Antibody Enhancer.
   - AP Polymer.
   - Fast Red Tablet.
   - Naphthol Phosphate Substrate.
9. UltraVision LP Detection System—HRP Polymer & DAB Plus Chromogen (Thermo Scientific). Store at 2–8 °C. Each component is stable for up to 18 months.
   - Hydrogen Peroxide Block.
   - Ultra V Block.
   - Primary Antibody Enhancer.
   - HRP Polymer.
   - DAB Plus Substrate.
   - DAB Plus Chromogen.
10. Harris–Hematoxylin (1:3) (Merck).
11. Acetone.
12. Ethanol.
13. Xylol.
14. Mounting medium (Dako).

2.7 DNA Assay

1. AllPrep DNA/RNA/Protein Mini Kit (Qiagen).
2. Ethanol.

2.8 GAG Assay

1. Blyscan Sulfated Glycosaminoglycan Assay (Biocolor).
2. Ethanol.

3 Methods

3.1 Heart Explantation

We used adult male Lewis rats of 250–350 g for the generation of acelluar whole-heart templates.

1. Anesthetize rats by intraperitoneal injection of 200 mg/kg BW Ketanest and 20 mg/kg BW xylazine.
2. Through median laparotomy gain access to the retroperitoneum by lifting the intestine package and shifting it aside.

3. Expose the v. cava inferior with two cotton swaps dissecting carefully through the retroperitoneal fat.
4. Use a 1 ml syringe with a 27 gauge needle to inject 1,000 0.2 ml of unfractionated heparin (5,000 IU/ml) into v. cava inferior. Wait 5 min allowing for systemic heparinization (*see* **Note 3**).
5. Transect the abdominal aorta and the inferior caval vein and let the rat exsanguinate.
6. Gain access to the mediastinum by median sternotomy, remove the retrosternal fat body and the thymus, and dissect the aortic arch.
7. After transection of the superior and inferior caval vein, the supra-aortic vessels, and the aorta at the transition from aortic arch to descending aorta, remove the heart from the chest cavity.
8. Insert a prefilled 14 G cannula into the thoracic aorta, ligate it proximal of the truncus brachiocephalicus, and rinse the heart with 20 ml of heparinized Ringer's solution (10 IU/ml heparin).

3.2 Whole-Heart Decellularization Through Coronary Perfusion

We developed a fully automated software-operated control system for whole-heart decellularization through automated long-term retrograde aortic perfusion of the explanted rat hearts that allows for coronary perfusion with a standardized constant perfusion pressure.

Therefore, the heart is inserted in a closed perfusion cycle consisting of a modified 100 ml glass flask, serving as perfusion chamber connected to a silicon tube system, with an additional volume of 20 ml. Coronary perfusion is enabled by retrograde aortic perfusion through connection of the thoracic aortic cannula to the tube system serving as perfusion inlet. During the decellularization process the explanted heart floats freely in the perfusate attached only at the perfusion inlet with the perfusate draining out of the heart trough the right atrium (*see* **Note 4**) (*see* Fig. 1). The tube system is clamped into a peristaltic pump that drives the perfusate circulation. For automated software-operated perfusion, a data acquisition device is connected to a pressure transducer that is connected in series to the perfusion inlet via an analog input module and to the peristaltic pump via an analog output module. Over an operational computer connected to the data acquisition device, an ad hoc-designed software is employed as control software, allowing the determination of a pressure set point for the coronary perfusion and operating the peristaltic pump online driving perfusate circulation with the determined perfusion pressure. Through a closed-loop control via a PID (proportional–integral–derivative) control algorithm embedded into the control software, the preset perfusion pressure is automatically kept constant during the entire

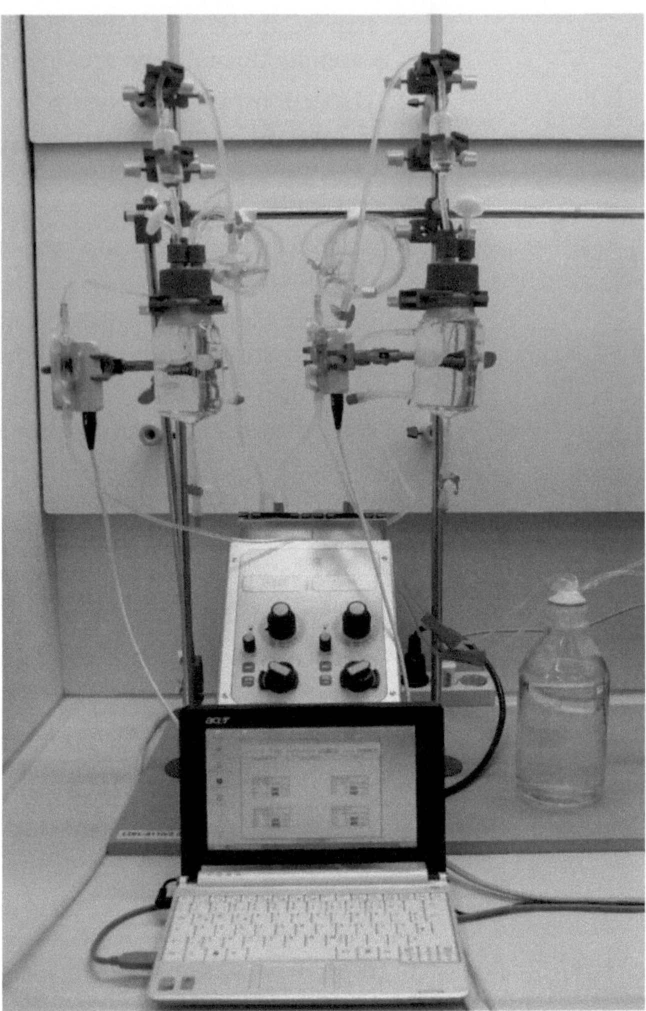

Fig. 1 Whole-heart decellularization through automated software-controlled coronary perfusion. The established system allows for independent pressure-controlled decellularization of individual hearts. Please refer to text for details

heart decellularization process through online adaption of the pump flow rate. This guarantees constant coronary perfusion pressure despite varying vascular tone along the process. For rat heart decellularization, a constant coronary perfusion between 75 and 80 mmHg has proven to be most efficient. Additionally, the control software visualizes all data online and records them as a .xlsx file for documentation and further analysis purposes. This allows to retrospectively exclude hearts from the experimental group before analysis, which most probably will show inefficient decellularization because of inconstant perfusion pressure, for example, because of aortic insufficiency or coronary burst.

1. Prefill the perfusion cycle with heparinized PBS (10 IU/ml Heparin) containing 10 mM adenosine.
2. Place the heart into the perfusion chamber by connecting the aortic cannula to the perfusion inlet. Close the perfusion chamber.
3. Start perfusate circulation with a coronary perfusion pressure of 77.5 mmHg manually or through the automatic software-operated control system. Perfusate is kept at room temperature unless otherwise stated.
4. Perfuse for 15 min with heparinized PBS (10 IU/ml Heparin) containing 10 mM adenosine (*see* **Note 5**).
5. Perfuse for 15 min with deionized water (*see* **Note 6**).
6. Perfuse for 12 h with 1 % SDS, 1 % DCA, and 0.05 % sodium azide in deionized water (*see* **Notes 7–9**).
7. Perfuse for 15 min with deionized water.
8. Perfuse for 12 h with 20 % glycerol, 0.05 % sodium azide, and 25 mM EDTA in 0.9 % NaCl solution.
9. Perfuse for 15 min with deionized water.
10. Perfuse for 12 h with 1 % saponin and 0.05 % sodium azide in deionized water.
11. Perfuse for 15 min with deionized water.
12. Perfuse for 12 h with 20 % glycerol, 0.05 % sodium azide, and 25 mM EDTA in 0.9 % NaCl solution.
13. Perfuse for 15 min with deionized water.
14. Perfuse for 12 h with 200 IU/ml DNase I and 50 mM MgCl in PBS at 37 °C (*see* **Note 10**).
15. Perfuse for 12 h with 100 IU/ml penicillin–streptomycin in PBS (*see* **Note 11**).
16. Remove the decellularized heart from the perfusion chamber and store in PBS supplemented with 100 IU/ml penicillin–streptomycin at 4 °C (*see* **Note 12**) (*see* Fig. 2).

3.3 H&E Staining

The quality of decellularization is validated by a number of different assays. As an initial analytic step, simple staining methods, such as hematoxylin and eosin (H&E) overview staining, may be used for visualization of residual cellular remnants (basophilic nuclei appear in blue/black and eosinophilic collagen and cytoplasm in red/pink color). For staining decellularized hearts are fixed in 4 % buffered formaldehyde solution and longitudinal cross sections resulting in tissue blocks of three different standardized regions (apical region, mid-ventricular region, and basal region) (*see* **Note 13**) are embedded in paraffin and cut with a microtome into histological sections of 5 μm thickness. Before staining deparaffinize and rehydrate specimens using standard protocols.

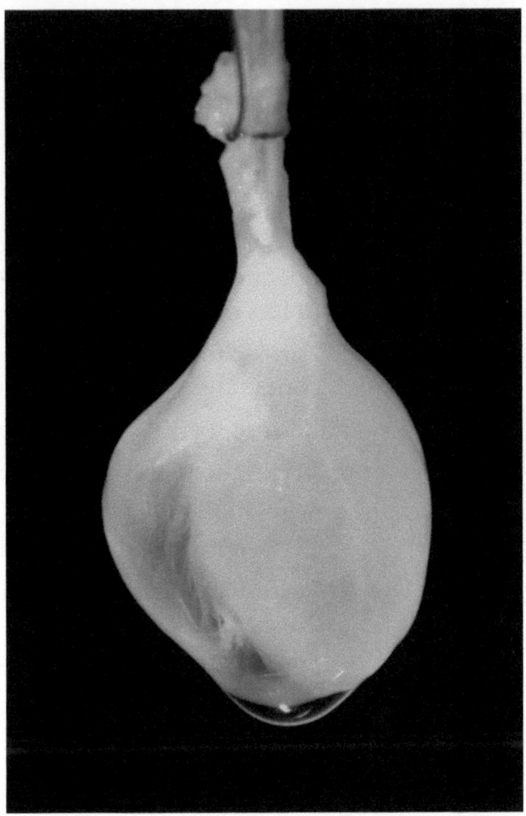

Fig. 2 Rat heart decellularized in toto with a simplified decellularization protocol. After removal of cellular components, the matrix turns transluminescent, while the decellularized heart as a whole preserves the basic anatomy, vascular network, and critical ECM characteristics of the native heart

The stain is performed as follows:

1. Fix sections of decellularized heart in acetone at –20 °C for 8–10 min.
2. Rehydrate in tap water.
3. Incubate in hematoxylin for 8 min.
4. Wash in tap water for 10 min.
5. Incubate in eosin for 5 min.
6. Rinse in tap water.
7. Dehydrate stepwise: 80 % ethanol (2 min), 90 % ethanol (2 min), and 100 % ethanol (2 min).
8. Differentiate in xylol.
9. Dry overnight, place a drop of Eukitt onto the slide before adding the coverslip and visualize in a bright field microscope.

3.4 Movat's Pentachrome Staining

The quality of matrix microstructure and composition is validated with Movat's pentachrome stain used for the differentiated visualization of ECM and cellular components (glycosaminoglycans appear in green/light blue, collagen fibers in yellow/orange, elastic fibers in dark light red/brown, nuclei in dark blue/black, and cytoplasm in dark red color) using samples as stated above. Before staining deparaffinize and rehydrate specimens using standard protocols.

The stain is performed as follows:

1. Rehydrate in tap water.
2. Stain in alcian blue (1 g alcian blue in 1 ml 99 % acetic acid and 100 ml aqua dest.) for 10 min.
3. Rinse in tap water.
4. Incubate in alkaline ethanol (10 ml 25 % ammonia in 90 ml 96 % ethanol) for 60 min.
5. Rinse in tap water.
6. Stain in Weigert's iron hematoxylin (1.16 g iron chloride, 1 ml 25 % HCL in 100 ml aqua dest., and 1 g hematoxylin in 100 ml 96 % ethanol) for 10 min.
7. Rinse in tap water.
8. Stain in brilliant crocein-acid fuchsin (0.08 g brilliant crocein and 0.02 g acid fuchsin in 0.5 ml 99 % acetic acid and 99.5 ml aqua dest.) for 10 min.
9. Wash in 0.5 % acetic acid for 2 min.
10. Wash in 5 % phosphotungstic acid for 20 min.
11. Wash in 0.5 % acetic acid for 2 min.
12. Dip 3× in 100 % ethanol.
13. Stain in Saffron du Gâtinais solution (6 g Saffron du Gâtinais in 100 ml 100 % ethanol).
14. Rinse in tap water.
15. Dehydrate stepwise: 80 % ethanol (2 min); 90 % ethanol (2 min); and 100 % ethanol (2 min).
16. Differentiate in xylol.
17. Air dry, place a drop of Eukitt onto the slide before adding the coverslip and visualize in a bright field microscope (*see* Fig. 3).

3.5 Immunohistochemical Staining for Cytoplasmatic Proteins Using Fast Red

Efficacy of cell removal is qualitatively assessed by exemplary immunohistochemical staining for sarcomeric α-actin using Fast Red validating removal of cytoplasmatic remnants. Use paraffin sections of 3 μm thickness from the samples as stated above.

1. Rehydrate in tap water.

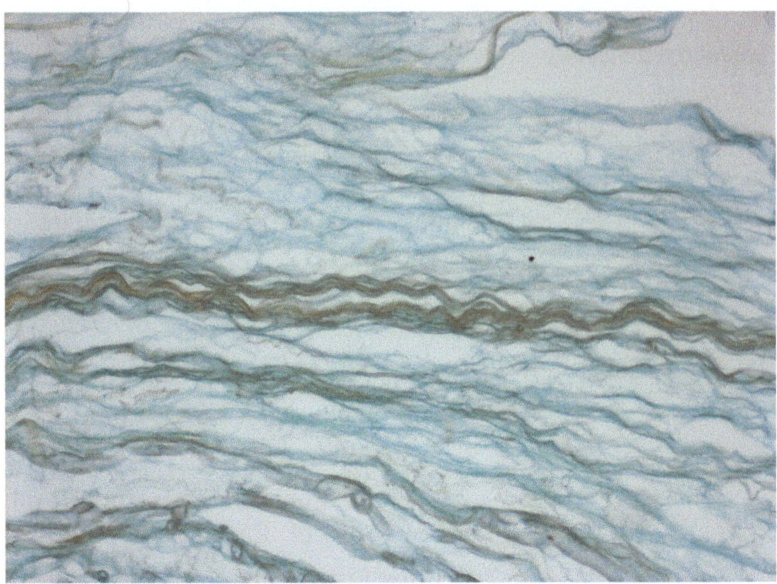

Fig. 3 Representative Movat staining showing cardial ECM of a decellularized whole heart. ECM remains integer with high amount of glycosaminoglycans, collagen, and elastic fibers. Please note that no nuclei (would appear in *blue*/*black*) or cytoplasmatic remnants (would appear in *red*) can be detected, indicative for complete decellularization (×100 magnification)

2. Heat in citrate buffer (pH 6) in a steamer for 20 min for epitope retrieval. Cool down to room temperature in ice bath.
3. Incubate in wash puffer for 10 min.
4. Block with *Ultra V* Block for 5 min or block in serum, of the same species as secondary antibody is derived from for 15 min to avoid unspecific binding.
5. Incubate with primary antibody against actin in dilution buffer (1:50) for 30 min at room temperature or overnight. Do not rinse sections between blocking step and primary antibody incubation (*see* **Notes 13** and **15**).
6. Rinse once in wash puffer.
7. Incubate with primary antibody enhancer in dilution buffer (1:50) for 15 min at room temperature.
8. Rinse once in wash puffer.
9. Incubate with *AP* Polymer for 30 min at room temperature.
10. Rinse twice in wash buffer.
11. Stain in Fast Red visualizing alkaline phosphatase for 10 min.
12. Rinse thrice in wash buffer.
13. Counterstain in Harris–Hematoxylin (1:3) for 10 min.
14. The results are visualized using a standard bright microscope.

3.6 Immunohistochemical Staining for Base Membrane Proteins Using DAB

Preservation of critical basal membrane components are qualitatively assessed by exemplary immunohistochemical staining for laminin and collagen IV using DAB (3,3′-Diaminobenzidine). Use paraffin sections of 3 μm thickness from the samples as stated above.

The stain is performed as follows:

1. Rehydrate in tap water.
2. Incubate in protease for 10 min at room temperature for epitope retrieval.
3. Incubate in wash puffer for 10 min.
4. Block endogenous peroxidase with hydrogen peroxide block for 5 min.
5. Block with *Ultra V* Block for 5 min or block in serum of the same species as secondary antibody is derived from for 15 min to avoid unspecific binding.
6. Incubate with primary antibody against either laminin antibody in dilution buffer (1:400) or collagen IV antibody in dilution (1:50) for 30 min at room temperature or overnight. Do not rinse sections between blocking step and primary antibody incubation (*see* **Notes 13** and **15**).
7. Rinse once in wash puffer.
8. Incubate with primary antibody enhancer in dilution buffer (1:50) for 15 min at room temperature.
9. Rinse once in wash puffer.
10. Incubate with *HRP* Polymer for 30 min at room temperature.
11. Rinse twice in wash buffer.
12. Stain in DAB as a chromogen for 10 min.
13. Rinse thrice in wash buffer.
14. Counterstain in Harris–Hematoxylin (1:3) for 10 min.
15. The results are visualized using a standard bright microscope (*see* Fig. 4).

3.7 DNA Assay

For further quantitative validation of cellular removal, efficacy specimens from the apex, septum, and left and right ventricle (*see* **Note 16**) of the decellularized heart are assessed for residual DNA content.

1. Cut decellularized specimens of 10–30 μg into small pieces.
2. Perform DNA extraction with the *AllPrep DNA/RNA/Protein Mini Kit* according to the instructions of the manufacturer.
3. For calculation of the DNA concentration, measure an aliquot at 260 nm for absorption in a photometer.

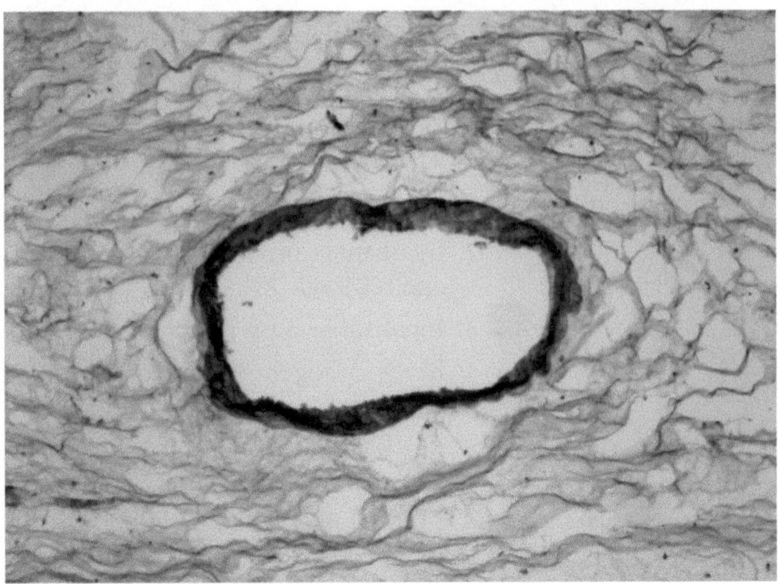

Fig. 4 Representative immunohistochemistry of cardial ECM of a decellularized whole heart showing the presence of laminin (*brown*, DAB) after decellularization. Laminin content remains particularly high at the basement membrane of the vascular system but is also discernible throughout the matrix (×100 magnification)

3.8 GAG Assay

For further quantitative validation of the degree of preservation of extracellular matrix composition specimens as stated above are assessed for overall glycosaminoglycan (GAG) composition.

1. Cut decellularized specimens of 10–30 μg into small pieces.
2. Perform GAG extraction with the *Blyscan Sulfated Glycosaminoglycan Assay* kit according to the instructions of the manufacturer.
3. For calculation of the GAG concentration, measure an aliquot at 656 nm for absorption in a photometer.

4 Notes

1. Perfusate can easily be exchanged through an additional outlet at the bottom of the perfusion chamber. Make sure to leave clamp the tube system and only exchange the perfusate in the perfusion chamber, this will prevent air getting into the perfusion cycle.
2. A bubble trap integrated into the perfusion cycle and connected immediately upstream of the perfusion inlet prevents air bubbles from entering the vascular system clogging the capillary system and influencing decellularization quality.

3. Systemic heparinization prior to explantation prevents clotting in the coronary system as soon as the heart is removed ex vivo.
4. A right atrial incision in the explanted heart will allow for better coronary drainage and thus optimizing perfusion outward flow.
5. Adenosine causes endothelial dependent relaxation of smooth muscle cells dilating coronary arteries and thus allowing for more efficient initial perfusion.
6. Washing cycles of the different decellularization steps should be performed with a hypotonic solution like deionized water instead of iso- or hypertonic tonic solutions like PBS, enhancing cell lysis by osmotic shock and ensuring the washing out of cell debris through a proper diffusion gradient.
7. All detergent solutions should be used after prior sterilization through microporous filtration. Although the *modus operandi* of detergents is the lysis of cell membranes and the solubilization of nuclear membranes therefore implicating a bactericide effect, sometimes we observed a suprainfection of the perfusate during the decellularization process. We do not recommend the sterilization of detergent solution in an autoclave since this may lead to chemical modification of the components.
8. Detergent solutions should always be prepared fresh and stored at room temperature prior to use. Inadequate long-term storage before processing may also influence the quality of decellularization.
9. Decellularization should be performed at room temperature (22–24 °C) unless otherwise stated. Lower temperatures (e.g., non-heated rooms) lead to crystallization of detergent solutions and may influence the quality of decellularization by inefficient detergent effect and by clogging of the vascular system.
10. For optimal effect of the DNase in the last decellularization step perform perfusion at 37 °C to enhance enzymatic activity using a simple heat exchanger connected in parallel to the perfusion inlet.
11. Testing decellularized heart templates for cytotoxicity we gained experimental evidence that after a final 12 h perfusion cycle with PBS the residual concentration of detergents does not provide any cytotoxic effect anymore.
12. Decellularized hearts can be stored in PBS supplemented with penicillin–streptomycin at 4 °C and are then ready to use. No additional sterilization processes are needed for in vitro or in vivo experiments.

13. Since decellularization efficacy appears to be perfusion pressure dependent and perfusion pressure may vary depending on the flow area without interfering with overall coronary perfusion pressure, decellularization efficacy control in different standardized areas is necessary.
14. Repeated freezing and thawing of antibodies are not recommended.
15. Specificity of the labeling (negative control) is confirmed by omission of the primary antibody and treating with the appropriate isotype IgG. Paraffin sections of respective native heart myocardium serve as a positive control. Negative and positive controls should be run simultaneously with all experimental specimens.

References

1. Song JJ, Ott HC (2011) Organ engineering based on decellularized matrix scaffolds. Trends Mol Med 17(8):424–432
2. Ng SL, Narayanan K, Gao S et al (2011) Lineage restricted progenitors for the repopulation of decellularized heart. Biomaterials 32(30):7571–7580
3. Badylak SF, Weiss DJ, Caplan A et al (2012) Engineered whole organs and complex tissues. Lancet 379(9819):943–952
4. Ott HC, Matthiesen TS, Goh SK et al (2008) Perfusion-decellularized matrix: using nature's platform to engineer a bioartificial heart. Nat Med 14(2):213–221
5. Akhyari P, Aubin H, Gwanmesia P et al (2011) The quest for an optimized protocol for whole-heart decellularization: a comparison of three popular and a novel decellularization technique and their diverse effects on crucial extracellular matrix qualities. Tissue Eng C Methods 17(9):915–926
6. Gilbert TW, Sellaro TL, Badylak SF (2006) Decellularization of tissues and organs. Biomaterials 27(19):3675–3683
7. Crapo PM, Gilbert TW, Badylak SF (2011) An overview of tissue and whole organ decellularization processes. Biomaterials 32(12):3233–3243
8. Keane TJ, Londono R, Turner NJ et al (2012) Consequences of ineffective decellularization of biologic scaffolds on the host response. Biomaterials 33(6):1771–1781
9. Gilbert TW, Freund JM, Badylak SF (2009) Quantification of DNA in biologic scaffold materials. J Surg Res 152(1):135–139
10. Badylak SF, Gilbert TW (2008) Immune response to biologic scaffold materials. Semin Immunol 20(2):109–116
11. Akhyari P, Kamiya H, Gwanmesia P et al (2010) In vivo functional performance and structural maturation of decellularised allogenic aortic valves in the subcoronary position. Eur J Cardiothorac Surg J Eur Assoc Cardiothorac Surg 38(5):539–546
12. Tudorache I, Cebotari S, Sturz G et al (2007) Tissue engineering of heart valves: biomechanical and morphological properties of decellularized heart valves. J Heart Valve Dis 16(5):567–573, discussion 574
13. Lichtenberg A, Cebotari S, Tudorache I et al (2007) Biological scaffolds for heart valve tissue engineering. In: Hauser H, Fussenegger M (eds) Methods in molecular medicine, 2nd edn. Tissue Eng 140:309
14. Lichtenberg A, Cebotari S, Tudorache I et al (2006) Flow-dependent re-endothelialization of tissue-engineered heart valves. J Heart Valve Dis 15(2):287–293, discussion 293–4
15. Lichtenberg A, Tudorache I, Cebotari S et al (2006) Preclinical testing of tissue-engineered heart valves re-endothelialized under simulated physiological conditions. Circulation 114(1 Suppl):I559–I565
16. Cebotari S, Lichtenberg A, Tudorache I et al (2006) Clinical application of tissue engineered human heart valves using autologous progenitor cells. Circulation 114(1 Suppl):I132–I137
17. Lichtenberg A, Breymann T, Cebotari S et al (2006) Cell seeded tissue engineered cardiac valves based on allograft and xenograft scaffolds. Prog Pediatr Cardiol 21(2):211–217

Chapter 15

Clinical Trials of Cardiac Repair with Adult Bone Marrow-Derived Cells

Vinodh Jeevanantham, Mohammad R. Afzal, Ewa K. Zuba-Surma, and Buddhadeb Dawn

Abstract

The past decade has witnessed a marked increase in the number of clinical trials of cardiac repair with adult bone marrow cells (BMCs). These trials included patients with acute myocardial infarction (MI) as well as chronic ischemic heart disease (IHD) and utilized different types of BMCs with variable numbers, routes of administration, and timings after MI. Given these differences in methods, the outcomes from these trials have been often disparate and controversial. However, analysis of pooled data suggests that BMC injection enhances left ventricular function, reduces infarct scar size, and improves remodeling in patients with acute MI as well as chronic IHD. BMC therapy also improves clinical outcomes during follow-up without any increase in adverse effects. Although the underlying mechanisms of heart repair are difficult to elucidate in human studies, valuable insights may be gleaned from subgroup analysis of key variables. This information may be utilized to design future randomized controlled trials to carefully determine the long-term safety and benefits of BMC therapy.

Key words Bone marrow, Stem cell, Clinical trial, Myocardial infarction, Myocardial repair, Cardiomyopathy, Coronary artery disease, Meta-analysis

1 Introduction

More than 16 million Americans suffer from coronary heart disease with an estimated 935,000 episodes of acute myocardial infarction (MI) per year [1]. The death of myocytes during MI leads to replacement of myocardial regions by noncontractile fibrous tissue, followed by progressive remodeling of the left ventricle (LV) with eventual development of ischemic cardiomyopathy [2, 3]. Unfortunately, the common medical and surgical options for MI and ischemic heart disease (IHD) are unable to replenish the lost myocardial tissue and thus cannot improve the overall prognosis of millions of patients with ischemic heart failure. Although cardiac transplantation offers a definitive therapy, the scarcity of donor hearts precludes its wider application. In light of this enormous clinical

Race L. Kao (ed.), *Cellular Cardiomyoplasty: Methods and Protocols*, Methods in Molecular Biology, vol. 1036, DOI 10.1007/978-1-62703-511-8_15, © Springer Science+Business Media New York 2013

burden, cell therapy for cardiac repair has attracted unprecedented attention among both basic and clinical cardiovascular researchers. Indeed, results from various animal models of MI and cardiomyopathy suggest that therapy with adult bone marrow cells (BMCs) improves LV function and attenuate LV remodeling. Based on these highly promising data, a number of clinical trials of cardiac repair with adult BMCs have already been completed in patients with acute MI as well as ischemic heart failure [4, 5].

These early trials of BMC therapy used diverse cell populations with highly variable cell numbers injected via different routes at different time intervals after MI in patients with acute MI, chronic IHD, and cardiomyopathy [4, 5]. Besides the differences in BMC types, the methodology for isolation and processing of cells also varied significantly among these studies [5–7]. Moreover, the investigators employed diverse techniques (left ventriculography, echocardiography, SPECT imaging, magnetic resonance imaging [MRI]) to assess cardiac outcome parameters [5]. Given these differences in study design and methods, it is not surprising that results from these BMC therapy trials have been often disparate and sometimes controversial. However, meta-analysis of pooled data has repeatedly shown that BMC transplantation results in modest improvements in various parameters of LV function and remodeling in patients with acute MI and chronic IHD [4, 5, 8, 9]. Such meta-analyses have also identified several important methodological variables that need further fine-tuning in order to maximize the benefits of BMC therapy for heart repair.

2 Clinical Trials of BMC Therapy for Cardiac Repair

The adult bone marrow contains many different types of hematopoietic and nonhematopoietic cells at various stages of development, ranging from very primitive stem/progenitors to mature cells that are ready to escape into the circulation. These cell types include mononuclear cells [10], mesenchymal stem cells (MSCs) [11], hematopoietic stem cells [12], side population cells [13], and very small embryonic-like stem cells (VSELs) [14–17], to name a few. The relatively easy availability of autologous BMCs in large numbers has made the bone marrow an attractive cellular source for clinical trials of cardiac repair. Table 1 provides the details of randomized controlled trials (RCTs) as well as cohort studies that examined the safety and efficacy of cardiac repair with various adult BMC populations in humans. The different types of cells used in these trials are described in brief below.

2.1 Bone Marrow Mononuclear Cells

Bone marrow mononuclear cells (BMMNCs) are highly heterogeneous and contain both hematopoietic as well as nonhematopoietic cells. BMMNCs are typically isolated by density gradient

Table 1
Controlled clinical trials of cardiac repair with various types of bone marrow-derived cells

Study	Trial design	Cell type	Number of cells	Route of injection	Type of IHD	Follow-up duration (months)	Results
Akar et al. [81]	Cohort	BMMNC	$1.29 \pm 0.09 \times 10^9$	IM during CABG	CIHD	18	LVEF ⇧; myocardial perfusion ⇧; wall motion ⇧; LVESVI ⇩; NYHA class ⇩
Ang et al. [107]	RCT	BMMNC	$85 \pm 56 \times 10^6$ (IM)	IM or IC during CABG	CIHD	6	No significant improvement in LVEF, regional thickening fraction, and LV volumes
Assmus et al. [30]	RCT	BMMNC and CPC	$205 \pm 110 \times 10^6$ (BMMNC) $22 \pm 11 \times 10^6$ (CPC)	IC	CIHD	6	BMMNC: LVEF ⇧; regional contractility ⇧ CPC: no significant improvement
Bartunek et al. [56]	Cohort	CD133+ BMC	$12.6 \pm 2.2 \times 10^6$	IC	AMI	4	In treated patients compared with baseline, global LVEF ⇧; regional function ⇧; infarct size ⇩; viability ⇧
Cao et al. [33]	RCT	BMMNC	$5 \pm 1.2 \times 10^7$	IC	AMI	48	LVEF ⇧; LVESV ⇩
Chen et al. [49]	RCT	MSC	$48–60 \times 10^9$	IC	AMI	6	LVEF ⇧; infarct wall motion ⇧; LVESV ⇩; infarct size ⇩; LVEDV ⇩
Chen et al. [50]	Cohort	MSC	5×10^6/ml	IC	CIHD	12	Perfusion ⇧; NYHA class ⇩; exercise tolerance ⇧
Choi et al. [73]	Cohort	PBSC	$2.03 \pm 0.69 \times 10^9$	IC	AMI	24	Compared with controls, no additional improvement in LV functional or structural parameters
Colombo et al. [58]	RCT	CD133+ cells from BM or PB	$5.9\ (4.9–13.5) \times 10^6$	IC	AMI	12	Myocardial blood flow ⇧ with BM-derived CD133+ cells; no significant change in LVEF, LV volumes, and infarct size

(continued)

Table 1 (continued)

Study	Trial design	Cell type	Number of cells	Route of injection	Type of IHD	Follow-up duration (months)	Results
Erbs et al. [65]	RCT	CPC	$69 \pm 14 \times 10^6$	IC	ICM	3	Global LVEF ⇧; infarct size ⇩; myocardial perfusion ⇧; coronary flow reserve ⇧
Ge et al. [25]	RCT	BMMNC	40×10^6	IC	AMI	6	LVEF ⇧; myocardial perfusion ⇧; LV dilation halted
Grajek et al. [97]	RCT	BMMNC	$2.34 \pm 1.2 \times 10^9$	IC	AMI	12	Myocardial perfusion ⇧; no significant change in LVEF and LV volumes; adverse events ⇩
Hare et al. [52]	RCT	MSC	0.5×10^6/kg –5×10^6/kg	IV	AMI	12	Ventricular arrhythmia ⇩; FEV1 ⇧; global symptom score improved; EF ⇧ in patients with anterior MI
Hendrikx et al. [26]	RCT	BMMNC	$60.25 \pm 31.35 \times 10^6$	IM during C ABG	CIHD	4	Regional wall thickening ⇧; no improvement in LVEF, LVESV, and LVEDV
Hirsch et al. [108]	RCT	BMMNC and PBMNC	$296 \pm 164 \times 10^6$ (BMMNC) $287 \pm 137 \times 10^6$ (PBMNC)	IC	AMI	4	No significant difference among group with regard to regional and global LV function, LV volumes, mass, and infarct size
Huang et al. [109]	RCT	BMMNC	NA	IC	AMI	6	LVEF ⇧; infarct size ⇩; no significant difference in LV volumes
Huikuri et al. [32]	RCT	BMMNC	$402 \pm 196 \times 10^6$	IC	AMI	6	LVEF ⇧
Janssens et al. [100]	RCT	BMSC	$172 \pm 72 \times 10^6$	IC	AMI	4	Infarct size ⇩; no improvement in LVEF, LVESV, and LVEDV

Kang et al. [71]	RCT	PBSC	$1.5 \pm 0.5 \times 10^9$	IC	AMI/CIHD	6	In patients with AMI: global LVEF ⇧; LVESV ⇩; infarct size ⇩; coronary flow reserve ⇧. In patients with OMI: coronary flow reserve ⇧
Katritsis et al. [51]	Cohort	MSC and EPC	$2–4 \times 10^6$	IC	AMI and CIHD	4	Myocardial perfusion ⇧; viability ⇧; no improvement in LVEF, LVESV, and LVEDV
Li et al. [72]	RCT	PBSC	$72.5 \pm 73 \times 10^6$	IC	AMI	6	Global LVEF ⇧; wall motion ⇧; no improvement in LVESV and LVEDV
Lipiec et al. [34]	RCT	BMMNC	$0.33 \pm 0.17 \times 10^6$ (CD133+) $3.36 \pm 1.87 \times 10^6$ (CD34+)	IC	AMI	6	Myocardial perfusion ⇧; significantly greater absolute improvement in infarct area wall motion; no significant difference in LVEF and volumes
Losordo et al. [68]	RCT	CD34+ BMC	5×10^4, 1×10^5, and 5×10^5 CD34+ cells/kg	IM (transendo-cardial)	CIHD	12	In cell-treated patients, angina frequency, nitroglycerin usage, exercise time, and CCS class showed trends toward greater improvement
Losordo et al. [69]	RCT	CD34+ BMC	1×10^5 or 5×10^5 CD34+ cells/kg	IM (transendo cardial)	CIHD	12	Weekly angina frequency and exercise tolerance improved significantly in low-dose group; improvements in high-dose group were not significant
Lunde et al. [29, 110–112]	RCT	BMMNC	$87 \pm 47.7 \times 10^6$	IC	AMI	36	No improvement in LVEF, infarct size, and LVEDV
Manginas et al. [59]	Cohort	CD133+ and CD133–CD34+ BMC	$16.9 \pm 4.9 \times 10^6$ (CD133+) $8 \pm 4 \times 10^6$ (CD133–CD34+)	IC	CIHD	10–40	In treated patients compared with baseline, LVEF ⇧; LVEDV ⇩; LVESV ⇩; myocardial perfusion ⇧

(continued)

Table 1 (continued)

Study	Trial design	Cell type	Number of cells	Route of injection	Type of IHD	Follow-up duration (months)	Results
Meluzin et al. [22, 96]	RCT	BMMNC	10×10^6 and 100×10^6	IC	AMI	12	In high-dose group, global LVEF ⇧; LVESV ⇩; earlier improvement in regional systolic function partially lost at 12 months
Meyer et al. [41–43, 113]	RCT	BMC	$24.6 \pm 9.4 \times 10^8$	IC	AMI	61	Early differences in global LVEF and regional wall motion between treated and control patients lost significance at 18 months; diastolic function improved; LVEF ⇧ in patients with infarct transmurality > median; major adverse events similar
Mocini et al. [27]	Cohort	BMMNC	$292 \pm 232 \times 10^6$	IM during CABG	CIHD	3	LVEF ⇧; wall motion ⇧
Nogueira et al. [114]	RCT	BMMNC	100×10^6	IC and cardiac vein	AMI	6	No significant improvement in LVEF; LVESV; LVEDV
Penicka et al. [19]	RCT	BMMNC	26.4×10^8 (IQR $19.6–33.0 \times 10^8$)	IC	AMI	4	No significant improvement in LVEF, infarct size, and LV volumes; study terminated due to lack of benefit and possible safety issues
Perin et al. [20, 23]	Cohort	BMMNC	$25.5 \pm 6.3 \times 10^6$	IM (transendocardial)	CIHD	12	Angina class ⇩; NYHA class ⇩; exercise capacity ⇧; myocardial perfusion ⇧; no improvement in global LVEF
Piepoli et al. [78]	RCT	BMMNC	Mean 418×10^6 (total BMC) 248.78×10^6 (mononuclear)	IC	AMI	12	LVEF ⇧; LVESV ⇩; LVEDV ⇩; VO2max ⇧; perfusion⇧; heart rate variability improved

Plewka et al. [86]	RCT	BMMNC	$144 \pm 49 \times 10^6$	IC	AMI	6	Compared with baseline, the absolute change in LVEF ⇧; diastolic function parameters improved in treated group
Pokushalov et al. [39]	RCT	BMMNC	$41 \pm 16 \times 10^6$	IM (transendo cardial)	CIHD	12	LVEF ⇧; LVESV ⇩; LVEDV ⇩; NYHA class ⇩; CCS class⇩; angina episodes ⇩; nitrate requirement ⇩
Quyyumi et al. [115]	RCT	CD34+ BMC	$5–15 \times 10^6$	IC	AMI	6	Myocardial perfusion ⇧ in ≥10 million cohort; trend toward improvement in LVEF in ≥10 million cohort
Rivas-Plata et al. [82]	Cohort	BMMNC	Mean $2,442 \times 10^6$	IM during CABG	CIHD	27	Absolute change in LVEF ⇧; significant decrease in NYHA functional class
Roncalli et al. [101]	RCT	BMC	$98.3 \pm 8.7 \times 10^6$	IC	AMI	3	Trend toward increase in percentage of patients with improved viability; no significant difference in LVEF and infarct size
Ruan et al. [44]	RCT	BMC	NR	IC	AMI	6	LVEF ⇧; segmental function in the infarct as well as viable area ⇧; LVESV ⇩; LVEDV ⇩
Schachinger et al. [28, 116, 117]	RCT	BMMNC	$236 \pm 174 \times 10^6$	IC	AMI	4	LVEF ⇧; regional wall motion ⇧; LVESV ⇩; coronary flow reserve ⇧; major adverse cardiovascular events ⇩; no improvement in LVEDV
Silva et al. [118]	RCT	BMMNC	100×10^6	IC or retrograde via coronary vein	AMI	6	In IC group, compared with baseline, LVEF ⇧
Srimahachota et al. [119]	RCT	BMMNC	$420 \pm 221 \times 10^6$	IC	AMI	6	No significant improvement in treated group

(continued)

Table 1 (continued)

Study	Trial design	Cell type	Number of cells	Route of injection	Type of IHD	Follow-up duration (months)	Results
Stamm et al. [60]	Cohort	CD133+	Median 7.19×10^6	IM during CABG	CIHD	62 ± 9	LVEF ⇧; myocardial perfusion improved; compared with baseline, LVEF improved in patients with LVEF of ≤40 %
Strauer et al. [18]	Cohort	BMMNC	$28 \pm 22 \times 10^6$	IC	AMI	3	Stroke volume index ⇧; regional wall motion ⇧; LV contractility index ⇧; infarct size ⇩; LVESV ⇩
Strauer et al. [24]	Cohort	BMMNC	90×10^6	IC	CIHD	3	LVEF ⇧; infarct wall motion ⇧; infarct size ⇩; viability ⇧; VO2max ⇧
Strauer et al. [40]	Cohort	BMMNC	$66 \pm 33 \times 10^6$	IC	CIHD	60	In treated patients, compared with baseline, LVEF ⇧; regional wall motion ⇧; infarct size ⇩; heart rate variability improved; VO2max ⇧; long-term mortality ⇩
Suarez de Lezo et al. [120]	RCT	BMMNC	$9 \pm 3 \times 10^8$	IC	AMI	3	In BMMNC-treated patients, LVEF ⇧; regional contractility ⇧
Tatsumi et al. [74]	Cohort	PBMNC	$4.92 \pm 2.82 \times 10^9$	IC	AMI	6	Global LVEF ⇧; wall motion ⇧; infarct size ⇩; LVESV index tended to be lower
Tendera et al. [35]	RCT	BMMNC or CD34+ CXCR4+ BMC	1.78×10^8 (BMMNC) 1.90×10^6 (CD34+ CXCR4+ BMC)	IC	AMI	6	In cell-treated patients with baseline LVEF of <37 %, LVEF improved compared with baseline
Traverse et al. [37]	RCT	BMMNC	100×10^6	IC	AMI	6	No significant difference in LVEF; LVESV ⇩

Traverse et al. [121]	RCT	BMMNC	$147 \pm 17 \times 10^6$	IC	AMI	6	No significant difference in LVEF, regional wall motion, LV volume indices, and infarct volume
Tse et al. [31]	RCT	BMMNC	$16.7 \pm 3.4 \times 10^6$ (low dose), $42 \pm 28 \times 10^6$ (high dose)	IM (transendocardial)	CIHD	6	LVEF ⇧; infarct wall thickening ⇧; LVESV ⇩; exercise time ⇧; NYHA class ⇩
Turan et al. [83]	Cohort	BMC	$101 \pm 20 \times 10^6$	IC	AMI	6	In treated patients, compared with baseline, LVEF ⇧; infarct size ⇩; infarct wall movement velocity ⇧; LVESV ⇩; NYHA class ⇩
Turan et al. [84]	RCT	BMC	$96 \pm 32 \times 10^6$	IC	AMI	12	Global LVEF ⇧; infarct wall movement velocity ⇧; infarct size ⇩; NYHA class ⇩; BNP levels ⇩; significant mobilization of BMCPCs existed 3, 6, and 12 months after cell therapy
van Ramshorst et al. [38, 87]	RCT	BMMNC	$98 \pm 6 \times 10^6$	IM (transendocardial)	CIHD	3	In treated patients, change in LVEF from baseline ⇧; improvement in CCS class and quality of life score; improved myocardial relaxation and filling pressures
Wohrle et al. [36]	RCT	BMMNC	$381 \pm 130 \times 10^6$	IC	AMI	6	No change in LVEF, LVESV, LVEDV, and infarct size
Yao et al. [85]	RCT	BMMNC	Estimated mean 384×10^6	IC	CIHD	6	No significant difference in LVEF, LV diameters, infarct size, and myocardial perfusion; diastolic parameter improved in treated patients compared with baseline

(continued)

Table 1 (continued)

Study	Trial design	Cell type	Number of cells	Route of injection	Type of IHD	Follow-up duration (months)	Results
Yao et al. [122]	RCT	BMMNC	$1.9 \pm 1.2 \times 10^8$ (single infusion) $2.0 \pm 1.4 \times 10^8$ (first infusion) $2.1 \pm 1.7 \times 10^8$ (second infusion)	IC	AMI	12	In patients receiving two injections, LVEF ⇧; infarct size ⇩
Yousef et al. [79]	Cohort	BMMNC	$61 \pm 39 \times 10^6$	IC	AMI	60	In treated patients, compared with baseline, LVEF ⇧; LVEDV ⇩; LVESV ⇩; infarct size ⇩; exercise capacity ⇧; mortality ⇩; quality of life improved
Zhao et al. [80]	RCT	BMMNC	$659 \pm 512 \times 10^6$	IM during CABG	CIHD	6	LVEF ⇧; infarct wall motion ⇧; perfusion ⇧; NYHA class ⇩; CCS class improved

AMI acute myocardial infarction, *BMC* bone marrow cell, *BMCPC* bone marrow-derived circulating progenitor cells, *BMMNC* bone marrow mononuclear cell, *BMSC* bone marrow stem cell, *CABG* coronary artery bypass graft, *CIHD* chronic ischemic heart disease, *CCS* Canadian Cardiovascular Society, *CPC* circulating progenitor cells, *EMM* electromechanical mapping, *EPC* endothelial progenitor cells, *IC* intracoronary, *ICM* ischemic cardiomyopathy, *IM* intramuscular, *LV* left ventricular, *LVEF* LV ejection fraction, *LVEDV* LV end-diastolic volume, *LVESV* LV end-systolic volume, *LVESVI* LVESV index, *MSC* mesenchymal stem cell, *NA* not available, *NYHA* New York Heart Association, *OMI* old myocardial infarction, *PB* peripheral blood, *PBMNC* PB-derived mononuclear cell, *PBSC* PB-derived stem cell, *PCI* percutaneous coronary intervention, *RCT* randomized controlled trial centrifugation using various commercially available formulations [10]. In the cohort study by Strauer et al. [18], intracoronary injection of autologous BMMNCs in patients with acute MI improved myocardial perfusion and regional function and reduced infarct size. Since this report, a large number of randomized controlled trials of BMMNC therapy in patients with acute MI, chronic IHD, and ischemic heart failure have been reported [19–37] (Table 1). Importantly, in the vast majority of these studies, BMMNC transplantation was associated with improvement in one or more parameters of global and regional myocardial function, perfusion, anatomy, infarct size, and viability (Table 1). In addition, improvement in New York Heart Association (NYHA) functional class, maximal oxygen uptake (VO2max), exercise capacity, anginal symptoms, and nitroglycerin intake has also been reported with BMMNC therapy [20, 23, 24, 31, 38–40].

A few other trials have injected relatively unselected nucleated BMCs via the intracoronary route [41–44]. In the study by Wollert et al. [41], significant improvement in global LVEF as well as regional wall motion was noted in BMC-treated patients after 6 months of follow-up. Interestingly, these differences in LVEF and other outcome parameters were no longer significant between control and BMC-treated patients after 18 months of follow-up, suggesting a transient nature of BMC-induced benefits [42]. Nonetheless, a more persistent improvement in diastolic function was noted in the same patients [42], indicating a broader range of benefits conferred by BMC therapy. In the study by Ruan et al. [44], the improvements in functional and anatomical parameters in BMC-treated patients did not change between 3 and 6 months of follow-up.

2.2 Mesenchymal Stem Cells

Bone marrow mesenchymal stem cells (MSCs) perform a supportive function in the stroma and give rise to nonhematopoietic cells. In addition, they are able to differentiate into osteocytic, chondrocytic, adipose, skeletal muscle, neural, and other lineages [11, 45]. Several reports suggest that MSCs also differentiate into cardiomyocytes under specific culture conditions in vitro and following myocardial transplantation in vivo [46–48]. From a feasibility standpoint, MSCs can be potentially harvested in advance, expanded in culture, and stored for use after an acute MI in the future. In clinical trials, intracoronary injection of bone marrow-derived MSCs resulted in improvement in global LVEF and regional wall motion, and reduction in infarct size, LVESV, as well as LVEDV in patients with acute MI [49]. In patients with ischemic cardiomyopathy, intracoronary injection of MSCs resulted in improved perfusion and improved exercise tolerance and NYHA class [50]. However, in the study by Katritsis et al. [51], intracoronary injection of two to four million MSCs enhanced myocardial perfusion and viability, but failed to improve global LVEF, LVESV, or LVEDV in patients with acute or old MI.

In the dose-ranging RCT by Hare and colleagues, intravenous administration of allogeneic MSCs after an acute MI increased LVEF in treated patients compared with baseline and resulted in reverse remodeling [52]. In a subsequent study comparing the efficacy of allogeneic vs. autologous MSCs in patients with ischemic cardiomyopathy, both MSC types reduced infarct size and the sphericity index, resulting in reverse remodeling, and autologous MSCs improved 6-min walk distance and quality of life compared with baseline [53]. Although no significant increase in EF was noted, LVESV and LVEDV improved with transendocardial MSC therapy with similar adverse event rates with both types of MSCs [53]. Together, these data indicate that in patients with ischemic heart failure, MSC injection favorably impacts patient functional capacity, quality of life, and LV remodeling.

2.3 AC133+ BMCs

Induction of angiogenesis in the periinfarct zone and infarcted myocardium has been advanced as a mechanism of cardiac repair by BMCs. Accordingly, the AC133+ subset of BMCs with angiogenic potential [54, 55] has been utilized for cardiac repair. Although intracoronary injection of AC133+ cells improved global LVEF and regional wall motion and reduced infarct size, spontaneous and inducible VT was noted in two cell-treated patients [56]. In addition, cell-treated patients experienced increased in-stent restenosis [56], and subsequent careful angiographic analysis revealed greater luminal narrowing in non-stented coronary arterial regions [57], suggesting potentially greater risk of atherogenesis with AC133+ BMC therapy. However, in a subsequent study by Colombo et al. [58], intracoronary injection of CD133+ cells in patients with large anterior MI resulted in improved myocardial blood flow by PET imaging without affecting other cardiac parameters significantly. In another study in patients with old anterior MI, intracoronary injection of CD133+ and CD133–CD34+ cells improved perfusion, LVEF, and remodeling [59].

CD133+ cells have also been used via the transepicardial route in patients undergoing CABG. In the study by Stamm et al. [60], intramyocardial injection of CD133+ BMCs along with CABG improved LVEF and myocardial perfusion compared with patients who underwent CABG alone. However, the differences in LVEF between cell-treated and control groups disappeared after 18 months, except in patients with baseline EF ≤40 % [61]. Moreover, patients who were operated on between 7 and 12 weeks after MI had greater chance of improvement with cell therapy compared with more delayed procedures. These data may suggest specific influence of myocardial milieu on the efficacy of CD133+ cells in cardiac repair.

2.4 Mobilized BMCs

In several clinical trials, the investigators transplanted BMCs harvested from the peripheral blood with or without prior mobilization with cytokines. Such use of mobilized progenitors circumvents the relatively invasive process of bone marrow aspiration in already sick patients.

2.4.1 Circulating Progenitor Cells (CPCs)

In the TOPCARE-AMI trial [62–64], intracoronary injection of peripheral blood-derived CPCs improved global LVEF and LVESV after 4 months. After 1 year of follow-up, MRI studies showed improved LVEF, smaller infarct size, and improved LV hypertrophy in CPC-treated patients [64]. In the study by Erbs et al. [65], intracoronary CPC delivery in the setting of recanalized chronic total occlusion reduced infarct size and the number of hibernating segments, increased coronary flow reserve, and improved regional wall motion and global LVEF. However, such benefits were absent in CPC-treated patients with previous MI, dysfunctional LV segments, and an open infarct-related artery in a subsequent RCT [30], perhaps indicating an important role played by the myocardial milieu in CPC-induced cardiac repair.

2.4.2 CD34+ Cells

It is well known that CD34+ cells from the peripheral blood as well as the bone marrow have angiogenic attributes [66, 67]. Consistently, transendocardial transplantation of autologous peripheral blood-derived CD34+ cells resulted in trends toward reduced angina frequency, reduced nitroglycerin usage, improved exercise time, and improvement in Canadian Cardiovascular Society (CCS) class in patients with refractory angina. [68]. These results were corroborated in a phase II study, in which transendocardial injection of CD34+ cells reduced weekly angina frequency and improved exercise time in patients with CCS class III–IV angina at enrollment [69]. Interestingly, these changes were more pronounced with a lower CD34+ cell dose (1×10^5 CD34+ cells/kg) compared with a higher (5×10^5 CD34+ cells/kg) dose [69].

2.4.3 Peripheral Blood Stem Cells

Peripheral blood-derived stem cells (PBSCs) [70–73] or mononuclear cells (PBMNCs) [74] have also been utilized for cardiac repair in several trials. Although the first RCT with G-CSF-mobilized PBSCs [70] was stopped due to increased in-stent restenosis, in a subsequent RCT [71] that used drug-eluting stents, intracoronary PBSC injection improved EF, reduced LVESV and infarct size, and improved coronary flow reserve in patients with acute MI. Other studies of intracoronary PBSCs and PBMNCs therapy in the setting of acute MI have also reported improvements in LV function and structure [72, 74]. However, the failure of PBSC therapy to improve LV function and remodeling in patients with ICM [71] suggests that myocardial characteristics (acute MI vs. chronic IHD) are important determinants of cardiac cell therapy outcomes. Regardless, these differences in outcomes and the potential risk of in-stent restenosis with cytokine-mobilized cell injection need to be carefully evaluated in larger RCTs.

3 Meta-analysis of Pooled Data on Effects of BMC Therapy

Although BMC therapy for heart repair has gained remarkable popularity in the recent past, the number of patients enrolled in each study has been rather small. Given the diversity in cell type, patient characteristics, study design, and outcomes assessed, results from these trials have often been discordant [4, 5, 75]. Therefore, several meta-analyses of pooled data from clinical trials of BMC therapy have been performed in the recent past [4, 8, 9, 76, 77]. Importantly, although each meta-analysis of BMC trials included somewhat different sets of studies, the results of these meta-analyses [4, 8, 9, 76, 77] have been generally concordant and show an overall beneficial impact of BMC therapy on cardiac function and structure in patients with acute MI as well as chronic IHD.

3.1 LV Ejection Fraction

The global LVEF reflects the overall contractile function of LV and has been reported in nearly all trials of BMC therapy. In our recent comprehensive meta-analysis that included 50 RCTs and cohort studies (a total of 2,625 patients) of BMC therapy for cardiac repair, BMC injection produced a 3.96 % greater increase in LVEF compared with controls [5]. The analysis of interaction indicated similar efficacy of BMC therapy in improving LVEF in patients with acute MI as well as chronic IHD [5]. The improvement in LVEF in BMC-treated patients compared with controls was 3.66 % in the meta-analysis by Abdel-Latif et al. [4], 4.21 % in the meta-analysis by Hristov et al. [9], 3 % in the meta-analysis by Lipinski et al. [8], 2.99 % in the meta-analysis by Martin-Rendon et al. [76], and 4.77 % in the meta-analysis by Zhang et al. [77]. These concordant findings from several meta-analyses indicate that BMC therapy is associated with a modest yet significant (2.99–4.21 %) improvement in LVEF compared with standard treatment [4, 8, 9, 76, 77].

3.2 Infarct Size

Infarct size is a reliable measure of the extent of cardiac repair induced by cell therapy and various techniques (SPECT, left ventriculogram, MRI) have been used in clinical trials for this purpose. In our recent meta-analysis of data from a total of 50 studies, a 4.03 % greater reduction in infarct size was noted in BMC-treated patients compared with controls [5]. In previous meta-analyses by Abdel-Latif et al. [4], Lipinski et al. [8], and Martin-Rendon et al. [76], infarct size reduction in BMC-treated patients was greater by 5.49 %, 5.6 %, and 3.5 %, respectively, compared with controls.

3.3 LV End-Systolic Volume

LVESV is a surrogate indicator of global LV systolic performance with unchanged LVEDV. In our recent meta-analysis [5], the reduction in LVESV was greater by 8.91 ml in BMC-treated patients compared with controls. Greater improvements in LVESV in BMC-treated patients were also reported in meta-analyses by

Abdel-Latif et al. (−4.80 ml) [4], Lipinski et al. (−7.4 ml) [8], and Martin-Rendon et al. (−4.74 ml) [76]. In this regard, although the reduction in LVEDV in BMC-treated patients was not significant in previous meta-analyses [4, 8, 76], our recent analysis showed a significantly greater reduction in LVEDV in BMC-treated patients, indicating improved remodeling [5]. Therefore, the reduction in LVESV with BMC therapy may reflect a combination of improved systolic performance as well as superior remodeling.

3.4 LV End-Diastolic Volume

After an MI, the LV undergoes remodeling with thinning of the infarct wall and hypertrophy of the viable myocardium [2, 3]. As a result, the LV chamber enlarges and the LVEDV gradually increases. Because LVEDV is an important indicator of LV remodeling, LVEDV was measured in many BMC trials, albeit with different techniques (echocardiography, MRI). In a meta-analysis that included trials with BMC injection within 14 days after acute MI, cell therapy was associated with a trend toward reduction in LVEDV [8]. In the largest meta-analysis that included data from patients with acute MI as well as chronic IHD [5], the reduction in LVEDV was greater by 5.23 ml in BMC-treated patients compared with controls, indicating remodeling benefits of BMC therapy. Although the exact mechanism remains unclear, the improved remodeling can result from myocyte salvage, reduced infarct expansion, salubrious paracrine effects on the matrix, or a combination of these. Future studies need to be conducted to assess the impact of BMC therapy on LVEDV as a function of the time interval between acute MI and BMC transplantation.

3.5 Other Outcome Parameters

Improvements in LV function and structure should logically result in improved patient symptoms and quality of life. Although symptomatic benefits are highly important clinical indicators of the overall efficacy of cell therapy, patient symptoms were reported in a relatively small number of early studies [23, 31, 50, 68]. Due to the differences in specific end points among studies and smaller number of patients for each parameter, analysis of pooled data could not be performed. However, the newer studies are increasingly employing a broader array of outcome measures and monitoring these patient-important variables. The parameters that have thus far been reported to improve with BMC therapy include: VO2max [24, 40, 78], exercise capacity or exercise time [23, 31, 50, 68, 69, 79], NYHA class [23, 31, 39, 50, 80–84], LV diastolic function [43, 85–87], angina frequency [23, 39, 68, 69], nitrate requirement [39, 68], CCS class [38, 39, 68, 80], FEV1 [52], and quality of life [38, 79]. Together, these observations suggest that the benefits of BMC transplantation extend well beyond the conventional measures of global LV function and volumes. These data also indicate that LV structure/function benefits of BMC therapy indeed translate into improved symptoms in patients with IHD.

4 Safety of BMC Transplantation

Along with the benefits, the potential side effects of BMC therapy have also been monitored in clinical trials, and the results from various meta-analyses indicate that BMC therapy does not increase the risk of adverse events compared with standard therapy [4, 8, 76]. Although only a few BMC trials reported "major adverse cardiovascular events" in a comprehensive fashion, results from earlier meta-analyses showed a similar incidence of mortality in BMC-treated and control patients [4, 8, 76]. However, in the largest meta-analysis, BMC therapy was associated with a reduced all-cause mortality and cardiac mortality, indicating an important survival benefit of BMC transplantation [5].

In addition, no increased incidence of ventricular or supraventricular arrhythmia, in-stent restenosis, and target vessel revascularization was noted in BMC-treated patients in meta-analyses of trials that enrolled patients with acute MI as well as chronic IHD [4, 5, 8, 76]. However, a reduced incidence of recurrent MI was noted in a meta-analysis of RCTs in patients with acute MI, along with a trend toward reduced hospitalization for heart failure [8]. In the recent analysis of RCTs as well as cohort studies, BMC therapy was associated with significantly lower incidence of recurrent MI and stent thrombosis, and trends toward reduced incidence of heart failure and cerebrovascular accident [5]. Nonetheless, potential adverse effects of BMC therapy continue to be monitored in large RCTs that are currently in progress.

5 Methodological Considerations

In earlier clinical trials of BMC therapy, vastly different cell numbers were injected via different routes and at various time points after MI in dissimilar patient populations. The methods of cell preparation were also quite different even for the same cell type. Although many of these issues still remain to be specifically answered in large RCTs, important insights have been gained from analysis of pooled data from completed trials.

5.1 Patient Characteristics

With the conduct of larger clinical trials, it has become increasingly apparent that clinical features of recipients are also important determinants of outcomes following BMC transplantation. Two key clinical characteristics are discussed below.

5.1.1 Type of Ischemic Heart Disease

Because the myocardial environment is vastly different in the setting of an acute MI when compared with chronic cardiomyopathy, the outcomes of BMC therapy may potentially differ in patients with these two broad clinical conditions. The results from preclinical studies suggest that BMC injection can also improve outcomes in models of cardiomyopathy [88, 89]. Consistently, in patients with chronic ischemic heart failure, BMC therapy was associated with improved regional wall motion [26, 27, 30, 65], perhaps reflecting the formation of new myocytes or enhanced preservation and augmented function of preexisting myocytes. The analysis of pooled data [5] showed no significant difference in improvements in LVEF and LVEDV with BMC therapy in patients with acute MI and chronic IHD [4, 5]. However, the reduction in LVESV was significantly greater in patients with chronic IHD compared with acute MI patients, and a trend toward greater reduction in infarct scar size was also noted in these patients [5]. However, very little is known at present with regard to retention, survival, and fate of transplanted BMCs in humans; and specific interactions of the myocardial milieu (acutely infarcted vs. chronic remodeled myocardium) with specific BMC types remain unknown. As an example of this cell-specific efficacy, BMMNCs but not CPCs were able to improve outcomes in patients with chronic cardiomyopathy in the TOPCARE-CHD trial [30]. However, CPC injection improved global LV function and regional wall motion in patients with chronic total occlusion in the study by Erbs et al. [65, 90]. Importantly, Erbs et al. injected larger number of CPCs (69 ± 14 million vs. 22 ± 11 million) at a shorter time interval after MI (7.5 ± 2.9 months vs. 77 ± 76 months) compared with the TOPCARE-CHD study [30], [65]. Thus, it will be important to determine whether specific BMC types are more suitable specifically for repairing remodeled myocardium.

5.1.2 LV Function at Baseline

Because having an acute ST-elevation MI was a primary criterion for many BMC trials, patients with relatively preserved LVEF despite MI were enrolled in several earlier trials. However, it is logical to predict that BMC injection would benefit hearts with more severe functional compromise compared with those with near-normal function. Consistent with this notion, in the REPAIR-AMI trial, a significant increase in LVEF was noted in patients with baseline LVEF of ≤48.9 % (the median), but not in those above the median [28]. Similar inverse relation of baseline LVEF with outcomes was noted in another study wherein BMC-treated patients with baseline LVEF of <35 % exhibited significantly greater increase in LVEF compared with those with baseline LVEF of ≥35 % [60]. Further, in the REGENT trial [35], patients with baseline LVEF of <37 %, but not those with LVEF of ≥37 %, receiving unselected or selected BMCs exhibited significant improvement with BMC therapy. The analysis of pooled data, however, did not show a significant interaction of baseline LVEF and improvement in LVEF or infarct size [5]. However, these subgroup analyses did show a significantly greater improvement in LVESV and LVEDV in patients with baseline LVEF of <43 % (the median) compared with those with baseline LVEF of ≥43 % [5], indicating superior remodeling benefits of BMC therapy in hearts with worse function at baseline.

5.2 BMC Number

After transplantation, a large number of BMCs are lost due to cell washout as well as cell death in the inflamed myocardium [91, 92], and reported data indicate that only a small percentage of injected cells is retained within the myocardium [21, 93–95]. In the study by Meluzin et al. [22, 96], only patients who received greater numbers of BMMNCs experienced sustained improvement in LVEF, suggesting a possible dose–response relationship. Accordingly, BMCs in considerably large numbers were injected in several clinical trials [19, 41, 49, 71, 73, 74, 81, 97], and the numbers of transplanted BMCs in trials thus far have ranged from 2 million to 60 billion. To determine the minimum number of BMCs required to produce the desired benefits, we compared the major outcomes (LVEF, infarct size, LVESV, LVEDV) from studies that used less than a certain number of BMCs with those from studies that used more. The results of such stepwise analysis showed that when less than 40 million BMCs were injected, cell therapy failed to improve significantly any of the four major outcome parameters, suggesting that at least 40 million BMCs need to be injected to induce effective cardiac repair. In another meta-analysis of data restricted to patients with acute MI, transplantation of more than 100 million BMCs was necessary to improve LVEF [76]. However, evidence from animal models suggests that a smaller number of selected BMCs may be more effective compared with unselected BMC population injected in larger numbers. This is exemplified in studies that reported superior cardiac reparative outcomes with CD34+ BMCs compared with unfractionated BMCs [98], and CD45− VSELs compared with a tenfold greater number of CD45+ hematopoietic stem cells [99]. The overall evidence therefore suggests that both cell type and number significantly influence the process of cardiac repair by BMCs.

5.3 Route of BMC Injection

In clinical trials, BMCs have been delivered successfully via intracoronary [18, 24, 25, 28, 30, 37, 40, 41, 44, 49, 50, 56, 83, 96, 100, 101], transepicardial (during CABG) [26, 27, 60, 80–82, 102], transendocardial [23, 31, 38, 39, 68, 69], as well as intravenous [52] routes. Each of these approaches presents specific advantages depending on the cell type and patient characteristics. Intracoronary BMC injection can be conveniently performed following PCI after an acute MI or during an elective catheterization in patients with known coronary artery disease. However, different types of BMCs may exhibit different abilities to cross the vascular wall and stay anchored in the myocardium. For example, the retention of CD34+ BMCs was greater compared with unselected BMCs with intracoronary delivery after acute MI [95]. Importantly, intracoronary injection of BMMNCs in patients with old MI [24] and CPCs in patients with revascularized chronic total occlusion [65] also resulted in improved LV function, indicating that intracoronary BMC delivery may be utilized even in the absence of myocardial vascular damage that would facilitate BMC egress in the setting of an acute MI.

In patients undergoing CABG, intramyocardial injection via transepicardial approach is both feasible and convenient. The advantage of a transendocardial injection using an electromechanical mapping system is the ability to direct BMC injection to viable myocardial areas. The intramyocardial route in general obviates issues related to restenosis and increased atheroma formation that have been noted with specific types of BMCs [56, 70]. Given the fundamental differences in approach and patient types, it is difficult to compare the merits and demerits of various routes. However, subgroup analysis of pooled data showed no significant difference in outcomes with intracoronary and intramyocardial routes in patients with chronic IHD [5]. Thus, a judicious selection of the delivery route based on the specific BMC type, patient characteristics, and logistics is necessary to improve the outcomes of cardiac repair with BMCs.

5.4 Timing of BMC Injection After Acute MI

Shortly after an acute MI, the inflamed state of the myocardium may potentially affect both BMC retention and survival. On one hand, greater expression of chemoattractants [103] and adhesion molecules [104] in the acutely infarcted heart may promote BMC retention, but on the other hand, the abundance of proinflammatory molecules may also cause excessive BMC death. In order to strike a balance between these effects, determining the optimal time for cell injection after MI is critically important. However, improvement in cardiac parameters has been reported with BMC injection across a broad range of timing after MI [4, 76]. In our earlier meta-analysis [4], injection of BMCs within the 5–30-day window after acute MI/PCI resulted in a trend toward greater infarct size reduction compared with BMC injection <5 days after MI/PCI. However, a greater improvement in LVEF with BMC injection >7 days after acute MI has also been reported in a meta-analysis of acute MI trials [76]. In yet another meta-analysis [105], BMC injection during 4–7 days after MI improved LVEF and LVESV, and reduced the incidence of revascularization, death, recurrent MI, restenosis, and arrhythmia. However, these benefits did not reach statistical significance when BMCs were transplanted within 24 h after acute MI [105]. In the largest meta-analysis [5], the reduction of LVEDV was significantly greater when BMCs were injected <7 days after acute MI, while other outcomes were similar with BMC injection during the 7–30-day interval after MI. Thus, specific molecular information regarding the kinetics of BMC retention and survival with transplantation at different intervals after MI in animal models will be necessary to arrive at an optimal time for transplantation in humans.

5.5 Methods of BMC Processing

Because of the differences in outcomes noted in clinical trials with seemingly similar BMC types [28, 29], the specific methods of

BMC processing have attracted closer scrutiny and analysis [6, 7]. Thus far, nearly all of the trials with BMMNCs have utilized a density gradient centrifugation method to isolate these cells. However, the precise formulations of various commercially available products (Lymphoprep, Ficoll-Paque, and such) vary to some extent, and subgroup analysis of outcomes of trials that used Lymphoprep with those using other products did not identify any significant interaction [5]. Additional analysis showed that when BMCs were resuspended in heparin-based solutions, the improvements in LVEF and LVESV were greater. However, heparin has been implicated in BMC dysfunction [106], and therefore, these findings from meta-analysis need to be validated in direct comparison.

6 Conclusions

The safety and efficacy of BMC therapy for cardiac repair have been evaluated in more than 50 clinical trials that used different BMC types and injected widely variable cell numbers via several distinct routes at variable intervals after MI in diverse patient populations. Despite these differences, several meta-analyses of pooled data consistently show that BMC therapy improves LV structure and function without any significant increase in adverse effects. BMC therapy also improves patient-important outcomes, including total and cardiovascular mortality and recurrent MI. These trials and analyses have identified several important methodological variables of BMC therapy that need further validation by direct comparison in large RCTs. Optimization of these methodological aspects is likely to further improve the benefits of this highly promising approach of myocardial repair.

Acknowledgments

This publication was supported in part by NIH grant R01 HL-89939. We gratefully acknowledge the expert secretarial assistance of Ms. Renee Falsken.

Conflict of Interest: None

References

1. Roger VL, Go AS, Lloyd-Jones DM, Benjamin EJ, Berry JD, Borden WB et al (2012) Heart disease and stroke statistics–2012 update: a report from the American Heart Association. Circulation 125: e2–e220
2. Pfeffer MA, Braunwald E (1990) Ventricular remodeling after myocardial infarction. Experimental observations and clinical implications. Circulation 81:1161–1172
3. Pfeffer MA, Pfeffer JM, Lamas GA (1993) Development and prevention of congestive

heart failure following myocardial infarction. Circulation 87:IV120–IV125

4. Abdel-Latif A, Bolli R, Tleyjeh IM, Montori VM, Perin EC, Hornung CA et al (2007) Adult bone marrow-derived cells for cardiac repair: a systematic review and meta-analysis. Arch Intern Med 167:989–997
5. Jeevanantham V, Butler M, Saad A, Abdel-Latif A, Zuba-Surma EK, Dawn B (2012) Adult bone marrow cell therapy improves survival and induces long-term improvement in cardiac parameters: a systematic review and meta-analysis. Circulation 126:551–568
6. Seeger FH, Tonn T, Krzossok N, Zeiher AM, Dimmeler S (2007) Cell isolation procedures matter: a comparison of different isolation protocols of bone marrow mononuclear cells used for cell therapy in patients with acute myocardial infarction. Eur Heart J 28: 766–772
7. Dawn B, Bolli R (2007) Bone marrow for cardiac repair: the importance of characterizing the phenotype and function of injected cells. Eur Heart J 28:651–652
8. Lipinski MJ, Biondi-Zoccai GG, Abbate A, Khianey R, Sheiban I, Bartunek J et al (2007) Impact of intracoronary cell therapy on left ventricular function in the setting of acute myocardial infarction: a collaborative systematic review and meta-analysis of controlled clinical trials. J Am Coll Cardiol 50: 1761–1767
9. Hristov M, Heussen N, Schober A, Weber C (2006) Intracoronary infusion of autologous bone marrow cells and left ventricular function after acute myocardial infarction: a meta-analysis. J Cell Mol Med 10:727–733
10. Ellis WM, Georgiou GM, Roberton DM, Johnson GR (1984) The use of discontinuous Percoll gradients to separate populations of cells from human bone marrow and peripheral blood. J Immunol Methods 66:9–16
11. Prockop DJ (1997) Marrow stromal cells as stem cells for nonhematopoietic tissues. Science 276:71–74
12. Spangrude GJ, Heimfeld S, Weissman IL (1988) Purification and characterization of mouse hematopoietic stem cells. Science 241: 58–62
13. Goodell MA, Brose K, Paradis G, Conner AS, Mulligan RC (1996) Isolation and functional properties of murine hematopoietic stem cells that are replicating in vivo. J Exp Med 183:1797–1806
14. Kucia M, Reca R, Campbell FR, Zuba-Surma E, Majka M, Ratajczak J et al (2006) A population of very small embryonic-like (VSEL) CXCR4(+)SSEA-1(+)Oct-4+ stem cells identified in adult bone marrow. Leukemia 20:857–869
15. Zuba-Surma EK, Kucia M, Abdel-Latif A, Dawn B, Hall B, Singh R et al (2008) Morphological characterization of very small embryonic-like stem cells (VSELs) by ImageStream system analysis. J Cell Mol Med 12:292–303
16. Zuba-Surma EK, Kucia M, Dawn B, Guo Y, Ratajczak MZ, Bolli R (2008) Bone marrow-derived pluripotent very small embryonic-like stem cells (VSELs) are mobilized after acute myocardial infarction. J Mol Cell Cardiol 44: 865–873
17. Zuba-Surma EK, Wojakowski W, Ratajczak MZ, Dawn B (2011) Very small embryonic-like stem cells: biology and therapeutic potential for heart repair. Antioxid Redox Signal 15:1821–1834
18. Strauer BE, Brehm M, Zeus T, Kostering M, Hernandez A, Sorg RV et al (2002) Repair of infarcted myocardium by autologous intracoronary mononuclear bone marrow cell transplantation in humans. Circulation 106: 1913–1918
19. Penicka M, Horak J, Kobylka P, Pytlik R, Kozak T, Belohlavek O et al (2007) Intracoronary injection of autologous bone marrow-derived mononuclear cells in patients with large anterior acute myocardial infarction: a prematurely terminated randomized study. J Am Coll Cardiol 49:2373–2374
20. Perin EC, Dohmann HF, Borojevic R, Silva SA, Sousa AL, Mesquita CT et al (2003) Transendocardial, autologous bone marrow cell transplantation for severe, chronic ischemic heart failure. Circulation 107: 2294–2302
21. Karpov RS, Popov SV, Markov VA, Suslova TE, Ryabov VV, Poponina YS et al (2005) Autologous mononuclear bone marrow cells during reparative regeneration after acute myocardial infarction. Bull Exp Biol Med 140:640–643
22. Meluzin J, Mayer J, Groch L, Janousek S, Hornacek I, Hlinomaz O et al (2006) Autologous transplantation of mononuclear bone marrow cells in patients with acute myocardial infarction: the effect of the dose of transplanted cells on myocardial function. Am Heart J 152:975.e9–15
23. Perin EC, Dohmann HF, Borojevic R, Silva SA, Sousa AL, Silva GV et al (2004) Improved exercise capacity and ischemia 6 and 12 months after transendocardial injection of autologous bone marrow mononuclear cells for ischemic cardiomyopathy. Circulation 110:II213–II218
24. Strauer BE, Brehm M, Zeus T, Bartsch T, Schannwell C, Antke C et al (2005) Regeneration of human infarcted heart muscle by intracoronary autologous bone marrow

cell transplantation in chronic coronary artery disease: the IACT Study. J Am Coll Cardiol 46:1651–1658

25. Ge J, Li Y, Qian J, Shi J, Wang Q, Niu Y et al (2006) Efficacy of emergent transcatheter transplantation of stem cells for treatment of acute myocardial infarction (TCT-STAMI). Heart 92:1764–1767
26. Hendrikx M, Hensen K, Clijsters C, Jongen H, Koninckx R, Bijnens E et al (2006) Recovery of regional but not global contractile function by the direct intramyocardial autologous bone marrow transplantation: results from a randomized controlled clinical trial. Circulation 114:I101–I107
27. Mocini D, Staibano M, Mele L, Giannantoni P, Menichella G, Colivicchi F et al (2006) Autologous bone marrow mononuclear cell transplantation in patients undergoing coronary artery bypass grafting. Am Heart J 151: 192–197
28. Schachinger V, Erbs S, Elsasser A, Haberbosch W, Hambrecht R, Holschermann H et al (2006) Intracoronary bone marrow-derived progenitor cells in acute myocardial infarction. N Engl J Med 355:1210–1221
29. Lunde K, Solheim S, Aakhus S, Arnesen H, Abdelnoor M, Egeland T et al (2006) Intracoronary injection of mononuclear bone marrow cells in acute myocardial infarction. N Engl J Med 355:1199–1209
30. Assmus B, Honold J, Schachinger V, Britten MB, Fischer-Rasokat U, Lehmann R et al (2006) Transcoronary transplantation of progenitor cells after myocardial infarction. N Engl J Med 355:1222–1232
31. Tse HF, Thambar S, Kwong YL, Rowlings P, Bellamy G, McCrohon J et al (2007) Prospective randomized trial of direct endomyocardial implantation of bone marrow cells for treatment of severe coronary artery diseases (PROTECT-CAD trial). Eur Heart J 28:2998–3005
32. Huikuri HV, Kervinen K, Niemela M, Ylitalo K, Saily M, Koistinen P et al (2008) Effects of intracoronary injection of mononuclear bone marrow cells on left ventricular function, arrhythmia risk profile, and restenosis after thrombolytic therapy of acute myocardial infarction. Eur Heart J 29:2723–2732
33. Cao F, Sun D, Li C, Narsinh K, Zhao L, Li X et al (2009) Long-term myocardial functional improvement after autologous bone marrow mononuclear cells transplantation in patients with ST-segment elevation myocardial infarction: 4 years follow-up. Eur Heart J 30:1986–1994
34. Lipiec P, Krzeminska-Pakula M, Plewka M, Kusmierek J, Plachcinska A, Szuminski R et al (2009) Impact of intracoronary injection of mononuclear bone marrow cells in acute myocardial infarction on left ventricular perfusion and function: a 6-month follow-up gated 99mTc-MIBI single-photon emission computed tomography study. Eur J Nucl Med Mol Imaging 36:587–593
35. Tendera M, Wojakowski W, Ruzyllo W, Chojnowska L, Kepka C, Tracz W et al (2009) Intracoronary infusion of bone marrow-derived selected CD34+CXCR4+ cells and non-selected mononuclear cells in patients with acute STEMI and reduced left ventricular ejection fraction: results of randomized, multi-centre Myocardial Regeneration by Intracoronary Infusion of Selected Population of Stem Cells in Acute Myocardial Infarction (REGENT) Trial. Eur Heart J 30:1313–1321
36. Wohrle J, Merkle N, Mailander V, Nusser T, Schauwecker P, von Scheidt F et al (2010) Results of intracoronary stem cell therapy after acute myocardial infarction. Am J Cardiol 105:804–812
37. Traverse JH, McKenna DH, Harvey K, Jorgenso BC, Olson RE, Bostrom N et al (2010) Results of a phase 1, randomized, double-blind, placebo-controlled trial of bone marrow mononuclear stem cell administration in patients following ST-elevation myocardial infarction. Am Heart J 160: 428–434
38. van Ramshorst J, Bax JJ, Beeres SL, Dibbets-Schneider P, Roes SD, Stokkel MP et al (2009) Intramyocardial bone marrow cell injection for chronic myocardial ischemia: a randomized controlled trial. JAMA 301: 1997–2004
39. Pokushalov E, Romanov A, Chernyavsky A, Larionov P, Terekhov I, Artyomenko S et al (2010) Efficiency of intramyocardial injections of autologous bone marrow mononuclear cells in patients with ischemic heart failure: a randomized study. J Cardiovasc Transl Res 3:160–168
40. Strauer BE, Yousef M, Schannwell CM (2010) The acute and long-term effects of intracoronary Stem cell Transplantation in 191 patients with chronic heARt failure: the STAR-heart study. Eur J Heart Fail 12:721–729
41. Wollert KC, Meyer GP, Lotz J, Ringes-Lichtenberg S, Lippolt P, Breidenbach C et al (2004) Intracoronary autologous bone-marrow cell transfer after myocardial infarction: the BOOST randomised controlled clinical trial. Lancet 364:141–148
42. Meyer GP, Wollert KC, Lotz J, Steffens J, Lippolt P, Fichtner S et al (2006) Intracoronary bone marrow cell transfer after myocardial infarction: eighteen months' follow-up data from the randomized, controlled BOOST (BOne marrOw transfer to enhance

ST-elevation infarct regeneration) trial. Circulation 113:1287–1294
43. Schaefer A, Meyer GP, Fuchs M, Klein G, Kaplan M, Wollert KC et al (2006) Impact of intracoronary bone marrow cell transfer on diastolic function in patients after acute myocardial infarction: results from the BOOST trial. Eur Heart J 27:929–935
44. Ruan W, Pan CZ, Huang GQ, Li YL, Ge JB, Shu XH (2005) Assessment of left ventricular segmental function after autologous bone marrow stem cells transplantation in patients with acute myocardial infarction by tissue tracking and strain imaging. Chin Med J (Engl) 118:1175–1181
45. Pittenger MF, Mackay AM, Beck SC, Jaiswal RK, Douglas R, Mosca JD et al (1999) Multilineage potential of adult human mesenchymal stem cells. Science 284:143–147
46. Makino S, Fukuda K, Miyoshi S, Konishi F, Kodama H, Pan J et al (1999) Cardiomyocytes can be generated from marrow stromal cells in vitro. J Clin Invest 103:697–705
47. Hattan N, Kawaguchi H, Ando K, Kuwabara E, Fujita J, Murata M et al (2005) Purified cardiomyocytes from bone marrow mesenchymal stem cells produce stable intracardiac grafts in mice. Cardiovasc Res 65:334–344
48. Pittenger MF, Martin BJ (2004) Mesenchymal stem cells and their potential as cardiac therapeutics. Circ Res 95:9–20
49. Chen SL, Fang WW, Ye F, Liu YH, Qian J, Shan SJ et al (2004) Effect on left ventricular function of intracoronary transplantation of autologous bone marrow mesenchymal stem cell in patients with acute myocardial infarction. Am J Cardiol 94:92–95
50. Chen S, Liu Z, Tian N, Zhang J, Yei F, Duan B et al (2006) Intracoronary transplantation of autologous bone marrow mesenchymal stem cells for ischemic cardiomyopathy due to isolated chronic occluded left anterior descending artery. J Invasive Cardiol 18: 552–556
51. Katritsis DG, Sotiropoulou PA, Karvouni E, Karabinos I, Korovesis S, Perez SA et al (2005) Transcoronary transplantation of autologous mesenchymal stem cells and endothelial progenitors into infarcted human myocardium. Catheter Cardiovasc Interv 65: 321–329
52. Hare JM, Traverse JH, Henry TD, Dib N, Strumpf RK, Schulman SP et al (2009) A randomized, double-blind, placebo-controlled, dose-escalation study of intravenous adult human mesenchymal stem cells (prochymal) after acute myocardial infarction. J Am Coll Cardiol 54:2277–2286
53. Hare JM, Fishman JE, Gerstenblith G, DiFede Velazquez DL, Zambrano JP, Suncion VY et al (2012) Comparison of allogeneic vs autologous bone marrow-derived mesenchymal stem cells delivered by transendocardial injection in patients with ischemic cardiomyopathy: the POSEIDON randomized trial. JAMA 308:2369–2379
54. Peichev M, Naiyer AJ, Pereira D, Zhu Z, Lane WJ, Williams M et al (2000) Expression of VEGFR-2 and AC133 by circulating human CD34(+) cells identifies a population of functional endothelial precursors. Blood 95:952–958
55. Bhatia M (2001) AC133 expression in human stem cells. Leukemia 15:1685–1688
56. Bartunek J, Vanderheyden M, Vandekerckhove B, Mansour S, De Bruyne B, De Bondt P et al (2005) Intracoronary injection of CD133-positive enriched bone marrow progenitor cells promotes cardiac recovery after recent myocardial infarction: feasibility and safety. Circulation 112:I178–I183
57. Mansour S, Vanderheyden M, De Bruyne B, Vandekerckhove B, Delrue L, Van Haute I et al (2006) Intracoronary delivery of hematopoietic bone marrow stem cells and luminal loss of the infarct-related artery in patients with recent myocardial infarction. J Am Coll Cardiol 47:1727–1730
58. Colombo A, Castellani M, Piccaluga E, Pusineri E, Palatresi S, Longari V et al (2011) Myocardial blood flow and infarct size after CD133+ cell injection in large myocardial infarction with good recanalization and poor reperfusion: results from a randomized controlled trial. J Cardiovasc Med (Hagerstown) 12:239–248
59. Manginas A, Goussetis E, Koutelou M, Karatasakis G, Peristeri I, Theodorakos A et al (2007) Pilot study to evaluate the safety and feasibility of intracoronary CD133(+) and CD133(-) CD34(+) cell therapy in patients with nonviable anterior myocardial infarction. Catheter Cardiovasc Interv 69:773–781
60. Stamm C, Kleine HD, Choi YH, Dunkelmann S, Lauffs JA, Lorenzen B et al (2007) Intramyocardial delivery of CD133+ bone marrow cells and coronary artery bypass grafting for chronic ischemic heart disease: safety and efficacy studies. J Thorac Cardiovasc Surg 133:717–725
61. Yerebakan C, Kaminski A, Westphal B, Donndorf P, Glass A, Liebold A et al (2011) Impact of preoperative left ventricular function and time from infarction on the long-term benefits after intramyocardial CD133(+) bone marrow stem cell transplant. J Thorac Cardiovasc Surg 142:1530–1539.e3
62. Assmus B, Schachinger V, Teupe C, Britten M, Lehmann R, Dobert N et al (2002) Transplantation of progenitor cells and regeneration enhancement in acute myocardial

infarction (TOPCARE-AMI). Circulation 106:3009–3017

63. Britten MB, Abolmaali ND, Assmus B, Lehmann R, Honold J, Schmitt J et al (2003) Infarct remodeling after intracoronary progenitor cell treatment in patients with acute myocardial infarction (TOPCARE-AMI): mechanistic insights from serial contrast-enhanced magnetic resonance imaging. Circulation 108:2212–2218
64. Schachinger V, Assmus B, Britten MB, Honold J, Lehmann R, Teupe C et al (2004) Transplantation of progenitor cells and regeneration enhancement in acute myocardial infarction: final one-year results of the TOPCARE-AMI Trial. J Am Coll Cardiol 44:1690–1699
65. Erbs S, Linke A, Adams V, Lenk K, Thiele H, Diederich KW et al (2005) Transplantation of blood-derived progenitor cells after recanalization of chronic coronary artery occlusion: first randomized and placebo-controlled study. Circ Res 97:756–762
66. Asahara T, Kawamoto A (2004) Endothelial progenitor cells for postnatal vasculogenesis. Am J Physiol Cell Physiol 287:C572–C579
67. Kawamoto A, Tkebuchava T, Yamaguchi J, Nishimura H, Yoon YS, Milliken C et al (2003) Intramyocardial transplantation of autologous endothelial progenitor cells for therapeutic neovascularization of myocardial ischemia. Circulation 107:461–468
68. Losordo DW, Schatz RA, White CJ, Udelson JE, Veereshwarayya V, Durgin M et al (2007) Intramyocardial transplantation of autologous CD34+ stem cells for intractable angina: a phase I/IIa double-blind, randomized controlled trial. Circulation 115:3165–3172
69. Losordo DW, Henry TD, Davidson C, Sup Lee J, Costa MA, Bass T et al (2011) Intramyocardial, autologous CD34+ cell therapy for refractory angina. Circ Res 109:428–436
70. Kang HJ, Kim HS, Zhang SY, Park KW, Cho HJ, Koo BK et al (2004) Effects of intracoronary infusion of peripheral blood stem-cells mobilised with granulocyte-colony stimulating factor on left ventricular systolic function and restenosis after coronary stenting in myocardial infarction: the MAGIC cell randomised clinical trial. Lancet 363:751–756
71. Kang HJ, Lee HY, Na SH, Chang SA, Park KW, Kim HK et al (2006) Differential effect of intracoronary infusion of mobilized peripheral blood stem cells by granulocyte colony-stimulating factor on left ventricular function and remodeling in patients with acute myocardial infarction versus old myocardial infarction: the MAGIC Cell-3-DES randomized, controlled trial. Circulation 114:I145–I151
72. Li ZQ, Zhang M, Jing YZ, Zhang WW, Liu Y, Cui LJ et al (2007) The clinical study of autologous peripheral blood stem cell transplantation by intracoronary infusion in patients with acute myocardial infarction (AMI). Int J Cardiol 115:52–56
73. Choi JH, Choi J, Lee WS, Rhee I, Lee SC, Gwon HC et al (2007) Lack of additional benefit of intracoronary transplantation of autologous peripheral blood stem cell in patients with acute myocardial infarction. Circ J 71:486–494
74. Tatsumi T, Ashihara E, Yasui T, Matsunaga S, Kido A, Sasada Y et al (2007) Intracoronary transplantation of non-expanded peripheral blood-derived mononuclear cells promotes improvement of cardiac function in patients with acute myocardial infarction. Circ J 71:1199–1207
75. Rosenzweig A (2006) Cardiac cell therapy–mixed results from mixed cells. N Engl J Med 355:1274–1277
76. Martin-Rendon E, Brunskill SJ, Hyde CJ, Stanworth SJ, Mathur A, Watt SM (2008) Autologous bone marrow stem cells to treat acute myocardial infarction: a systematic review. Eur Heart J 29:1807–1818
77. Zhang SN, Sun AJ, Ge JB, Yao K, Huang ZY, Wang KQ et al (2009) Intracoronary autologous bone marrow stem cells transfer for patients with acute myocardial infarction: a meta-analysis of randomised controlled trials. Int J Cardiol 136:178–185
78. Piepoli MF, Vallisa D, Arbasi M, Cavanna L, Cerri L, Mori M et al (2010) Bone marrow cell transplantation improves cardiac, autonomic, and functional indexes in acute anterior myocardial infarction patients (Cardiac Study). Eur J Heart Fail 12:172–180
79. Yousef M, Schannwell CM, Kostering M, Zeus T, Brehm M, Strauer BE (2009) The BALANCE Study: clinical benefit and long-term outcome after intracoronary autologous bone marrow cell transplantation in patients with acute myocardial infarction. J Am Coll Cardiol 53:2262–2269
80. Zhao Q, Sun Y, Xia L, Chen A, Wang Z (2008) Randomized study of mononuclear bone marrow cell transplantation in patients with coronary surgery. Ann Thorac Surg 86:1833–1840
81. Akar AR, Durdu S, Arat M, Kilickap M, Kucuk NO, Arslan O et al (2009) Five-year follow-up after transepicardial implantation of autologous bone marrow mononuclear cells to ungraftable coronary territories for patients with ischaemic cardiomyopathy. Eur J Cardiothorac Surg 36:633–643
82. Rivas-Plata A, Castillo J, Pariona M, Chunga A (2010) Bypass grafts and cell transplant in

heart failure with low ejection fraction. Asian Cardiovasc Thorac Ann 18:425–429

83. Turan RG, Bozdag-Turan I, Ortak J, Akin I, Kische S, Schneider H et al (2011) Improvement of cardiac function by intracoronary freshly isolated bone marrow cells transplantation in patients with acute myocardial infarction. Circ J 75:683–691
84. Turan RG, Bozdag TI, Turan CH, Ortak J, Akin I, Kische S et al (2012) Enhanced mobilization of the bone marrow-derived circulating progenitor cells by intracoronary freshly isolated bone marrow cells transplantation in patients with acute myocardial infarction. J Cell Mol Med 16:852–864
85. Yao K, Huang R, Qian J, Cui J, Ge L, Li Y et al (2008) Administration of intracoronary bone marrow mononuclear cells on chronic myocardial infarction improves diastolic function. Heart 94:1147–1153
86. Plewka M, Krzeminska-Pakula M, Lipiec P, Peruga JZ, Jezewski T, Kidawa M et al (2009) Effect of intracoronary injection of mononuclear bone marrow stem cells on left ventricular function in patients with acute myocardial infarction. Am J Cardiol 104:1336–1342
87. van Ramshorst J, Antoni ML, Beeres SL, Roes SD, Delgado V, Rodrigo SF et al (2011) Intramyocardial bone marrow-derived mononuclear cell injection for chronic myocardial ischemia: the effect on diastolic function. Circ Cardiovasc Imaging 4:122–129
88. Olivares EL, Ribeiro VP, Werneck de Castro JP, Ribeiro KC, Mattos EC, Goldenberg RC et al (2004) Bone marrow stromal cells improve cardiac performance in healed infarcted rat hearts. Am J Physiol Heart Circ Physiol 287:H464–H470
89. Nagaya N, Kangawa K, Itoh T, Iwase T, Murakami S, Miyahara Y et al (2005) Transplantation of mesenchymal stem cells improves cardiac function in a rat model of dilated cardiomyopathy. Circulation 112: 1128–1135
90. Kendziorra K, Barthel H, Erbs S, Emmrich F, Hambrecht R, Schuler G et al (2008) Effect of progenitor cells on myocardial perfusion and metabolism in patients after recanalization of a chronically occluded coronary artery. J Nucl Med 49:557–563
91. Zhang M, Methot D, Poppa V, Fujio Y, Walsh K, Murry CE (2001) Cardiomyocyte grafting for cardiac repair: graft cell death and anti-death strategies. J Mol Cell Cardiol 33:907–921
92. Suzuki K, Murtuza B, Beauchamp JR, Smolenski RT, Varela-Carver A, Fukushima S et al (2004) Dynamics and mediators of acute graft attrition after myoblast transplantation to the heart. FASEB J 18:1153–1155
93. Barbash IM, Chouraqui P, Baron J, Feinberg MS, Etzion S, Tessone A et al (2003) Systemic delivery of bone marrow-derived mesenchymal stem cells to the infarcted myocardium: feasibility, cell migration, and body distribution. Circulation 108:863–868
94. Dow J, Simkhovich BZ, Kedes L, Kloner RA (2005) Washout of transplanted cells from the heart: a potential new hurdle for cell transplantation therapy. Cardiovasc Res 67:301–307
95. Hofmann M, Wollert KC, Meyer GP, Menke A, Arseniev L, Hertenstein B et al (2005) Monitoring of bone marrow cell homing into the infarcted human myocardium. Circulation 111(17):2198–2202
96. Meluzin J, Janousek S, Mayer J, Groch L, Hornacek I, Hlinomaz O et al (2008) Three-, 6-, and 12-month results of autologous transplantation of mononuclear bone marrow cells in patients with acute myocardial infarction. Int J Cardiol 128:185–192
97. Grajek S, Popiel M, Gil L, Breborowicz P, Lesiak M, Czepczynski R et al (2010) Influence of bone marrow stem cells on left ventricle perfusion and ejection fraction in patients with acute myocardial infarction of anterior wall: randomized clinical trial: impact of bone marrow stem cell intracoronary infusion on improvement of microcirculation. Eur Heart J 31:691–702
98. Kawamoto A, Iwasaki H, Kusano K, Murayama T, Oyamada A, Silver M et al (2006) CD34-positive cells exhibit increased potency and safety for therapeutic neovascularization after myocardial infarction compared with total mononuclear cells. Circulation 114:2163–2169
99. Dawn B, Tiwari S, Kucia MJ, Zuba-Surma EK, Guo Y, Sanganalmath SK et al (2008) Transplantation of bone marrow-derived very small embryonic-like stem cells attenuates left ventricular dysfunction and remodeling after myocardial infarction. Stem Cells 26:1646–1655
100. Janssens S, Dubois C, Bogaert J, Theunissen K, Deroose C, Desmet W et al (2006) Autologous bone marrow-derived stem-cell transfer in patients with ST-segment elevation myocardial infarction: double-blind, randomised controlled trial. Lancet 367: 113–121
101. Roncalli J, Mouquet F, Piot C, Trochu JN, Le Corvoisier P, Neuder Y et al (2011) Intracoronary autologous mononucleated bone marrow cell infusion for acute myocardial infarction: results of the randomized multicenter BONAMI trial. Eur Heart J 32: 1748–1757
102. Donndorf P, Kundt G, Kaminski A, Yerebakan C, Liebold A, Steinhoff G et al (2011)

Intramyocardial bone marrow stem cell transplantation during coronary artery bypass surgery: a meta-analysis. J Thorac Cardiovasc Surg 142:911–920

103. Kucia M, Dawn B, Hunt G, Guo Y, Wysoczynski M, Majka M et al (2004) Cells expressing early cardiac markers reside in the bone marrow and are mobilized into the peripheral blood following myocardial infarction. Circ Res 95:1191–1199

104. Kukielka GL, Hawkins HK, Michael L, Manning AM, Youker K, Lane C et al (1993) Regulation of intercellular adhesion molecule-1 (ICAM-1) in ischemic and reperfused canine myocardium. J Clin Invest 92:1504–1516

105. Zhang S, Sun A, Xu D, Yao K, Huang Z, Jin H et al (2009) Impact of timing on efficacy and safety of intracoronary autologous bone marrow stem cells transplantation in acute myocardial infarction: a pooled subgroup analysis of randomized controlled trials. Clin Cardiol 32:458–466

106. Seeger FH, Rasper T, Fischer A, Muhly-Reinholz M, Hergenreider E, Leistner DM et al (2012) Heparin disrupts the CXCR4/SDF-1 axis and impairs the functional capacity of bone marrow-derived mononuclear cells used for cardiovascular repair. Circ Res 111:854–862

107. Ang KL, Chin D, Leyva F, Foley P, Kubal C, Chalil S et al (2008) Randomized, controlled trial of intramuscular or intracoronary injection of autologous bone marrow cells into scarred myocardium during CABG versus CABG alone. Nat Clin Pract Cardiovasc Med 5:663–670

108. Hirsch A, Nijveldt R, van der Vleuten PA, Tijssen JG, van der Giessen WJ, Tio RA et al (2011) Intracoronary infusion of mononuclear cells from bone marrow or peripheral blood compared with standard therapy in patients after acute myocardial infarction treated by primary percutaneous coronary intervention: results of the randomized controlled HEBE trial. Eur Heart J 32:1736–1747

109. Huang RC, Yao K, Zou YZ, Ge L, Qian JY, Yang J et al (2006) Long term follow-up on emergent intracoronary autologous bone marrow mononuclear cell transplantation for acute inferior-wall myocardial infarction. Zhonghua Yi Xue Za Zhi 86:1107–1110

110. Beitnes JO, Hopp E, Lunde K, Smith HJ, Solheim S, Arnesen H et al (2008) Long-term follow-up of left ventricular function after acute myocardial infarction treated with intracoronary injection of autologous bone marrow cells. The ASTAMI study. Circulation 118:S_863

111. Beitnes JO, Hopp E, Lunde K, Solheim S, Arnesen H, Brinchmann JE et al (2009) Long-term results after intracoronary injection of autologous mononuclear bone marrow cells in acute myocardial infarction: the ASTAMI randomised, controlled study. Heart 95:1983–1989

112. Lunde K, Solheim S, Forfang K, Arnesen H, Brinch L, Bjornerheim R et al (2008) Anterior myocardial infarction with acute percutaneous coronary intervention and intracoronary injection of autologous mononuclear bone marrow cells: safety, clinical outcome, and serial changes in left ventricular function during 12-months' follow-up. J Am Coll Cardiol 51:674–676

113. Meyer GP, Wollert KC, Lotz J, Pirr J, Rager U, Lippolt P et al (2009) Intracoronary bone marrow cell transfer after myocardial infarction: 5-year follow-up from the randomized-controlled BOOST trial. Eur Heart J 30: 2978–2984

114. Nogueira FB, Silva SA, Haddad AF, Peixoto CM, Carvalho RM, Tuche FA et al (2009) Systolic function of patients with myocardial infarction undergoing autologous bone marrow transplantation. Arq Bras Cardiol 93: 374–379, 367–372

115. Quyyumi AA, Waller EK, Murrow J, Esteves F, Galt J, Oshinski J et al (2011) CD34(+) cell infusion after ST elevation myocardial infarction is associated with improved perfusion and is dose dependent. Am Heart J 161: 98–105

116. Erbs S, Linke A, Schachinger V, Assmus B, Thiele H, Diederich KW et al (2007) Restoration of microvascular function in the infarct-related artery by intracoronary transplantation of bone marrow progenitor cells in patients with acute myocardial infarction: the Doppler Substudy of the Reinfusion of Enriched Progenitor Cells and Infarct Remodeling in Acute Myocardial Infarction (REPAIR-AMI) trial. Circulation 116: 366–374

117. Schachinger V, Erbs S, Elsasser A, Haberbosch W, Hambrecht R, Holschermann H et al (2006) Improved clinical outcome after intracoronary administration of bone-marrow-derived progenitor cells in acute myocardial infarction: final 1-year results of the REPAIR-AMI trial. Eur Heart J 27: 2775–2783

118. Silva SA, Sousa AL, Haddad AF, Azevedo JC, Soares VE, Peixoto CM et al (2009) Autologous bone-marrow mononuclear cell transplantation after acute myocardial infarction: comparison of two delivery techniques. Cell Transplant 18:343–352

119. Srimahachota S, Boonyaratavej S, Rerkpattanapipat P, Wangsupachart S, Tumkosit M, Bunworasate U et al (2011) Intra-coronary bone marrow mononuclear cell transplantation in patients with ST-elevation myocardial infarction:

a randomized controlled study. J Med Assoc Thai 94:657–663

120. Suarez de Lezo J, Herrera C, Pan M, Romero M, Pavlovic D, Segura J et al (2007) Regenerative therapy in patients with a revascularized acute anterior myocardial infarction and depressed ventricular function. Rev Esp Cardiol 60:357–365
121. Traverse JH, Henry TD, Ellis SG, Pepine CJ, Willerson JT, Zhao DX et al (2011) Effect of intracoronary delivery of autologous bone marrow mononuclear cells 2 to 3 weeks following acute myocardial infarction on left ventricular function: the LateTIME randomized trial. JAMA 306:2110–2119
122. Yao K, Huang R, Sun A, Qian J, Liu X, Ge L et al (2009) Repeated autologous bone marrow mononuclear cell therapy in patients with large myocardial infarction. Eur J Heart Fail 11:691–698

Chapter 16

Clinical Study Using Adipose-Derived Mesenchymal-Like Stem Cells in Acute Myocardial Infarction and Heart Failure

Ilia Alexander Panfilov, Renate de Jong, Shin-ichiro Takashima, and Henricus J. Duckers

Abstract

Adipose tissue represents an abundant, accessible source of regenerative cells that can be easily obtained in sufficient amount for therapy. Adipose-derived regenerative cells (ADRC) are comprised of leukocytes, smooth muscles, endothelial cells, and mesenchymal stem cells. In contrast to bone-marrow-derived MSC, the abundance of adipose tissue in patients and the higher frequency per unit mass of regenerative cells allow for the isolation of cells in therapeutic meaningful amounts in less than 2 h after donor tissue acquisition.

Harvest of adipose tissue can thus follow primary PCI, allowing efficient treatment within 24 h. This obviates the need for extensive cell culturing in GMP clean room facilities and makes ADSCs a promising and practical autologous cell source. In the following chapter, we will describe the liposuction procedure for stem cell harvest, two cell delivery techniques, and pressure/volume loop analysis for the follow-up of our patients enrolled in the clinical studies.

Key words ADSC, ADRC, Liposuction, Intracoronary infusion, Intramyocardial injection, Myocardial infarction, Heart failure, Stem cell therapy

1 Introduction

The clinical utility of cardiovascular stem cell therapy passed the phase of proof-of-concept. After 14 years of research, this field is now entering phase III clinical trials to treat ischemic heart disease. Previous work in animal models shows the potential to improve tissue regeneration by neoangiogenesis, and more recently neomyogenesis. The promise of this therapy is high, with multiple disciplines working on cardiovascular ischemic models in the regenerative medicine field [1].

In particular, mesenchymal stem cells (MSC) appear to have many features that we specifically look for in an ideal stem cell for cardiovascular disease. Preclinical and clinical studies showed that these cells are highly proliferative in cell culture, and that they are

Race L. Kao (ed.), *Cellular Cardiomyoplasty: Methods and Protocols*, Methods in Molecular Biology, vol. 1036, DOI 10.1007/978-1-62703-511-8_16, © Springer Science+Business Media New York 2013

capable of mediating cardiovascular regenerative effects [2, 3], through paracrine mechanisms that target resident cardiomyocytes and vascular cells [4]. Long-term follow-up of patients, who received BM MSC stem cell therapy for the treatment of acute myocardial infarction, showed a sustained improvement of global LVEF by 3.9 % and decreased infarct size at 5-year follow-up [5].

The technique of isolating and subculturing autologous MSC stem cells is however logistically challenging. Patients first have to undergo bone marrow puncture (40 cm^3). The bone marrow aspirate is then transported to a GMP-certified facility, where the BM-derived mesenchymal stem cell population is selected by plastic adherence isolation [6, 7]. For a therapeutic relevant amount, a bone marrow graft of 40 cm^3 has to be subcultured for 6–12 weeks. The culturing of allografts for a prolonged period of time is inherently associated with an increased risk of graft failure and contamination.

One of the abundant sources of stem cells in adults is multipotent mesenchymal-like stem cells that have been isolated from subcutaneous adipose tissue. First identified by Zuk [8], these mesenchymal-like stem cells act through their paracrine effects to improve angiogenesis, reduce ischemic-induced apoptosis, modulate inflammation, and enhance progenitor cell recruitment and differentiation. One of the major benefits of adipose tissue is the ability to harvest ADRC in clinically relevant amounts that would not require additional cell culture to generate sufficient numbers of stem cells [9, 10]. Within 2 h after liposuction, from as little as 200 g of lipoaspirate, 40–60 million ADRCs can be isolated by simple centrifugation to separate the buoyant adipocyte fraction and the non-buoyant vascular stromal fraction. Feasibility and safety of ADRC therapy has been demonstrated in a multicenter, randomized, placebo-controlled trial in humans with STEMI (APOLLO) and congestive heart failure (PRECISE) [11].

2 Materials

To perform liposuction under aseptic conditions, use a Toomey cannula with a standard tip up to 15 cm long and a 4–6 mm inner diameter. For infiltration of the targeted liposuction regions in the periumbilical region, use a Toomey syringe and a 14 gauge, blunt LAMIS infiltrator to inject tumescent fluid composition. We advise when removing fat in periumbilical region to do this symmetric, keeping the overall area of aspiration as small as possible (*see* **Note 1**).

2.1 Liposuction

1. Check Hb and aPTT before initiation of the procedure for prevention or early detection of bleeding (*see* **Note 2**).
2. Always employ monitoring of ECG vital signs and blood pressure (every 5–10 min) during procedure.

3. Prepare a sterile field in around the periumbilical region.
4. Anesthetize the location of incision with a local injection of lidocaine (2 %).
5. Make an approximately 0.5 cm stab skin incision.
6. Infiltrate tumescent solution using a blunt LAMIS infiltrator and a volume ratio of 1:1 of tumescent solution (*see* **Note 3**) to the selected fat for harvesting.
7. After 20–30 min, the fat is harvested using the Toomey aspiration cannula attached to the 50 cm^3 syringe.
8. After the syringe is filled (complete filling is not required), the syringe is capped and ready for transportation to isolation facility.
9. Continue liposuction until desired volume is achieved.
10. Close surgical incision with appropriate suture.
11. Apply standard elastic pressure corset immediately upon conclusion of tissue harvest.
12. Check Hb and aPTT every hour for a minimum of 8 h after the procedure.

2.2 ADRC Isolation

The Celution system is essentially designed to automatically process lipoaspirate tissue and separate the ADRCs from the adipose tissue by enzymatic digestion of the tissue using centrifugation to separate the non-buoyant ADRCs from the buoyant lipid adipocytes. The abundance of adipose tissue in human subjects and the higher concentration of adult regenerative cells per unit mass of adipose tissue allow for the isolation of an efficacious number of cells without having to subculture them in a laboratory.

3 Methods

3.1 Intracoronary Infusion

1. Place the therapeutic 7 Fr coronary guiding catheter into the culprit main vessel.
2. Infuse 200 μg of nitroglycerin through guiding catheter.
3. Record fluoroscopy of target vessel in LAO and RAO projection with at least 90° difference to quantify by online QCA.
4. Record TIMI flow of the culprit vessel.
5. Place 0.014 in. soft-tipped CFR wire (Volcano, Cordova, CA) into the culprit vessel distal to stent edge.
6. Perform coronary flow reserve measurement using adenosine continuous infusion at a rate of 140 μg/kg/min.
7. Place over the wire the infusion catheter in the stent in the culprit vessel.
8. Remove flow wire from microinfusion catheter.

9. Attach infusion syringe to central lumen of infusion catheter (*see* **Note 4**).
10. Start infusion (*see* **Note 5**) of ADRC cells at 2.5 ml/min.
11. After 30 % of the total cell suspension volume is infused, the infusion pump is stopped and contrast dye is injected into the guiding catheter vessel to evaluate and record TIMI coronary flow.
12. Repeat **step 11** after 60 % of total cell suspension volume has been infused.
13. After completion of the cell injection, insert coronary flow wire through the microinfusion catheter.
14. Perform coronary flow reserve measurement using adenosine continuous infusion at a rate of 140 μg/kg/min.
15. Measure maximal coronary flow during adenosine hyperemia (*see* **Note 6**).
16. Remove flow wire.
17. Inject 200 μg of nitroglycerin through guiding catheter.
18. Record coronary angiography of the culprit vessel with two views, with at least 60° difference to LAO recording for QCA analysis.
19. Evaluate and record level TIMI coronary flow in target vessel.

3.2 Intramyocardial Injection by Use of the Helix Catheter ™ (BioCardia Inc., San Carlos)

1. Place an 8 Fr sheath into femoral artery.
2. Perform LV gram in LAO and RAO projection (with at least 90° difference to the LAO recording).
3. Trace endocardial borders on transparencies overlaying the on-screen images during end-diastole and end-systole of the LV gram cycle.
4. Mark noncontractile myocardial segments on the transparent.
5. Place a guidewire in left ventricle.
6. Advance the BioCardia Morph steerable catheter over the wire into the left ventricle and remove the wire.
7. Advance the Helic Infusion Catheter (HIC) through the Morph catheter. Advance the HIC perpendicular to the targeted endoventricular wall under fluoroscopic guidance.
8. Engage the myocardium by three turns clockwise of the Helic Catheter.
9. Confirm intramyocardial engagement by flush of contrast through the HIC against the intramyocardial tissue.
10. Start injection of 0.2 ml stem cell suspension by slow infusion over 30 s.
11. After injection, allow 30 s of dwelling time.

12. Disengage the catheter by three counterclockwise turns.
13. Repeat **steps 7–12** until a total of 15 injections with 0.2 ml suspension are injected in the target zone.

3.3 Pressure-Volume Loop

1. Use a ≥7 Fr arterial and an ≥8 Fr venous sheath in the femoral artery/venae.
2. Place a Swan-Ganz thermodilution catheter in the pulmonary artery.
3. Place conductance catheter along the long axis of the left ventricle under fluoroscopic guidance.
4. Optimize conductance catheter position based on online PV signals.
5. Determine blood resistivity by drawing 5 ml blood into cuvette.
6. Perform thermodilution CO measurements three times, and record pressure-volume loops during CO measurements.
7. Perform hypertonic saline injections (3×, 7 ml, 10 % saline) via the distal port of the thermodilution catheter, and record pressure-volume loops during injections (preferably during breath-holding at end-expiration).
8. Remove Swan-Ganz catheter.
9. Place balloon occlusion catheter into inferior vena cava.
10. Record positioning with cinegram without contrast.
11. Record baseline pressure-volume loops during breath-holding at end-expiration (approximately 10 s).
12. Inflate balloon in vena cava position to reduce preload to LV and record pressure-volume loops during LV unloading until systolic pressure drops by approximately 20 mmHg (preferably with breath-holding at end-expiration).
13. Deflate balloon.
14. Repeat once **steps 11–13**.

4 Notes

1. Patient must have the ability to undergo liposuction to obtain a minimum of 220 ml adipose tissue.
2. Liposuction must not be performed on patient that previously received any IIb/IIIa glycoprotein inhibitor within 7 days preceding the liposuction, or those who have received any anticoagulant within 1 h of liposuction and have an aPTT result of ≥1.8 times the control value.
3. Prepare tumescent fluid with 1 mg epinephrine and 20 ml 2 % lidocaine in 500 ml Ringer's lactate.

4. Make sure no blood or air bubbles reside in connector, and flush with small amounts of saline if necessary.
5. For use in AMI, ADRCs suspended in a standard 20 ml/cc lactated Ringer's solution may be infused into the coronary artery via an angioplasty catheter or microinfusion catheter with Twin-Pass.
6. To investigate the effect on hemodynamic changes during the measurements, both resting and hyperemic conditions should be measured twice.

Acknowledgement

This work was supported by VIDI grant of Henricus J. Duckers, BioCardia Inc. (San Carlos), and Cytori Therapeutics Inc. (San Diego, California).

References

1. Caplan AI, Correa D (2011) The MSC: an Injury Drugstore. Cell Stem Cell 9:11–15. doi:10.1016/j.stem.2011.06.008
2. Amado LC, Saliaris AP, Schuleri KH et al (2005) Cardiac repair with intramyocardial injection of allogeneic mesenchymal stem cells after myocardial infarction. Proc Natl Acad Sci U S A 102:11474–11479. doi:10.1073/pnas.0504388102
3. Toma C (2002) Human mesenchymal stem cells differentiate to a cardiomyocyte phenotype in the adult murine heart. Circulation 105:93–98. doi:10.1161/hc0102.101442
4. Gnecchi M, Zhang Z, Ni A, Dzau VJ (2008) Paracrine mechanisms in adult stem cell signaling and therapy. Circ Res 103:1204–1219. doi:10.1161/CIRCRESAHA.108.176826
5. Clifford DM, Fisher SA, Brunskill SJ et al (2012) Stem cell treatment for acute myocardial infarction. Cochr Data System Rev (Online) 2:CD006536, doi: 10.1002/14651858.CD006536.pub3
6. Friedenstein AJ, Chailakhjan RK, Lalykina KS (1970) The development of fibroblast colonies in monolayer cultures of guinea-pig bone marrow and spleen cells. Cell Tissue Kinet 3:393–403
7. Pittenger MF (1999) Multilineage potential of adult human mesenchymal stem cells. Science 284:143–147. doi:10.1126/science.284.5411.143
8. Zuk PA, Zhu M, Ashjian P et al (2002) Human adipose tissue is a source of multipotent stem cells. Mol Biol Cell 13:4279–4295. doi: 10.1091/mbc.E02-02-0105
9. Caplan AI (2009) Why are MSCs therapeutic? New data: new insight. J Pathol 217:318–324. doi:10.1002/path.2469
10. Fraser JK, Schreiber R, Strem B et al (2006) Plasticity of human adipose stem cells toward endothelial cells and cardiomyocytes. Nat Clin Pract Cardiovasc Med 3(Suppl 1):S33–S37. doi:10.1038/ncpcardio0444
11. Houtgraaf JH, den Dekker WK, van Dalen BM et al (2012) First experience in humans using adipose tissue-derived regenerative cells in the treatment of patients with ST-segment elevation myocardial infarction. J Am Coll Cardiol 59:539–540. doi: 10.1016/j.jacc.2011.09.065

INDEX

Race L. Kao (ed.), *Cellular Cardiomyoplasty: Methods and Protocols*, Methods in Molecular Biology, vol. 1036, DOI 10.1007/978-1-62703-511-8, © Springer Science+Business Media New York 2013

MIX
Papier aus verantwortungsvollen Quellen
Paper from responsible sources
FSC® C105338

If you have any concerns about our products,
you can contact us on
ProductSafety@springernature.com

In case Publisher is established outside the EU,
the EU authorized representative is:
Springer Nature Customer Service Center GmbH
Europaplatz 3, 69115 Heidelberg, Germany

Printed by Libri Plureos GmbH
in Hamburg, Germany